PEDIATRIC NEPHROLOGY

DEVELOPMENTS IN NEPHROLOGY

VOLUME 3

Also in this series:

1. CHEIGH JS, STENZEL KH, RUBIN AL eds: Manual of clinical nephrology of the Rogosin Kidney Center. 1981. ISBN 90-247-2397-3

2. NOLPH KD ed: Peritoneal dialysis. 1981. ISBN 90-247-2477-5

Series ISBN 90-247-2428-7

PEDIATRIC NEPHROLOGY

Proceedings of the Fifth International
Pediatric Nephrology Symposium, held in
Philadelphia, PA, October 6-10, 1980

edited by

ALAN B. GRUSKIN, MD
St. Christopher's Hospital for Children,
Philadelphia, PA,
USA

and

MICHAEL E. NORMAN, MD
Children's Hospital of Philadelphia,
Philadelphia, PA,
USA

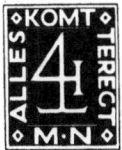

1981

MARTINUS NIJHOFF PUBLISHERS
THE HAGUE / BOSTON / LONDON

Distributors:

for the United States and Canada
Kluwer Boston, Inc.
190 Old Derby Street
Hingham, MA 02043
USA

for all other countries
Kluwer Academic Publishers Group
Distribution Center
P.O.Box 322
3300 AH Dordrecht
The Netherlands

This volume is listed in the Library of Congress Cataloging in Publication Data

ISBN-13:978-94-009-8321-2   e-ISBN-13:978-94-009-8319-9
DOI: 10.1007/978-94-009-8319-9

PREFACE

The Proceedings of the Fifth International Pediatric Nephrology Symposia are dedicated to those who make the writing possible: the delegates; those who wanted to attend, but could not, and to our colleagues, families and friends who helped organize the meeting.

With the advent of certification of pediatric nephrologists in the USA and the increasing numbers of pediatric nephrologists contributing to and practicing this specialty throughout the world, it is appropriate that we begin to record our international symposia in order to periodically document the State of the Art of pediatric nephrology and to share new information in a timely fashion with colleagues who care for children.

Four previous international pediatric nephrology symposia have been sponsored by the International Pediatric Nephrology Association. These meetings were held in Guadalajara, Mexico, 1968, Paris, France, 1971, Washington, DC, USA, 1974 and Helsinki, Finalnd, 1977.

This is the first time that it has been possible to organize the publication of the proceedings of a symposium. The enclosed manuscripts represent more than seventy percent of the symposia presentations delivered at the Fifth International Pediatric Symposia (October 6-10, 1980, Phila., PA) which was co-hosted by St. Christopher's Hospital for Children and The Children's Hospital of Philadelphia representing the Departments of Pediatrics of Temple University School of Medicine and The University of Pennsylvania School of Medicine.

The material presented touches upon most areas of pediatric nephrology and is organized in the manner in which the symposia were presented. The manuscripts have been prepared by the individual authors using the technique of camera ready copy. Thus, there is some variation in the style of presentations amongst the manuscripts and no editing has been done. By preparing and reproducing the proceedings in this fashion the time between the meeting and publication is sufficiently shortened so as to make the material available to interested individuals quickly and economically. The total program and free paper abstracts presented at the meeting may be found in Pediatric Research, Volume 14, August, 1980.

Alan B. Gruskin, M.D., President
Michael E. Norman, M.D., Secretary General
Fifth International Pediatric Nephrology Symposium

FIFTH INTERNATIONAL PEDIATRIC NEPHROLOGY SYMPOSIUM

6-10 OCTOBER 1980

OFFICERS

President   Alan B. Gruskin, Philadelphia, U.S.A.
Secretary-General   Michael E. Norman, Philadelphia, U.S.A.

Sponsored by the International Paediatric Nephrology Association
Secretary-General   G.C. Arneil, Glasgow, Scotland
Treasurer   O. Oetliker, Berne, Switzerland
Assistant S-cretaries O. Oetliker, Berne, Switzerland
                    J. Lewy, New Orlenas, U.S.A.
                    T. Sakai, Kanagawa, Japan

COUNCILLORS

1974-80	1977-83
P.L.Calagno, Washington, U.S.A.	A. Adeniyi, Ibadan, Nigeria
J. de la Cruz, Bogota, Colombia	L.B. Travis, Galveston, USA
P. Grossmann, Berlin, D.D.R.	G. Gordillo, Mexico City, Mexico
A.F. Michael, Jr., Minneapolis,USA	J. Brodehl, Hannover, B.R.D.
J.G. Mongeau, Montreal, Canada	M.A. Holliday, San Francisco, USA
K.L. Lam, Kuala Lumpur, Malaysia	M. Ignatova, Moscow, U.S.S.R.
R.H.R. White, Birmingham, England	D. A. McCredie, Victoria, Australia
J. Winberg, Stockholm, Sweden	M. Broyer, Paris, France

ORGANIZING COMMITTEES

International

G. Arbus (Toronto)
G. Arneil (Glasgow)
C. Gianantonio (Buenos Aires)
I. Greifer (New York)
R. Habib (Paris)
I. Houston (Manchester)
H. Olbing (Essen)
T. Sakai (Kanagawa-Ken)

Philadelphia

J. Baluarte	M. Polinsky
D. Cornfeld	J. Prebis
M. Cote	W. Schwartz
J. Duckett	
B. Faulkner	
J. Foreman	
R. Gottlieb	
L. Hiner	

PROGRAM CONTENT COMMITTEE

A. Aperia (Stockholm)	D. McCredie (Melbourne)
T. Barratt (London)	A. Michael (Minneapolis)
H. Boichis (Tel Hashomer)	O. Oetliker (Bern)
P. Jose (Washington)	J. Pascual (San Juan)
J. Lewy (New Orleans)	D. Potter (San Francisco)

TABLE OF CONTENTS

SYMPOSIA PRESENTATIONS

SYMPOSIA PRESENTATIONS

SYMPOSIA PRESENTATIONS

SYMPOSIA PRESENTATIONS

CURRENT PROBLEMS IN THE PATHOGENESIS OF GLOMERULONEPHRITIS

J. STEWART CAMERON, Renal Unit, Department of Medicine, Guy's Hospital, London SE1 9RT, U.K.

INTRODUCTION

If we are to make progress in the conquest of glomerulonephritis, the commonest cause of renal failure, we must first identify clearly the areas of ignorance in this study; choosing those for examination in which techniques available or foreseeable allow the construction of crucial experiments. In the study of glomerulonephritis, as in science as a whole, this enquiry may be hindered by assumptions, often unstated, and by hypotheses which become accepted uncritically as dogma, so that we cease to enquire of the data for new ideas. In this essay I wish to examine some areas in which questions are asked rather infrequently, and in which the lack of questioning may impede our understanding. I wish to disturb, not reassure, and to discuss not what we know, but what we think we know. I wish to explore what the limits of our ignorance may be, and identify areas in which unwarranted assumptions pass unquestioned. As put by Josh Billings: "it ain't what we don't know that makes us ignorant, it's what we know that ain't so".

Philosophic speculation about the process of acquiring knowledge in science has usually been the prerogative of philosophers, historians - even social scientists - rather than practicing scientists themselves. Above all, clinical investigators rarely undertake any structural examination of what they are actually about in clinic and laboratory. The classical, Socratic view of the acquisition of knowledge or ideas pictures the process as a voyage of discovery into the world, in which world ideas, processes and objects are already present, awaiting our attention. Today this view has been supplanted by the views of philosophers such as Popper, and we now give the accolade of "fact" simply to those hypotheses which still successfully resist the assault of attempted refutation by reason or experiment. A new hypothesis becomes necessary when observations not explicable by the old hypothesis arise, and each new hypothesis subsumes and expands the previous hypothesis, explaining both the old and the new discordant facts. On occasion this may require a radical change in direction of thinking, a point much emphasised by Kuhn, but whether the process is a gradual step-by-step process, or largely discontinuous, makes little difference for the present discussion. It is interesting that the English word for "fact" comes from the Latin for "make", not "discover", "reveal" or "find". New ideas are constructs, models of the world, to be progressively amplified and refined.

The importance of this philosophic diversion to my present essay becomes apparent when we examine ignorance. In the Socratic view, ignorance is simply the result of incomplete or defective exploration. In the modern, Popperian view, it is the result of faulty or inadequate constructs. Moreover, a Gresham's law of ideas seems to operate: sloppy or unquestioned constructs often act to block the introduction of testing of more complete or appropriate ideas. Ignorance may not therefore be passive process only, but has its own genesis, and in many areas (such as politics and sociology) can be used as a powerful manipulative tool. With this in mind, I propose to examine a series of questions in the study of glomerulonephritis, some the common daily debate of interested laboratories, others less often raised, and therefore more necessary to pose and discuss.

1. Is all glomerulonephritis an immune disorder?

Like most tissues, the kidney has only a limited repertoire of responses to injury, however this may come about. We must be on our guard, therefore, when we see patterns of injury in the glomerulus in human disease which we know can be mimicked by immunological manipulation not to assume too readily, or without collateral evidence, that immunological events may underlie the immune disease. For example, evidence is accumulating that the renal and other manifestations of Alport's syndrome are the result of an inherited metabolic disorder of basement membrane synthesis. Yet the glomerular scarring lesions can mimic exactly those of idiopathic focal segmental glomerulosclerosis, and proliferation within and without the tuft may be seen amounting to crescents in occasional glomeruli. Only study of the basement membranes under electron microscopy allows us to identify relatively specific appearances of splitting and granularity. What if these were not available to us at ultrastructural level?

The late lesions found in the course of patients with a haemolytic

uraemic syndrome may resemble glomerulonephritis on both optical and
electron microscopic examination; yet we believe the initial injury to
have been unrestrained intravascular platelet aggregation on a non-immune
basis. Immunoglobulins of IgG or IgM may also be present together with
complement components. These may also be found in the glomeruli in later
stages of the injury produced by the chemical agent puromycin aminonucleoside,
and there is no doubt that the finding of other immunoglobulins or complement
components does not permit the implication of immune involvement in the
pathogenesis of the disease, especially when IgM and/or C3 are the
components found in isolation. It is possible, but unlikely, that this
fixation is the result of secondary recruitment of immune reactions after
an initial non-immunologic injury but this seems unlikely.

Purely non-immunologic events may operate in the induction of both
the minimal change lesion and focal segmental glomerulosclerosis. The
majority of the phenomena relating to disordered lymphocyte function in
patients with minimal change disease can be proved to arise, either from
the effects of immediate or remote treatment, or from the nephrotic state
induced, and present therefore in nephrotic syndromes from many other
causes. I have discussed elsewhere the possibility that focal segmental
glomerulosclerosis might be the glomerular component of a non-immunologic
microvascular injury, and the scars, as Renee Habib has argued, may be the
result of podocyte injury from a variety of causes. Why do we have to
try to think of either of these conditions as the result of immunologic
events? Many other non-immunologic agents may be capable of disturbing
the structural or electrical microarchitecture of the glomerular capillary
filter and lead to proteinuria, which of itself has been shown to be
capable of damaging the podocyte.

2. To what extent can we extrapolate from animal experiments to man?

Although the first observations relating to the genesis of nephritis
were made in human beings, one of the most fruitful areas of investigation
has been the exploration of spontaneous and experimentally-induced
glomerulonephritis in laboratory animals. Usually, in interpreting these
data, at most a brief ritual genuflection is made to the altar of species
difference, and the issue is then ignored thereafter. One limitation has
been that until very recently the data concerned very few antigens and
even fewer species. If Klaus Thurau could complain that the bulk of renal
physiology was known as it applied to the left kidney of the anaesthetised

albino rat, immunologists should also be aware that the majority of their
conclusions about glomerulonephritis concerned only the injection of
bovine serum albumin in New Zealand rabbits.

Most animals suffer spontaneous nephritis. Indeed, it begins to
look as though man is a relatively nephritis-free animal, perhaps for
genetic reasons, perhaps because he has improved his immune responses by
good nutrition and eliminated many potential pathogens from his environment.
The studies of animals should make us cautious on extrapolation for two
reasons: strain differences within animals, and differences between species
in the ability to induce nephritis. One of the most striking of these
interspecies differences is the differing ease with which glomerular
proliferation can be induced in rabbits and rodents. In the rabbit, most
forms of immunological manipulation designed to produce nephritis will
induce nephritis with ease, with abundant crescent and periglomerular
proliferation. In contrast it is rather difficult to induce glomerular
proliferation at all in rodents, other than a mild increase in mesangial
cellularity. In contrast, in rodents, immune complexes formed in vitro '
and then injected intravenously localise rather readily in the glomeruli
at mesangial or subendothelial site (although not at subepithelial sites).
The resultant disease, if any, is rather mild. In the rabbit this passive
model fails to result in glomerular localisation of complexes and disease
is never seen, unless the animal is manipulated to induce local or general
inflammation. As a result of these early observations by Benacerraf and
others, the importance of the leucocyte-PAF system in rabbits was worked
out by Cochrane, Henson and their colleagues. Although PAF has now been
characterised as an acetylglyceryl phosphoryl choline, and it is present
in man, its significance for immune complex deposition in humans is quite
unknown. It appears that rodents - and perhaps man - can localise immune
complexes without its aid. Examination of the rabbit platelet, so important
in immune complex localisation in that animal, reveals two very important
differences from human platelets which suggest caution is extrapolating to
man. The first is that rabbit platelets contain more than 30 times the
quantity of vasoactive amines and ADP than human platelets do. The second
is that (in common with rodents and other common laboratory animals) its
platelets bear the immune adherence receptor for C3b, which human platelets
do not. As a result of this receptor, rabbit platelets can participate
in any situation where C3b is generated, whereas human platelets bear only

an Fc receptor which can react directly with the antibody in immune complexes and is inhibited by complement.

Within species the strain variation of susceptibility to nephritis varies greatly. In some strains of rabbit, it is very difficult to induce severe nephritis by the injection of heterologous anti-glomerular basement membrane nephritis. However, the best studied variations are in mice and rats. Some strains of mice regularly produce nephritis in response to chronic viral infection or malarial parasitisation, others do not. In rats, some strains are very susceptible to the induction of nephritis by the injection of kidney extracts containing the tubular antigen FXla, whilst others are almost totally resistant; Steinglen and colleagues showed by cross breeding that this susceptibility was under genetic control. It is a big step from inbred rats to outbred man, but susceptibility to some forms of human nephritis does appear to be linked to the HLA locus particularly the D and DR antigens, which is now thought to be closely associated with genes modulating some immune responses in man.

Finally, there are no morphological animal counterparts, either spontaneous or experimental, to a number of forms of human glomerular disease: IgA nephropathy, intramembranous dense deposit disease, or minimal change nephritis. In others, for example membranous nephropathy, we are fortunate to have both experimental and spontaneous models: Heymann nephritis in the rat and spontaneous membranous nephropathy in cats. Occasionally we have only the spontaneous model, as in murine and canine SLE. Anti-GBM nephritis has only been noted, besides man, in the horse, despite the ease with which it may be induced in sheep by injection of heterologous GBM antigens, or passively by injection of antibody in rabbits. There are tantalising "near misses", which mimic human disease in some respects but differ from it in important respects, such as the spontaneous, genetically controlled hypocomplementemic mesangiocapillary disease of newborn landrace lambs.

All this should make us very cautious in interpreting any data derived from inbred strains of laboratory animal which apparently throw light on the pathogenesis of human disease.

3. Is most human glomerulonephritis the result of glomerular fixation of circulating soluble immune complexes formed in antigen excess?

A few years ago an elegant and useful hypothesis had become accepted dogma: that the great majority - perhaps 95% - of human glomerulonephritis

was the result of the formation, circulation and glomerular localisation
of rather small, soluble immune complexes formed in antigen excess, giving
a granular appearance of immune "deposits" on immunofluorescent staining;
whilst the remaining 5% resulted from fixation of antibody on the GBM,
giving a linear fluorescence. It now appears that some forms of animal
nephritis, and probably in some human disease, glomerular injury may result
from the combination of free circulating antibody with antigen fixed or
"planted" in the glomerulus. The antithesis between anti-GBM glomerulonephritis and "soluble complex" nephritis was blurred by the realisation
that, on the one hand the glomerular injury (as opposed to transient
proteinuria) in the anti-GBM model depended, not upon the fixation of the
injected anti-GBM antibody, but the fixation of secondary autologous
antibody to the "planted" anti-GBM IgG, which now functioned an an
immunising antigen for the host animal. On the other hand, work on the
Heymann model of nephritis showed that passive fixation of antibody to
discontinuous antigens in the GBM could lead to a granular appearance on
immunofluorescence. The new concepts are both more complete and more
satisfying, but will doubtless be discarded in their turn, having provoked,
as all good hypotheses should, a further series of experiments. We still
do not know whether in situ combination of low avidity antibody and small
antigens in the subepithelial space is the proximate cause of human
membranous nephropathy, although this seems likely. Couser has reviewed
the evidence on in situ complex elsewhere in this volume, and I will not
discuss this topic further. I would, however, like to comment further on
the nature and formation of complexes in the subendothelial-mesangial
space of the glomerular capillaries.

The suggestion that these are the result of complexes formed in
antigen excess has its origin in studies of the "single shot" model of acute
serum sickness in rabbits. In this model free antigen is present in the
circulation after injection of a large dose, at first alone, then in
company with immune complexes containing the antigen, when antigen, antibody
and complement in that order are observed to appear in the kidney with a
varying degree of inflammation and functional disturbance. Only when the
antigen has disappeared, and the complexes likewise, does free antibody
appear and persist.

In experiments involving repeated injections of foreign protein the
situation is rather different. The message from these experiments of

Germuth, Dixon and their colleagues, that a single antibody-antigen system could, by suitable manipulation, give rise to most of the appearances of human glomerulonephritis, is and remains a crucial piece of evidence. However, some of the detailed interpretation of the mechanisms may need re-examination. All the animals in these studies are likely to have swung from antibody excess to antigen excess and back again throughout the 24 hours when they received a single daily injection of BSA. In general, they will have been in modest antibody excess near equivalence, which with a multivalent antigen like BSA must have led to the formation of insoluble complexes. In passing, we can note that the antibody assays used, being functional, would have expressed equally antibody avidity as antibody quantity. The only experiments using the chronic BSA model in which all animals were kept in antigen excess throughout, those of Boyns and Hardwicke, resulted in no disease at all.

In contrast, Stilmant and Couser have shown that ferritin, in the presence of antibody excess, will lead to a mesangial-subendothelial deposit nephritis. Gabbiani using the rabbit, and Clark in the pig have shown that infusion of ferritin into the renal artery of animals previously immunised with ferritin will lead to first a focal glomerulonephritis and then, in the pig, an appearance similar to mesangiocapillary glomerulonephritis, with subendothelial deposits in the true peripheral capillary rather than the paramesangial area. In these experiments forming, rather than pre-formed, complexes are present in the renal circulation, and may play a part in the disease, since, even allowing for the short life of poorly soluble complexes in the circulation the kidneys receive 10% of the cardiac output and must receive some complexes of this type even though they do not persist. Also, reticuloendothelial blockade may be induced and perpetuated by the elimination of such complexes and lead to a prolongation of the life in the circulation of the remainder.

Turning to human disease, one of the best studied antigen-antibody systems is the DNA-anti-DNA system. This remains in antibody excess, without free circulating DNA but abundant anti-DNA antibody, for more than 99% of the time in most patients; and sudden falls in the titre of DNA antibody in the circulation can be observed just before clinical exacerbations. When (after clotting artefacts have been eliminated) small amounts of free DNA are found in the circulation the patient usually suffers cutaneous vasculitis or cerebral disease rather than nephritis. Data are not yet

available for the HB_e-anti-HB_e system in membranous nephropathy, but appear
from preliminary material from Japan presented in this Congress to be in
antigen excess; this might be expected, given the epimembranous site of
the deposits. Studies in the rarer mesangiocapillary glomerulonephritis
found in association with $HB_{\underline{e}}$ might be expected to show antibody excess,
if the above speculations are correct.

Evidence has accumulated that the formation, circulation and renal
trapping of small soluble complexes is a normal part of immune elimination
and that the kidney acts as an immunoabsorbent for these complexes. This
elimination is not accompanied by disease, or at most transient mild
proteinuria, and is a feature of many febrile infectious diseases (so-called
"febrile" protinuria). Thus, we are quite likely to find this material
present in the kidney in disease, even if it has no pathogenetic
significance; indeed, because of local inflammation these complexes may
be present in excess and mislead us to think that their presence has
initiated or perpetuated the disease.

Thus, at least some forms of human glomerulonephritis appear to arise
from differential penetration of low molecular antigen and (usually) low
avidity antibody into the capillary wall or mesangium, there they combine.
Others may arise from poorly-soluble or insoluble complexes at equivalence
or in antibody excess deposited in the mesangium or subendothelial space.
Yet others may be the result of the trapping of small, soluble antigen-
excess complexes, usually in the peripheral capillary wall and usually
without much inflammation; but probably a minority of human disease arises
from this route and most such complexes may be non-toxic.

4. What can we learn from the study of immune complexes in the serum of
   patients with glomerulonephritis?

The discussion above leads naturally into a consideration of what,
if anything, we can learn from the immune complexes which can be found in
the circulation. We can suggest three possibilities:

   (i)   circulating complexes are depositing in the tissues and
         represent a true sample of the injurious material on its way
         to fixation and initiation of injury. They may persist in
         the circulation because of reticuloendothelial blockade which
         thus increases their potential toxicity.

   (ii) they are poorly-fixing, poorly-phagocytosed complexes which
         are left in the circulation after localisation of any toxic

       complexes in tissues

(iii) a combination of (i) and (ii)

(iv) circulating complexes are epiphenomena of the immune events which lead to tissue injury and have no direct relation to this injury.

Consideration of section 3 above leads to the immediate conclusion that circulating complexes at best, can only give a distorted reflection of what is going on in the tissues. The correlations of immune complexes in the circulation with clinical events, patterns of histopathological damage or severity in systemic lupus are in general very poor, although striking correlations may be seen, especially in untreated, early active disease. Equally striking dissociations of activity and pattern are seen more frequently, but find their way into the literature less often!

One set of difficulties with immune complex assays is technical. Over forty methods are now available, each dependent upon some biological or physical property of the immune complex. None detects all species of complexes, and all react with material(s) which are not immune complexes. Many are interfered with by other immune reactants present in the plasma or bound to the complex; for example, Clq or antiglobulins ("rheumatoid" factors). In idiopathic glomerulonephritis, other than acute post-infectious types, methods which detect complement-binding complexes (such as the Clq fluid or solid phase assays or the Raji cell assay) find few or no complexes present. In contrast, non-complement-dependent assays, such as platelet aggregation, K-cell assays or rheumatoid factor IgG assays, find abundant material, including in paients with membranous nephropathy. On the other hand, in SLE the Raji cell assay is usually strongly positive in most patients, even those on immunosuppression. On closer examination, however, the great majority of this material is monomer IgG reacting with surface and nuclear antigens of the Raji cell, and not immune complexes at all. Finally, in many diseases - neoplastic disease and rheumatoid arthritis are two - immune complexes are present in the serum in abundance, and yet nephritis is almost unknown.

At the moment we cannot identify those complexes important in initiating or perpetuating glomerulonephritis with any certainty. A further problem arises in that, as well as entering the tissues from the circulation, there is good evidence that this is a reversible phenomenon and that especially in states of low avidity antibody, complexes or their components may re-enter the circulation from the tissues. (The role of complement in this solubilisation is discussed below.) Complexes in solution in the circulation are probably in variable equilibrium with complexes in the tissue, with free antibody and/or antigen, and with other species of complex, as in Steensgaard's in vitro experiments. Removal of one species of complex could lead to re-equilibration within the circulation. Thus, sampling the plasma at one instant and trying from this to guess from it what may be going on in the tissues is like a bad Xerox copy of a single frame from a movie which is being run in another room.

A final, strikingly discordant observation which should make us question the value of immune complex measurements (and their role in pathogenesis) is the absence of reports of recurrence in transplanted kidneys of the "archetypal immune complex disease" - SLE. Worldwide, over 300 grafts have been performed successfully in patients with SLE, but no case of recurrent disease has been documented. The suggestion that this is because many patients in renal failure have "burnt out" SLE, or that the immunosuppression after transplantation is somehow effective in inhibiting the disease in a fashion which was not evident before transplantation, seem to me inadequate. We have transplanted one patient with active disease, requiring immunosuppression and with complexes inthe circulation by three assays, without recurrence. In contrast, membranous nephropathy has been recorded on a dozen or more occasions!

5. How is the glomerulus damaged in human glomerulonephritis?

Much work has been done on the mediation of injury in the glomerulus, and I can only glance at this problem here. The relevance of any studies in this area will, of course, depend upon the relevance of the model chosen to human disease. The complement-polymorph system of injury is the best known, and is probably relevant to acute (and usually reversible) injury; its participation in chronic injury, in animals of man, is doubtful. Much of our information on injury has been obtained in the rabbit, an animal particularly unsuitable for extrapolation to man, and much of it concerns acute, predominantly extracapillary injury. In human disease, we seek the causes of chronic, mostly endocapillary scarring. It must be admitted that we have little idea how this may come about.

Evidence is accumulating that both cells, particularly monocytes, and coagulation mechanisms, particularly platelets, play a central role in the mediation of chronic injury. This arises through the interaction of

damaged endothelium with both cells (leucocytes, monocytes, platelets) and
humoral plasma factors concerned with what is usually termed the coagulation
system. It has become clear that on the one hand platelets have a role in
the induction of inflammation and the removal of foreign material; and
that on the other, leucocytes have a role in both coagulation and fibrinolysis
The arbitrary separation of "systems" such as inflammatory, kinin, prostaglandin, complement and coagulation systems lies rather with the methods
of their dissection ex vivo, rather than their mode of operation in vivo
in health or disease.

One point worth comment is the usual assumption that agents capable
of injury found at the site of injury are necessarily injurious. It is
well known that policemen may be found at the scene of crimes; few would
suggest that they were always responsible for the events! Complement, as
well as being capable of inducing inflammation through anaphylatoxins
and chemotaxis, is also capable (as Nussenzweig has pointed out) of
solubilising complexes through intercalation of C3b generated by the
alternative pathway into the complex. On the cellular side, monocytes and
polymorphs, although experimental studies confirm their ability to generate
inflammation in both acute serum sickness and in anti-GBM injury, are also
capable of removing antigens, complexes and immune reactants. In this
particular movie, it is not always easy to distinguish the good guys from
the bad guys; and some of the actors may on occasion play a double role.

Finally, we must seek an explanation for the many observations which
suggest that deposition of complexes, antibody or complement is often not
associated with injury. In several forms of nephritis these agents may
be diffusely distributed, but the damage is focal and segmental; SLE and
Henoch-Schonlein purpura come to mind. This may simply be an effect of
local difference in concentrations of immune reactants which is inapparent
by conventional techniques such as immunofluorescence. However, the
clinical histories suggesting activation of such latent disease by non-
specific events (immunisation by unrelated antigens, infections, or drugs)
suggests that other modulators of injury are present which we do not
yet understand.

6. What determines chronicity and progression in glomerulonephritis?

One of the major questions which remains unanswered is just what
determines resolution of injury on the one hand, or the destruction of the
glomerulus on the other.

It is clear that what destroys the filtering surface of the glomerulus is not usually acute injury with inflammation (although necrosis plays ist part in some patients) but subsequent scarring: paradoxically, it is the healing, not the injury which eventually destroys the kidney in glomerulonephritis. What is the difference between a "one shot" disease with healing and chronic disease with scarring? A conventional answer would be that continued deposition of freshly-formed immune complexes into the kidney leads to continued inflammation with consequent scarring. This concept can easily be extended to include in situ complex formation, and there is evidence to support it, from patients in whom the offending antigen could be identified and eliminated. In these patients with infections, tumours or drug-induced nephropathies, a remarkable resolution usually takes place, sometimes even from renal failure requiring dialysis. However, in each case identification of the antigen as the putative agent depends upon its being found in the glomerular lesions, which seems to be an unusual finding in glomerulonephritis as a whole. It may be that these instructive cases are unusual exceptions of antigen overload, rather than typical examples of the type of genetically-determined nephritis now seen in the Western world.

One can note here that records suggest that the cases seen today in Europe and North America represent the residue of a twenty-fold greater incidence one hundred years ago, comparable to that found in tropical areas today. It is possible that the cases now seen in developed countries are those which depend upon subtle inherited deficiencies in immune elimination, and the strong associations of Goodpasture's syndrome and membranous nephropathy with individual HLA-DR antigens supports this idea. Association of immune responses with the HLA locus are now well established in man, to the point where human immune response genes analagous to those described in mice may be postulated. Gross deficiencies of the immune system, particularly the complement system (known to be carried on the same 6th chromosome as the HLA locus) are well known to be associated with a much higher incidence of immune complex disease than normal. In contrast, the majority of patients with glomerulonephritis in the Third World may be largely dependent upon a nutritionally-compromised immune system, overwhelmed by chronic infection or parasitoses.

If continuing antigen deposition is the mechanism for continuing disease, then the antigen should be detectable in the lesions late in the disease, as well as at the onset. For years, many laboratories all over the world have sought antigens in human nephritis, and the result has been a miserable few cases, whom antigen and/or antibody could be identified, many of whom have had acute disease. In the great majority of forms of chronic nephritis, no antigen could be found. This has been variously explained by reason of the small amounts of complex deposited, the possible masking of the antigen sites by IgG or complement, or scarring with removal of the complexes and disappearance of the antigen.

The simplest explanation appears to have been overlooked: that in most forms of chronic nephritis in man there are no exogenous antigens present in the lesions. This suggestion implies that some secondary mechanism takes over and leads to progression, possibly after an exogenous antigen has initiated the disease. What possible mechanisms could do this? Three emerge, all of which might operate together, or in different individuals.

The first is that the initial assault leads to acute soluble complex disease and that this depresses reticuloendothelial function so that previously "normal" circulating immune complexes can deposit in the kidney. This would result in the antigens of the secondary phase being either autologous or banal, and supposes that the R.E. defect, once established, persists as a vicious circle by reason of the persistence of the immune complexes in the circulation. The work on the extraordinarily rapid reversal of depressed clearance of heat-damaged red cells by plasmapheresis could be interpreted in this light.

The second possible mechanism is that the initial injury renders autologous antigens immunogenic, and that in essence the chronic phase of most forms of nephritis is an autoimmune disease. The work of the late Rawle Mackintosh on the enhanced immunogenicity of IgG whose sialic acid had been removed by bacterial neuraminidase supports this idea, and recent observations of DNA and anti-DNA antibody in cryoprecipitable material from patients with "idiopathic" nephritis may be relevant. In this view, the offending antigens perpetuating disease in chronic nephritis are autologous. One identified pathogen whose elimination does not appear to lead to arrest or resolution of the nephritis is p.malariae. The problem here is to know for how long parasite antigen might persist in the reticuloendothelial system and be released slowly. However, there is evidence that the perpetuating antigens in the experimental nephritis induced in mice treated with p.berghei are not malarial. Initially, both malarial antigen and anti-malarial antibody can be detected in the immune deposits within the kidney, but whilst the deposits persist for months, this antigen-antibody system becomes undetectable after only a few weeks. In the chicken infected with p.gallinaceum, the persisting antigen is tentatively identified as a serum protein leached off infected red cells.

The third mechanism is to a certain extent a variation on the second, and was the first to be proposed. This suggests that the deposited material in the glomerulus evokes a secondary antibody repsonse, and that this antibody response to the "planted" material continues the damage after initial deposition of complexes, including exogenous antigens, has initiated the injury. Alternatively, local damage to glomerular structures renders autologous glomerular antigens immunogenic.

None of these explanations is exclusive, and continued deposition of complexes may also occur in some individuals, as it almost certainly does in patients with shunt nephritis or subacute bacterial endocarditis.

7. Conclusion

It is a platitude that progress in any field of study can be made only by generating new hypotheses for testing. We can only generate these new hypotheses if we first identify the questions which require answer. This requires a certain boldness, which is often lacking amidst the process of grant allocation, and even at the point where original and "controversial" work is considered for publication. This behaviour is capable of generating and perpetuating ignorance, just as contrasting behaviour can foster the increase of knowledge.

"Compared to the pond of knowledge, our ignorance remains Atlantic"

Duncan and Weston Smith.
The Encyclopedia of Ignorance.

DEVELOPMENTAL RENAL PHYSIOLOGY

C.M. EDELMANN,JR.

In 1940, Barnett(1) demonstrated by inulin clearance that the rates
of glomerular filtration in neonates were considerably lower than levels
found in older children and adults, thus launching the field of developmental renal physiology. This observation has been confirmed repeatedly.
Barnett also suggested that with birth, the rate of increase in renal
function that proceeds in utero is markedly accelerated, even in premature infants, permitting the kidney to assume excretory and regulatory
functions in the absence of the placenta. This phenomenon has been
demonstrated nicely by Guignard and associates(2), who studied low-birth-
weight infants during the first 72 hours after birth and over the subsequent three weeks. The increase in GFR between the 28th and 35th week of
gestation was more rapid than during the subsequent five weeks, but a
striking acceleration after birth was apparent.

Over the next quarter century numerous investigators examined renal
blood flow, clearances of electrolytes, concentrating and diluting mechanisms, and acid-base control in infants of various ages, as well as to
a limited extent in experimental animals. Important observations were
made characterizing the functional immaturity of the kidney of the neonate
and pointing out the consequent decrease in homeostatic limits. These
studies had immediate relevance to newborn care. The healthy full-term
infant grows and develops with little concern over his immature kidneys.
The sick infant and the low-birth-weight infant readily demonstrate the
importance of their limitations in renal function when stressed by disease
or the personnel caring for them.

Although the observations made during this early period were of extreme importance, and laid the foundation necessary for the further study
of developmental renal physiology, they did not provide an understanding
of what was biologically different in the immature state to account for
the functional differences that were observed. In the last two decades

it has been possible to apply increasingly powerful tools to the study of
the kidney, and in the past ten years we have seen many of these applied
to the study of development. There has been a literal explosion of knowledge, with an ability to get closer and closer to fundamental understanding of the biology of maturation.

Recently, more than 150 nephrologists gathered in New York for a three
day workshop on developmental renal physiology[*]. The exchange of ideas
among basic scientists, clinical investigators, and clinicians was truly
exciting. In my address today, I would like to summarize work in a few
selected areas of developmental renal physiology in which there has been
significant progress. I am indebted to many of the participants at the
recent workshop for permitting me to include their studies.

GLOMERULAR FILTRATION RATE

In some of our early studies, we noted striking increases in GFR during
the course of maneuvers such as the induction of volume expansion. This
suggested to us that the GFR was being regulated at a low level, and was
not obligated. It now appears that this is correct, and we shall go into
possible reasons for this later on. Let us consider first the factors
that control GFR and analyze them on a developmental scale.

The rate of glomerular filtration depends on the pressure available to
provide the energy for ultrafiltration, the area of the membrane through
which filtration can take place, and permeability characteristics of that
membrane. This is summarized in the equation: $SNGFR = P_{UF}ks$. This indicates that the rate of filtration in a single nephron is dependent upon
the pressure for ultrafiltration, P_{UF}, the hydraulic conductivity of the
membrane, in this case, the glomerular capillary wall, k, and the total
area of capillary through which filtration takes place, S. We shall examine each of these individually.

As summarized in the equation $P_{UF} = P_{GC} - (\Pi_{GC} + P_{PT})$, the pressure
for filtration is the resultant of the hydrostatic pressure within the
glomerular capillary, P_{GC}, the opposing force of the oncotic pressure
within the capillary (Π_{GC})[**], and the opposing force of the hydrostatic
pressure within the proximal tubule (P_{PT}).

*1st International Workshop on Developmental Renal Physiology, N.Y.,
Oct. 2-4, 1980.
**Since the concentration of protein in the glomerular filtrate is
close to zero, it will be disregarded in this discussion.

Spitzer and Edelmann(3) measured these forces in newborn guinea pigs, using micropuncture techniques. They found a small increase in pressure for ultrafiltration that could account for an increase in filtration rate with maturation of about 10%.

In order to study the permeability of the glomerular capillaries, Goldsmith and associates(4) studied the renal clearance of dextrans of varying molecular size, relative to the clearance of inulin, comparing one-week-old and six-week-old puppies. A small but real increase in permeability was noted in the older animals. This increased permeability by itself could account for an increase in filtration rate of about 5%. That permeability does not seem to be a limiting factor is supported by the work of Ichikawa et al.(5) in the Munich Wistar rat. Let us consider the changes that take place in the forces that underly filtration along the length of the glomerular capillary. At the proximal end of the capillary, the hydrostatic force favoring filtration is greater than the oncotic force opposing it, and filtration takes place. As filtration proceeds, the concentration of protein within the capillary increases progressively, so that at some point the hydrostatic force favoring filtration and the oncotic force opposing it may become equal. This condition is termed filtration equilibrium, and is accompanied by cessation of filtration. On the other hand, the hydrostatic force may remain greater than the oncotic force along the entire course of the capillary, in which case filtration will continue throughout. In Ichikawa's studies(5), in which these forces were measured directly, filtration equilibrium was present in the immature animal. Therefore, the permeability of the capillary membrane could not be considered a limiting factor at any given stage of development.

Let us turn now to the final regulator of glomerular filtration, surface area. In the study of Fetterman and associates(6), it was shown that in the immature kidney the glomeruli, although small, are relatively larger than the tubules, as compared to older infants and children. This was shown by the high values of the ratio of glomerular surface area to proximal tubular volume in infants compared to older subjects. This study suggested that from birth to maturity there is relatively little increase in glomerular size—not enough to account for the striking increase in filtration rate. The interpretation, however, failed to take into account the fact that with maturation there is increasing complexity of the capillary network within the glomerulus, so that not only the overall size of the glomerulus but the number and density of capillary loops contained there-in must be considered.

In order to examine this, John, Goldsmith and Spitzer(7) studies the kidneys of puppies 1,3 and 6 weeks of age and adult dogs, injected with Microfil. The renal vasculature was perfused in vivo, and the volume of Microfil filling the glomerular capillaries was measured utilizing a neutron activation technique. From measurement of glomerular capillary diameter the surface area for filtration could be calculated. A marked increase in both cortical and juxtamedullary glomerular capillary surface area took place with advancing age, which could account for an 8-fold in-crease in filtration rate.

It is of interest that in measurements in rats, using an electron microscopic technique and computer analysis, Larsson(8) demonstrated a 28-fold increase in the area of glomerular capillary basement membrane, during a period in which glomerular filtration increased by a factor of 22, supporting the conclusions of John et al.(7), using a different ex-perimental technique and a different species.

If we put together all these observations, we can account completely for the 20 to 25-fold increase in filtration rate that has been noted to occur between the newborn and the adult state in the rat, dog, guinea pig and human. The major factor, as noted, is the increase in glomerular cap-illary surface area.

At any given stage of development, as suggested by the studies of Ichikawa et al.(5) surface area and permeability do not seem to be limit-ing factors, at least in the Munich-Wistar rat, since filtration equilib-rium pertains. The hydrostatic pressure for filtration, therefore, must be the dominant factor. The fact that filtration pressure is far less than systemic pressure reflects the high resistance of the renal vascular bed. In studies reported by Gruskin et al.(9) in piglets, a very high renal vascular resistance was found in the youngest animals, with a pro-gressive fall with age. This was accompanied by a reciprocal increase in renal blood flow.

It would appear then that glomerular filtration rate is limited by regulation of the vascular supply to the glomeruli, which in turn con-trols the rate of glomerular perfusion. We still must ask the question why.

GLOMERULAR-TUBULAR BALANCE

Some years ago we(10) suggested that the rate of glomerular filtration
in the immature kidney was kept at a low level in order to avoid deliver-
ing excessive amounts of filtrate to immature tubules. This was based on
available data, including the demonstration of a low filtration fraction,
low bicarbonate threshold, aminoaciduria, and a low capacity to reabsorb
glucose relative to the filtration rate. This concept of glomerular-tubular imbalance, with a gradual rise in filtration rate as tubules enlarge
and mature, provided an attractive explanation for many of the characteristics of the immature kidney. The hypothesis began to fail, however, as
additional studies appeared. It became clear that the aminoaciduria of
the infant was selective, not generalized, and seemed to relate to differential rates of maturation of specific transport mechanisms(11,12).

In the studies of Arant et al.(13) in puppies and Brodehl et al.(14)
in infants and children, the maximal capacity to reabsorb glucose relative to GFR was not found to be low, as previously reported. In micropuncture studies by Spitzer and Brandis(15) and Horster and Valtin(16),
TF/P inulin in the proximal tubule, a measure of fractional reabsorption,
was not found to increase with age, as might have been expected if the
tubules initially were being overwhelmed. And finally, Spitzer and
Brandis(15) showed that the filtration rate in single nephrons was proportional to the length of the proximal tubule, providing further evidence for glomerular-tubular balance.

As other studies appeared, however, things became less clear. Evidence
was presented by Aperia et al.(17), Kleinman(18), Spitzer and Schoeneman
(19) and others that the fraction of filtered sodium reabsorbed in the
proximal tubule of the immature kidney was less than in the mature state.
For example, Kleinman(18) administered saline to puppies and showed that
they had a limited natriuretic response. The value of 99.7% of the
filtered sodium reabsorbed during the control period fell to only 98.5%
after administration of saline. When he gave diuretic agents to block
distal reabsorption of sodium, however, almost 50% of the filtered sodium
was excreted in the urine, indicating that at least that amount had been
delivered to the distal nephron, a surprisingly high fraction. Rodriguez-
Soriano et al.(20) performed studies in infants and children during hypotonic saline diuresis, permitting him to use the clearance of free water
plus the clearance of sodium as an index of distal delivery, and the

clearance of free water alone as a measure of distal reabsorption. The highest values for distal delivery were obtained in the youngest subjects, with a progressive fall with increasing age. However, at any given rate of distal delivery, reabsorption at that site was the same for all age groups. Although these studies suggest a very different set for glomerulo-tubular balance in the immature kidney, it must be recognized that they were carried out under states of volume expansion and may not characterize accurately the more basal or usual state. More studies will be needed to clarify this. However, some other interesting observations may be pertinent. Kotchen et al.(21) have measured changes in plasma renin levels with age. Strikingly high values were observed in young infants. Similarly, Kowarski and co-workers(22) found extraordinarily high levels of plasma aldosterone in neonates.

The characteristics of sodium handling described above, together with the elevated plasma levels of renin and aldosterone, led Spitzer(23) to propose that immediately after birth, while filtration rate remains low, sodium is effectively reabsorbed in the proximal and distal portions of the nephron. With an increase in GFR and increased delivery of sodium into the nephron, increased reabsorption of sodium takes place primarily in the distal portion, as a consequence of increased stimulation by aldosterone. Subsequent to this, with further maturation of the proximal tubule and increased capacity for sodium reabsorption, less is delivered distally, less needs to be reabsorbed distally, and this is reflected in a fall in aldosterone concentration.

Sulyok(24) has shown in low-birth-weight infants an inability to conserve sodium and to remain in sodium balance. In a study of Siegel(25), fractional excretion of sodium measured in infants during the second day of life fell from 6% in the most immature infants to 0.3 to 0.7% in the full-term. All infants 26 to 29 weeks gestational age were in negative sodium balance, in contrast to only 14% of those with gestational age 40 weeks. Of great interest is the recent study of Sulyok et al.(26) in which infants of low gestational age received supplements of sodium chloride. These infants did not go into negative sodium balance, did not develop hyponatremia, and did not show elevated levels of plasma renin. A further observation, which remains unexplained, is that the supplemented infants also maintained higher values of blood bicarbonate than nonsupplemented infants.

THE CENTRIFUGAL PATTERN OF RENAL DEVELOPMENT

A striking feature of the immature kidney is that it develops in a centrifugal pattern, so that at any given stage, the most mature nephrons lie in the deep cortex and the most immature are in the outer cortex. This pattern is reflected in the distribution of blood flow to various parts of the kidney, as shown by a number of studies, employing the distribution of microspheres and xenon wash-out curves(27-30). The changes found from the pattern in the newborn with relatively little flow to the outer cortex and a rich supply to the inner cortex, to the pattern of the adult, with an approximately equal distribution, is striking. As would be expected, a similar pattern of distribution has been found by Jose et al.(31) for filtration rate, using the Hanssen technique. They observed an increasing ratio of outer cortical to inner cortical glomerular filtration rate with age, reflecting the progressively increasing rate of filtration in the more superficial glomeruli. This pattern mimicked the outer cortical to inner cortical rate of blood flow, as measured by microspheres in the same study.

NATRIURETIC RESPONSE

Despite these intriguing observations, it has been difficult to relate the centrifugal pattern of development to functional characteristics of the immature kidney. Goldsmith et al.(32) studied the response of puppies to saline loading, speculating that the limited response of the immature kidney might relate to the fact that the outer cortex is undeveloped and thus cannot participate fully in natriuresis. As the outer cortex matures, one might anticipate an increasing natriuretic response. Although the smallest response was noted in the youngest animals, the response of 9 to 15-day-old animals was almost as great as that of the adults, and significantly greater than that of 19 to 24-day-olds. Moreover, studies of blood flow distribution did not show a change from hydropenia to salt loading in any age group studied, suggesting that an inability to perfuse the outer cortex at a higher rate could not be the explanation for the limited natriuresis.

The phenomena underlying the limited diuretic response of the immature kidney thus remain to be fully elucidated. Of interest, although adding complexity, is a recent observation of Solomon and associates(32). Infant rats expanded with blood from littermates excreted 20% of their volume load, in contrast to adult animals that excreted 85% in the same period of time. However, when infant animals were expanded with blood from adults, they excreted 42% of the load. This observation suggests that the presence of some factor in adult blood may be necessary to mount a full diuretic response.

CONCENTRATING MECHANISMS

Let us turn to another area, the renal concentrating mechanism. Although it has been recognized for decades that the concentrating capacity of the immature kidney of many species is less than that of the adult, the reasons for this are not clear.

In studies in infants, Edelmann et al.(34) were able to show that a major limitation related to the low rate of excretion of urea, as a consequence of the infant being in a strongly anabolic state and utilizing most of the dietary nitrogen intake for growth. When a high protein diet was offered, urinary concentrating capacity rose markedly, the increase being entirely attributable to increased urinary urea. Of note, however, is the fact that this response was observed only when blood levels of urea rose to a striking degree. Provision of small amounts of urea as a dietary supplement, which had been shown to enhance concentrating capacity in adult animals, had no effect in infants(35). It is thought that urea enhances concentrating capacity by being concentrated in the medulla of the kidney in a process of recirculation. Urea is delivered to the medulla through the loops of Henle that arise from outer cortical glomeruli. Edwards et al.(36) examined the anatomical arrangement of the loops of Henle in young rats. The progressive increase in the length of the loops, penetration into the medulla, and incorporation into the vascular bundles were found to occur as a function of age. An increase in the concentration of urea in the renal papilla correlated precisely with the penetration of the outer cortical loops of Henle into the medulla.

This beautiful study demonstrates nicely the importance of relating anatomical and functional studies in an organ whose architecture is changing rapidly. It provides one of the few situations in which the centrifugal pattern of development can be related to a functional characteristic.

The urinary concentrating mechanism is dependent upon deposition of solute in the medulla to produce a hypertonic interstitium against which fluid in the collecting duct can equilibrate, when the collecting duct epithelium has been rendered permeable to water by the action of antidiuretic hormone. Solute is concentrated in the medulla by the active transport of sodium chloride in the thick ascending limb of Henle and by the passive deposition of urea. In examining this aspect of the urinary concentrating mechanism, Horster(37) measured the capacity of isolated segments of cortical thick ascending limb to transport sodium. Although the hydraulic conductivity of the thick ascending limb was the same in immature and mature animals, a six-fold increase in capacity to transport sodium was observed. This was accompanied by a six-fold increase in Na-K-ATPase in that segment, although it is not known whether a cause-and-effect relationship obtains.

A great deal is now known concerning the action of antidiuretic hormone at a cellular and subcellular level. It has been shown that ADH binds to the cell membrane at specific receptor sites, and activates adenyl cyclase within the membrane to convert ATP to cyclic AMP(cAMP). How cAMP acts to increase cellular permeability to water, urea, and sodium, is not known. Phosphodiesterase serves to destroy cAMP, providing feedback control. Schlondorf et al.(38) have shown that newborn rats have a smaller response in terms of adenylate cyclase activation to administration of sodium fluoride, parathormone, or vasopressin. Other studies suggest less binding of vasopressin to membrane receptor sites(39), and greater activity of phosphodiesterase. It is apparent, then, that studies of the renal concentrating mechanism, dependent on both renal and extra-renal factors, must take into account physiologic, anatomic, and hormonal factors, and must extend from the whole organ to the subcellular level.

RENAL METABOLISM

To a great extent, the metabolism of the kidney and the changes that take place with maturation have been ignored. Major differences exist between various levels of the kidney, and it is likely that further differences are present at various stages of development.

Oxygen consumption is at its highest in the cortex, which is comprised mostly of proximal tubular segments. This corresponds to a high rate of blood flow, cells rich in mitochondria, and abundant Krebs cycle enzymes. Gluconeogenesis is present and fatty acids serve as the major source of energy. Other metabolic substrates include lactate, glutamine and citrate.

Gluconeogenesis seems to occur exclusively in the cells of the proximal tubule, the segment in which substrates of gluconeogenesis are reabsorbed. This is the only site in the kidney in which are present enzymes essential for gluconeogenesis: e.g., phosphoenolpyruvate carboxykinase, glucose-6-phosphatase, and fructosebiphosphatase. Gluconeogenesis and glycolysis use many of the same enzymes, with reactions that proceed in opposite directions. Therefore, the two processes cannot occur simultaneously within the same cell. If an important function of the proximal tubule is to carry out gluconeogenesis, it cannot depend on glycolysis as an energy source for active transport.

The outer medulla, which contains most of the thick portion of the loops of Henle, and portions of the collecting ducts, also depends mainly on oxidative metabolism. In this area, however, in which gluconeogenesis does not occur, glucose is used increasingly as an energy source. The enzymes that are involved in glycolysis but not in gluconeogenesis, e.g. pyruvate kinase, hexokinase, and phosphofructokinase, are found in increasing concentration as one proceeds distally along the course of the nephron. Nevertheless, glucose remains only a minor energy source in the outer medulla, most of the energy requirement being provided by free fatty acids, as in the cortex.

Major differences in metabolism are observed as one moves into the inner medulla and papilla. Here energy derives from anaerobic glycolysis. Despite a high rate of anaerobic glycolysis, some oxidative metabolism does take place and has been shown, for example, to be essential for the operation of the concentrating mechanism. How do these observations apply to the immature kidney? As noted earlier, the fetal kidney develops in a centrifugal pattern. One might predict, therefore, that glycolysis, a characteristic of the inner medulla, might be more highly developed in the immature kidney than gluconeogenesis, an activity confined to the cortex. Few data are available. In the rat, e.g., the activities of some of the enzymes that are important in glycolysis are in fact at fully mature levels at the time of birth[40]. Phosphofructokinase activity falls abruptly just before birth in this species and continues to decline slowly thereafter, perhaps reflecting a changeover from anaerobic glycolytic activity before birth to aerobic metabolism after birth. It should be apparent that the developmental study of renal metabolism and correlation of metabolic and functional characteristics remains a fertile area for investigation[41].

CONCLUSION

The study of developmental renal physiology has gone from performance of clearance studies in infants and experimental animals to investigation of single nephron function, measurements in isolated nephron segments, investigation of renal cells grown in tissue culture, and studies of isolated cellular membranes. Increasingly, we must see the collaboration of the anatomist, the biochemist, and the physiologist, in addition to the clinical investigator and the clinician. The ultimate goal of an increased understanding of all aspects of renal function is our ability to offer improved care to infants in health and disease.

REFERENCES

1. Barnett, H.L. Renal physiology in infants and children. I. Method for estimation of glomerular filtration rate. Proc. Soc. Exp. Biol. Med. 44: 654, 1940.
2. Guignard, J.-P., Torrado, A., Feldman, H., and Gautier, E. Assessment of glomerular filtration rate in children. Helv. Paediat. Acta 35: 437, 1980.
3. Spitzer, A., and Edelmann, C.M., Jr. Maturational changes in pressure gradients for glomerular filtration. Amer. J. Physiol. 221: 1431, 1971.
4. Goldsmith, D.I., Jodorkovsky, R.A., Kleinman, S.R., Sherwinter, J., and Spitzer, A. Changes in glomerular capillar permeability to dextrans during development. Ped. Res. 13: 1126, 1974.
5. Ichikawa, I., Maddox, D.A., Brenner, B.M. Maturational development of glomerular ultrafiltration in the rat. Amer. J. Physiol. 236: F465, 1979.
6. Fetterman, G.H., Shuplock, N.A., Philipp, F.J., and Gregg, H.S. The growth and maturation of human glomeruli and proximal convolutions from term to adulthood: Studies by microdissection. Pediatrics 35: 601, 1965.
7. John, E., Goldsmith, D.I., and Spitzer, A. Developmental changes in glomerular vasculature: physiologic implications. Clin. Res. 28: 450A, 1980.
8. Larsson, L. Discussion. First International Workshop on Developmental Renal Physiology, N.Y., 1980.
9. Gruskin, A.B., Edelmann, C.M., Jr., and Yuan, S. Maturational changes in renal blood flow in piglets. Pediatr. Res. 4: 7, 1970.
10. Edelmann, C.M., Jr. Maturation of the neonatal kidney. Proc. 3rd. International Congress of Nephrology, Wash. D.C., 1966, Vol. 3; pp.1-12.
11. Segal, S., and Smith, I. Delineation of cystine and cysteine transport systems in rat kidney cortex by developmental patterns. Proc. Natl. Acad. Sci. U.S.A. 63: 926, 1969.
12. Baerlocker, K.E., Scriver, C.R., and Mohyuddin, F. Ontogeny of iminoglycine transport in mammalian kidney. Proc. Natl. Acad. Sci. U.S.A. 65: 1016, 1970.
13. Arant, B.S., Jr., Edelmann, C.M., Jr., and Nash, M.A. The renal reabsorption of glucose in the developing canine kidney. A study of glomerulotubular balance. Pediatr. Res. 8: 638, 1974.

14. Brodehl, J., Franken, A., and Gellissen, K. Maximal tubular reabsorption of glucose in infants and children. Acta Paediatr. Scand. 61: 413, 1972.

15. Spitzer, A., and Brandis, M. Functional and morphologic maturation of the superficial nephrons. Relationship to total kidney function. J. Clin. Invest. 53: 1, 1974.

16. Horster, M., and Valtin, H. Postnatal development of renal function: Micropuncture and clearance studies in the dog. J. Clin. Invest. 50: 779, 1971.

17. Aperia, A., Broberger, O., Thodenius, K., and Zetterström, R. Development of renal control of salt and fluid homeostasis during the first year of life. Acta Paediatr. Scand. 64: 393, 1975.

18. Kleinman, L.I. Renal sodium reabsorption during saline loading and distal blockade in newborn dogs. Amer. J. Physiol. 228: 1403, 1975.

19. Spitzer, A., and Schoeneman, M. The role of the kidney in sodium homeostasis during maturation. Submitted for publication.

20. Rodriguez-Soriano, J., Vallo, A., Castillo, G., and Oliveros, R. Renal handling of water and sodium in infancy and childhood. A study using clearance methods during hypotonic saline diuresis. J. Ped. Neph. Urol., in press.

21. Kotchen, T.A., Strickland, A.L., Rice, T.W., and Walters, D.R. A study of the renin-angiotensin system in the newborn infant. J. Ped. 80: 938, 1972.

22. Kowarski, A., Katz, H., and Migeon, C.J. Plasma aldosterone concentration in normal subjects from infancy to adulthood. J. Clin. Endo. Metab. 38: 489, 1974.

23. Spitzer, A.S. Renal Physiology and Functional Development, in Pediatric Kidney Disease, C.M. Edelmann, Jr.(Ed.), Little, Brown N.Y. , pp.25-128.

24. Sulyok, E. The relationship between electrolyte and acid-base balance in premature infants during early post-natal life. Biol. Neonate 17: 227, 1971.

25. Siegel, S.R. Effects of low sodium diet and impaired sodium conservation in the newborn. First International Workshop on Developmental Renal Physiology, N.Y. 1980.

26. Sulyok, E., Nemeth, M., Tenyi, I., Csaba, I.F., Varga, L., and Varga, F. The relationship between the postnatal development of renin-angiotensin-aldosterone system and electrolyte and acid-base status of the sodium chloride supplemented premature infants. First International Workshop of Developmental Renal Physiology, N.Y. 1980.

27. Jose, P.A., Logan, A.G., Slotkoff, L.M., Lillienfield, L.S., Calcagno, P.L., and Eisner, G.M. Intrarenal blood flow distribution in canine puppies. Pediatr. Res. 5: 335, 1971.

28. Kleinman, L.I., and Reuter, J.H. Maturation of glomerular blood flow distribution in the newborn dog. J. Physiol. (Lond.) 228: 91, 1973.

29. Aschinberg, K.C., Goldsmith, D.I., Olbing, H., Spitzer, A., Edelmann, C.M., Jr., and Blaufox, M.D. Neonatal changes in renal blood flow distribution in puppies. Amer. J. Physiol. 228: 1453, 1975.

30. Olbing, H., Blaufox, M.D., Aschinberg, L.C., Silkalns, G.I., Bernstein, J., Spitzer, A., and Edelmann, C.M., Jr. Postnatal changes in renal blood flow distribution in puppies. J. Clin. Invest. 52: 2885, 1973.

31. Jose, P.A., Pelayo, J.C., Felder, R.E., Tavani, N., Montgomery, S.B., Calcagno, P.L., and Eisner, G.M. Maturation of single nephron filtration rate in the canine puppy: The effect of saline loading. First International Workshop on Developmental Renal Physiology, N.Y. 1980.

32. Goldsmith, D.I., Drukker, A., Blaufox, M.D., Edelmann, C.M., Jr, and Spitzer, A. Hemodynamic and excretory responses of the neonatal canine kidney to acute volume expansion. Amer. J. Physiol. 237: F392, 1979.

33. Solomon, S., Hathaway, S., and Curb, D. Evidence that the renal response to volume expansion involves a blood-borne factor. Biol. Neonate 35: 113, 1979.

34. Edelmann, C.M., Jr., Barnett, H.L., and Troupkou, V. Renal concentrating mechanisms in newborn infants: Effect of dietary protein and water content, role of urea, and responsiveness to antidiuretic hormone. J. Clin. Invest. 39: 1062, 1960.

35. Edelmann, C.M., Jr., Barnett, H.L., and Stark, H. Effect of urea on concentration of urinary nonurea solute in premature infants. J. Appl. Physiol. 21: 1021, 1966.

36. Edwards, B.R., Mendel, D.B., LaRochelle, F.T., Jr., Stern, P., and Valtin, H. Postnatal development of urinary concentrating ability in rats. Changes in renal anatomy and neurohypophysical hormones. First International Workshop on Developmental Renal Physiology, N.Y. 1980.

37. Horster, M. Discussion. First International Workshop on Developmental Renal Physiology, N.Y. 1980.

38. Schlondorff, D., Weber, H., Trizna, W., and Fine, L.G. Vasopressin responsiveness of renal adenylate cyclase in newborn rats and rabbits. Amer. J. Physiol. 234: F16, 1978.

39. Rajerison, R.M., Butlen, D., and Jard, S. Ontogenetic development of antidiuretic hormone receptors in rat kidneys: comparison of hormonal binding and adenylate cyclose activation. Mol. Cell. Endocrin. 4: 271, 1976.

40. Burch, H.B., Kuhlman, A.M., Skerjance, J., and Lowry, O.H. Changes in patterns of enzymes of carbohydrate metabolism in the developing rat kidney. Pediatrics 47: 199, 1971 (supplement).

41. Metcoff, J. Synchrony of organ development contributing to water and electrolyte regulation in early life. Clin. Neph. 1: 107, 1973.

RENAL TUBULAR ACIDOSIS

J. RODRIGUEZ-SORIANO, Department of Pediatrics, Hospital Infantil de la
Seguridad social and University School of Medicine, Bilbao, Spain

Renal tubular acidosis (RTA) represents a clinical syndrome characterized by
a state of renal tubular insufficiency with regard to the reabsorption of bicarbonate, the excretion of net hydrogen ion, or both, and includes a large
number of etiologies. In this condition, in contradistinction to the so-called
glomerular acidosis, glomerular function is normal or is comparatively less impaired than tubular function.

On clinical and pathophysiological grounds RTA is actually classified into
several categories (1,2):

   I. Primary defect in bicarbonate reabsorption (Proximal RTA; Type 2).

  II. Primary defect in distal net hydrogen ion secretion:

     1. Inability to maximally acidify the urine (Distal RTA; Type 1).

     2. Combined defects in bicarbonate reabsorption and hydrogen ion
        secretion (Hybrid RTA; Type 3)

     3. Secondary to hyperkalemia and hypoammoniuria (Type 4).

In this presentation we will briefly review the pathogenetic and clinical
aspects of each type of renal tubular acidosis.

PROXIMAL RENAL TUBULAR ACIDOSIS

The pathophysiological characteristics of proximal RTA are well known.
Patients with this disorder present a diminished renal bicarbonate threshold
that leads to the excretion of a large amount of filtered bicarbonate at normal
palsma bocarbonate concentration. When an appropriate degree of systemic acidosis is reached the urine is acidic and bicarbonate-free and may contain net
acid in an amount equivalent to the estimated endogenous load of approximately
1.5 to 2 mEq/Kg/day in infants and children and of 1 mEq/Kg/day in adults (3).
In our personal concept of proximal RTA the best definition of this type of
tubular acidosis is given by the demonstration of a low bicarbonate threshold
with normal urinary acidification at plasma bicarbonate concentrations below
this level. It must be understood that we have proposed the terms proximal and
distal with a pathophysiological and not a topographic meaning, that is
without implying an exclusive role of either the proximal or the distal tubule
in the origin of the disorder. In this sense, we believe that the demonstration
of a urinary excretion of more than 15% of the filtered amount of bicarbonate

at normal plasma bicarbonate levels is not a necessary requirement to establish the diagnosis.

The pathogenetic factors involved in the impairment of bicarbonate reabsorption are various and of different significance. Alteration of either intrinsic or extrinsic renal factors participating in the tubular reclamation of filtered bicarbonate may be implicated, depending on the specific etiology. In most cases proximal RTA is observed in the context of a proximal tubular dysfunction and thus is observed in the clinical context of the Fanconi syndrome, but other circumstances leading to a decreased tubular reabsorption of bicarbonate such as chronic renal insufficiency, hyperkalemia, extracellular fluid volume expansion or a state of secondary hyperparathyroidism should always be considered as modulating factors of the primary renal tubular defect. The role of phosphate depletion, a situation that is present in many proximal tubular disorders, remains controversial. Gold and coworkers (4) suggested that phosphate depletion caused an impairment of bicarbonate reabsorption in the dog, but other investigators found a defect in ammonia secretion when such depletion was introduced in the rat (5). As pointed out by Arruda and Kurtzman (5) it is possible that the site of the nephron involved and the defect of urinary acidification present may vary according to the species studied and the degree of phosphate depletion induced. Finally, some drugs may cause an experimental type of proximal RTA. The effects of acetazolamide and maleic acid are well known. Recently it has been shown that the infusion of dibasic amino acids (lysine, arginine, ornithine) may impair selectively the tubular reabsorption of bicarbonate, probably by interfering with hydrogen ion secretion at the level of the proximal tubule, the only site where these amino acids can be concentrated intracellularly (6).

It is important to recognize that bicarbonate reabsorption along the nephron is not only dependent on hydrogen ion secretion but is also interrelated with sodium reabsorption: a bicarbonate specific ATPase plays an important role in sodium reabsorption and it should be expected that a defect in bicarbonate reabsorption be associated with a simultaneous defect in sodium reabsorption. We have examined, by the use of clearance methodology during hypotonic saline diuresis, water and sodium reabsorption in 17 normal children, in 9 children with proximal RTA, associated in all but one with the Fanconi syndrome, and in 5 children with primary distal RTA (7). Patients with proximal RTA presented mainly an impaired reabsorption of sodium in the proximal tubule, which was in great part, but not completely, compensated by an absolute increase in distal sodium reabsorption. Patients with distal RTA showed normal reabsorption of sodium in the proximal tubule but they were unable to reabsorb completely the load of sodium escaping proximal reabsorption due to a defect of sodium reabsorption in the distal diluting segments. Our results indicate that the classification of RTA into proximal and distal types is also valid according to the differences found in the tubular handling of water and sodium.

Clinical spectrum of proximal RTA. (Table 1). Proximal RTA can be observed, although not frequently, as a primary entity. There is a sporadic form, observed in infants, which depends on a transient defect of bicarbonate reabsorption (8,9) but there are also cases persistent in nature and of familial presentation. Brenes et al (10) have reported a family of 9 members with growth failure as the only clinical presentation of proximal RTA and have suggested an autosomal dominant type of hereditary transmission. There is also an autosomal recessive type associating severe proximal RTA with growth and mental retardation and ocular abnormalities such as nystagmus, corneal opacities, cataracts and glaucoma (11,12). The secondary forms of proximal RTA are well known and in most cases are observed in the context of the Fanconi syndrome.

TABLE I.   CLINICAL SPECTRUM OF PROXIMAL RTA

    I. PRIMARY PROXIMAL RTA

        1. Sporadic (transient in infancy)

        2. Familial (persistent)

           -Dominant transmission

           -Recessive transmission

    II. SECONDARY PROXIMAL RTA

        1. Associated with Fanconi syndrome

        2. Associated with other clinical entities

           -Hyperparathyroidism

           -Vitamin D deficiency and dependency

           -Leigh's syndrome

           -Metachromatic leukodystrophy

           -Cyanotic heart disease

           -Osteopetrosis

           -Some hyperkalemic states

DISTAL RENAL TUBULAR ACIDOSIS

In distal RTA the urine pH is inappropriately high, usually greater than 6.0, net acid excretion is low and a small bicarbonaturia is present despite the presence of a severe degree of systemic acidemia. At normal levels of plasma bicarbonate the urinary excretion of bicarbonate remains low, generally less than 5% of the amount filtered. These pathophysiological characteristics are always present in older children and adults but infants and young children with distal RTA usually excrete larger amounts of bicarbonate.

The pathogenetic factors able to cause an inability to maximally acidify the urine are shown in Table II. In the first place distal RTA may depend on a diminished distal delivery of sodium to the distal sites of sodium/hydrogen ion exchange,   as has been demonstrated to occur in decompensated hepatic cirrhosis (13). We have shown that the same situation occurs in nephrotic children during relapses of proteinuria and in the phase of edema formation. An appropriate dose of ammonium chloride was administered 8 hours before the study to induce systemic acidemia. In 6 nephrotic patients the mean urinary pH was 6.09 and the mean hydrogen ion excretion was 59 $\mu Eq/min/1.73m^2$ at the time when the urine was practically without sodium (mean excretion:4 $\mu Eq/min/1.73m^2$).

After the intravenous administration of furosemide, urine pH dropped abruptly to a mean value of 4.8 and net hydrogen ion excretion increased to a value of 185 $\mu Eq/min/1.73m^2$ simultaneously with an increase of sodium excretion to a mean value of 800 $\mu Eq/min/1.73m^2$. This exchange type of distal RTA has not been previously recognized in the pediatric literature.

TABLE II. PATHOGENETIC FACTORS IN DISTAL RTA

INABILITY TO MAXIMALLY ACIDIFY THE URINE
- Diminished distal delivery of sodium (exchange defect)
- Inability to secrete hydrogen ion (secretory defect)
- Increased back-diffusion of hydrogen ion (gradient defect)
- Abolition of electrical gradient for hydrogen ion secretion (short-circuit or voltage defect)

The other pathogenetic types of distal RTA have been mainly elucidated by means of experimental studies: post-ureteral obstruction causes a true secretory defect in hydrogen ion secretion, amphotericin B increases tubular back-diffusion of hydrogen ion and drugs such as amiloride or lithium abolish the electrical gradient necessary for hydrogen ion secretion. These important advances in the understanding of the different mechanisms involved in the development of a defect in urinary acidification have been derived by the application of techniques such as the measurement of urinary pCO_2 during alkaline diuresis or after the administration of neutral sodium phosphate and the study of urinary pH after the infusion of sodium sulfate. In the so-called secretory defect all maneuvers are unable to stimulate distal secretion of hydrogen ion: urine pH remains high under sulfate infusion and urinary pCO_2 remains low in alkaline urine or during neutral phosphate infusion. In the so-called gradient defect, due to an enhanced back-diffusion of hydrogen ion, the response may vary according to whether the increased membrane permeability of the distal nephron is only present for hydrogen ion or is also present for carbonic acid. In our limited experience with a case of distal RTA secondary to the administration of amphotericin B, urinary pCO_2 reached the low level of normal during alkali administration and urinary pH decreased only moderately during sulfate infusion. Furosemide administration during systemic acidemia provoked, however, an important drop in urinary pH. Finally in the short-circuit or voltage defect the effect of sulfate and phosphate infusions on urinary pH and urinary pCO_2 respectively, will depend on the degree of correction of the electrical gradient induced by those functional maneuvers. In the experimental defect induced by lithium the response is adequate but in the defect provoked by the administration of amiloride a negative response is obtained probably because neither sulfate nor phosphate can overcome the defect in distal sodium reabsorption caused by the drug (14).

This functional approach to the study of patients with distal RTA has been rarely reported in humans. In 5 children with primary distal RTA we have shown low values of urinary pCO_2 during bicarbonate administration or during neutral phosphate administration and no decrease of urinary pH during sodium sulfate infusion. These results suggest a true secretory defect in hydrogen ion excretion, as proposed first by Halperin et al (15), and not the presence of a gradient defect as it was previously believed. The intimal nature of that se- secretory defect remains unknown although in some cases a deficiency in the en- zyme carbonic anhydrase B has been suggested.

Clinical spectrum of distal RTA. (Table III). Although distal RTA can be ob- served as both a primary or a secondary condition, most cases observed in in- fants and children correspond to the primary or idiopathic form. It must be emphasized that most primary forms are persistent in time even when the diag- nosis of distal RTA is performed as early as the first months of life. The association with nerve deafness constitutes a separate entity, transmitted by an autosomal recessive gene, and although in some cases a deficiency in car- bonic anhydrase B has been suspected, this deficiency has not been confirmed in other studies.

When the diagnosis of primary distal RTA is established later in childhood the known symptomatology of growth retardation, polyuria, nephrocalcinosis and bone lesions is present. Although adequate alkali therapy can improve the cli- nical picture the renal damage induced by the nephrocalcinosis can not be re- versed. It must be, however, recognized that primary distal RTA is a heredi- tary disorder that can be often diagnosed very early in life, before irrever- sible renal damage has occurred. In the light of the personal experience of 5 cases of primary distal RTA diagnosed during the first months of life the following observations can be made relating to a new natural history of the disease based on early diagnosis and treatment:

a) An associated renal bicarbonate wasting is almost invariably present during the first years of life (16,17). The excessive bicarbonaturia seems to depend on a concomitant defect in proximal tubular reabsorption of bicarbonate and is transient in nature tending to progressively disappear after 2-3 years of age.

b) The dose of bicarbonate needs to compensate both for the endogenous pro- duction of hydrogen ion and the associated bicarbonate loss. During the first months of life therapeutic requirements of bicarbonate (or citrate) may be as high as 10-14 mEq/Kg/day, and become progressively lower during childhood. The previously recommended dose of 2 mEq/Kg/day is probably adequate only beyond 5- 6 years of age, that is when the associated bicarbonate wasting has already disappeared.

c) When the diagnosis of primary distal RTA is established soon after birth and correct alkali therapy is instituted, progressive nephrocalcinosis can be prevented, normal glomerular function is maintained and normal growth and development is attained. A correct dosage of alkali therapy should aim not only to normalize the blood acid-base equilibrium but also to maintain the urinary excretion of calcium and citrate in the range of normal. McSherry and coworkers (18) have also proposed the study of plasma lysyl-oxydase, an enzyme regulating collagen synthesis, as a useful marker of adequate alkali therapy since values rapidly increase when bicarbonate dosage is below the level appropriate to promote maximal growth.

TABLE III. CLINICAL SPECTRUM OF DISTAL RTA

I. PRIMARY DISTAL RTA

   1. Persistent
      -Adult or "classic" type
      -Incomplete
      -With bicarbonate wasting
           -in infancy
           -with secondary hyperparathyroidism
      -With nerve deafness

   2. Transient
      -In infancy ?

II. SECONDARY DISTAL RTA

   1. Disorders of mineral metabolism
      -Primary hyperparathyroidism
      -Hyperthyroidism with nephrocalcinosis
      -Vitamin D intoxication
      -Idiopathic hypercalciuria with nephrocalcinosis
      -Hypomagnesemia-hypercalciuria with nephrocalcinosis

   2. Hyperglobulinemic states
   3. Hyponatriuric states
   4. Drugs
      -Amphotericin B, amiloride, lithium

   5. Renal diseases
      -Renal transplantation
      -Medullary sponge kidney
      -Obstructive uropathy

   6. Genetic diseases
      -Hereditary fructose intolerance with nephrocalcinosis
      -Ehlers-Danlos syndrome
      -Hereditary elliptocytosis
      -Sickle-cell anemia
      -Wilson's disease
      -Osteopetrosis
      -Carbonic anhydrase B deficiency ?

7. Endocrine disorders
    -Hypothyroidism

TYPE 4 RENAL TUBULAR ACIDOSIS

This type of renal tubular acidosis has been recently recognized by Sebastian and Morris in a group of patients with hyperkalemia (2).

The pathogenetic factors involved in this syndrome are various: impairment of bicarbonate reabsorption, impairment of distal hydrogen ion secretion and decreased renal production of ammonia. The defect in bicarbonate reabsorption is less important than that observed in the usual type of proximal RTA: Bicarbonate loss at normal plasma bicarbonate levels rarely attains 10% of the amount filtered. Although hyperkalemia per se could reduce the tubular reclamation of bicarbonate, another important factor is the existance of a functional defect in the distal "cation-exchange" segment with reduced secretion of hydrogen ion and potassium. Aldosterone deficiency is the most frequent cause of such a distal defect but it may also depend on tubular unresponsiveness to aldosterone or an intrinsic tubular abnormality. Finally hypoammoniuria is pre sent either because of the inhibitory effect on the glutaminase system of the hyperkalemia itself or because of the reduction in nephron mass present in many patients with this syndrome.

Clinical spectrum of Type 4 RTA (Table IV). The clinical spectrum of Type 4 RTA includes mainly patients with isolated hypoaldosteronism or with hyporeninemic-hypoaldosteronism associated with various etiologies of chronic renal failure. The frequency of distal tubular disorders causing this type of RTA is limited in pediatrics to rare cases of Spitzer's syndrome or some cases of pseudohypoaldosteronism. Finally a brief comment should be made about the existance of a transient type of Type 4 RTA observed in infancy and of unknown etiology. McSherry et al (19) have reported 13 patients aged between 2 and 23 months with primary Type 4 RTA. Hyporeninemic-hypoaldosteronism was not present and all abnormalities disappeared at about 3-5 years of age. This new type of transient RTA should be differentiated from transient cases of proximal RTA already commented upon in this brief review.

TABLE IV. CLINICAL SPECTRUM OF TYPE 4 RTA

I. ALDOSTERONE DEFICIENCY, WITHOUT RENAL DISEASE
1. Combined mineralocorticoid deficiency
    -Addison's disease
    -Congenital adrenal hyperplasia with salt wasting
2. Isolated hypoaldosteronism
    -Familial hypoaldosteronism

II. HYPORENINEMIC-HYPOALDOSTERONISM IN PATIENTS WITH CRF
    -Diabetic nephropathy

-Pyelonephritis

-Interstitial nephritis

-Nephrosclerosis

III.   DISTAL TUBULAR DISORDERS

1.   Primary

-Pseudohypoaldosteronism

-Spitzer's syndrome

-Hyperkalemia-hypertension-hyporeninemia syndrome

2.   Secondary

-"Salt-wasting" syndrome

-Renal amyloidosis

-S.L.E.

-Drugs (methicillin)

IV.   UNDETERMINED

-Transient in infancy·

REFERENCES

1. Rodriguez-Soriano J. 1978. Renal tubular acidosis. In Edelmann CM (ed): Pediatric Kidney Disease. Boston: Little, Brown and Co. p. 995.
2. Sebastian A, Morris RC Jr. 1977. Renal tubular acidosis. Clin Nephrol 7: 216-230.
3. Chan JCM. 1980. Acid-base and mineral disorders in children: A review. Int J Pediat Nephrol 1:54-63.
4. Gold LW, Massry SG, Arieff L, Coburn JW. 1973. Renal bicarbonate wasting during phosphate depletion. A possible cause of altered acid-base homeostasis in hyperparathyroidism. J Clin Invest 52:2556-2561.
5. Arruda JAL, Kurtzman NA. 1980. Hyperparathyroidism and metabolic acidosis. A complex interaction of multiple factors. Nephron 26:1-6.
6. Gougoux A, Vinay P, Lemieux G, Richardson RMA, Siu-Cheng Tam, Goldstein MB, Stinebaugh BJ, Halperin ML. 1980. Effect of blood pH on distal nephron hydrogen ion secretion. Kidney Int 17:615-621.
7. Rodriguez-Soriano J, Vallo A, Castillo G, Oliveros R. 1980. Renal handling of water and sodium in children with proximal and distal renal tubular acidosis. Nephron 25:193-198.
8. Rodriguez-Soriano J, Boichis H, Stark H, Edelmann CM Jr. 1967. Proximal renal tubular acidosis. A defect in bicarbonate reabsorption with normal urinary acidification. Pediat Res 1:81-98.
9. Nash MA, Torrado A, Greifer I, Spitzer A, Edelmann CM Jr. 1972. Renal tubular acidosis in infants and children. Clinical course, response to treatment and prognosis. J Pediat 80:738-748.
10. Brenes LG, Brenes JN, Hernandez MM. 1977. Familial proximal renal tubular acidosis. Amer J Med 63:244-252.
11. Donckerwolcke RA, Van Stekelenburg GJ, Tiddens HA. 1970. A case of bicarbonate-losing renal tubular acidosis with defective carboanhydrase activity. Arch Dis Child 45:769-773.
12. Winsnes A, Monn E, Stokke O, Feyling T. 1979. Congenital persistent proximal type renal tubular acidosis in two brothers. Acta Paediatr Scand 68:861-868.

REFERENCES

13. Better OS, Goldschmid Z, Chaimovitz C, Alroy GG. 1972. Defect in urinary acidification in cirrhosis. The role of excessive tubular reabsorption of sodium in its etiology. Arch Intern Med 130:77-83.

14. Kurtzman NA. 1980. "Short-circuit" renal tubular acidosis. J.Lab Clin Med 95:633-636.

15. Halperin ML, Goldstein MB, Haig A, Johnson MD, Stinebaugh BJ. 1974. Studies on the pathogenesis of type I (distal) renal tubular acidosis as revealed by the urinary Pco_2 tensions. J Clin Invest 53:669-677.

16. McSherry E, Sebastian A, Morris RC Jr. 1972. Renal tubular acidosis in infants: the several kinds, including bicarbonate-wasting classic renal tubular acidosis. J Clin Invest 51:499-514.

17. Rodriguez-Soriano J, Vallo A, Garcia-Fuentes M. 1975. Renal tubular acidosis in infancy: a bicarbonate-wasting state. J Pediat 86:524-532.

18. Griger C, Siegel R, McSherry E. 1978. The effect of acidosis on plasma lysyl oxidase activity in children with renal tubular acidosis. (Abstr) Kidney Int 14:652.

19. McSherry E, Portale A, Gates J. 1978. Non-azotemic, non-hyporeninemic type 4 renal tubular acidosis observed in early childhood (Abstr). Kidney Int 14:769.

MECHANISMS OF IMMUNE COMPLEX INJURY

W.G. COUSER, D.J. SALANT, M.P. MADAIO, AND S. ADLER. EVANS MEMORIAL
DEPARTMENT OF CLINICAL RESEARCH AND THE DEPARTMENT OF MEDICINE, UNIVER-
SITY HOSPITAL, BOSTON UNIVERSITY MEDICAL CENTER, BOSTON, MA 02118

There has been a marked resurgence of interest in the general topic
of immune complex glomerulonephritis in the past two to three years.
Several factors account for this phenomenon, including the recent availability of assays for circulating immune complexes in human renal disease,
but the major reason is that several basic observations made in the laboratory have prompted important revisions in the way we now think about
immune complex nephritis. These changes have occurred particularly in
two areas. First, there have been important changes in the concepts of
how these granular deposits form in glomeruli. Secondly, there have
also been some new discoveries with respect to the mechanisms by which
these deposits mediate glomerular injury. This presentation will review some of these observations and give you some idea, at least from
our prospective, of current thinking about the pathogenesis of immune
complex glomerulonephritis.

To review the conventional schema we have all been taught about
immune complex nephritis, it states that antibody combines with free
antigen in the circulation to form a circulating, soluble immune complex.
These complexes are deposited on the glomerular capillary wall by a passive
process of glomerular filtration or trapping. Activation of the complement
system by the deposited complex results in release of chemotactic factors,
attraction of neutrophils and complement-neutrophil mediated glomerular
injury (1). With respect to several types of glomerular immune deposits
there is now good evidence to suggest that much of this schema is probably
incorrect (2).

The first thing that must be clearly appreciated in discussing immune
complex nephritis is that immune complex deposits form at several different
sites within the glomerulus. It is probably the site of deposit formation

as much as any other single factor which determines the type and severity
of the glomerular lesion which results. Deposits at different sites are
associated with quite different clinical and pathologic manifestations.
It is also becomming clear that deposits at different sites probably
form by different mechanisms. Mesangial deposits are characteristic of
many glomerular diseases but particularly the focal forms of glomerulonephritis seen in lupus, Henoch-Schönlein purpura and IgG-IgA nephropathy.
Deposits along the subendothelial surface of the glomerular capillary
wall are seen in diffuse proliferative lupus nephritis and in Type I
membranoproliferative glomerulonephritis. There are two distinct types
of subepithelial immune deposits: the widely spaced subepithelial "humps"
that are characteristic of poststreptococcal glomerulonephritis and the
very finely granular deposits that begin initially in filtration slit
pores and are characteristic of membranous nephropathy. While all of
these deposits have in the past been believed to result from a single
mechanism, that is the glomerular filtration and trapping of circulating
soluble immune complexes, it is now clear that this mechanism alone cannot account for the variety of different deposits seen or the markedly
different clinical and histologic lesions they produce.

The hypothesis that all of these deposits represent glomerular trapping of circulating immune complexes is based almost entirely on studies
carried out in the BSA-serum sickness models of immune complex nephritis.
In acute serum sickness one sees immune deposits and glomerular lesions
that closely resemble those seen in man. In the now classic studies of
the serum sickness models by Germuth and Dixon, it was shown that the
major determinant of the site of deposit formation was the degree of antibody response in the immunized animal (3-5). Animals with a high antibody
response developed only large molecular weight, antibody excess aggregates
of over 2 million daltons which were taken up primarily by the extra-renal
reticuloendothelial system with only occassional mesangial deposits.
Animals with a moderate antibody response formed smaller complexes near
equivalence, in the 1-2 million molecular weight range, and deposits developed in the mesangium and along the subendothelial surface with a proliferative glomerulonephritis. Animals with a poor antibody response
formed small immune complexes of 300-500,000 daltons, in antigen excess,
and deposits developed in a subepithelial distribution with a membranous

lesion. It was further noted that if one measured the antibody response weekly and re-injected enough antigen to maintain persistent antigen excess, the so-called chronic serum sickness model, that deposits would develop almost exclusively in the subepithelial space, regardless of the level of antibody response (5). It is also known that production of low avidity antibodies, another condition which would favor free circulating antigen, also favors subepithelial deposit formation (6). However, the principal determinant of the site of complex formation, and hence of the type of glomerular lesion produced, seemed to be immune complex size as determined primarily by antigen-antibody ratio rather than the extent of the immune response per se.

Many subsequent studies have attempted to further define the factors regulating glomerular immune complex localization by making pre-formed immune complexes of various types in the test tube, injecting them under controlled conditions into animals and studying their renal deposition (7, 8). A number of additional factors which influence glomerular complex localization have been defined by such studies. The primary determinant still appears to be immune complex size, as determined primarily by antigen-antibody ratio, and the ability of immune complexes to form lattices. Other factors include immune complex charge, plasma immune complex levels and renal blood flow, reticuloendothelial function and vasoactive amine activity which have all been shown to influence the quantity of passively administered immune complexes which deposit in the glomerulus (9-12).

In interpreting the data derived from pre-formed immune complex infusion studies, it is important to recognize that the subepithelial deposits characteristic of chronic serum sickness and membranous nephropathy have generally not been produced by infusion of pre-formed immune complexes regardless of the size or dose of the immune complexes used (2). The one exception to this summary of a rather large literature is a study by Germuth and associates in which subepithelial deposits were observed using very low avidity pre-formed complexes (13). Since such low avidity complexes dissociate extensively *in vivo*, however, it is not certain that the deposits observed actually represented intact, circulating immune complexes. The inability to produce subepithelial deposits by pre-formed complex infusion has always been difficult to reconcile with the hypothesis that these deposits represent circulating complex trapping. This problem has only recently been clarified, largely by studies carried out in a different model of immune complex glomerulonephritis, the so-called Heymann nephritis model of experimental membranous nephropathy in rats.

In Heymann nephritis, rats immunized with an antigen derived from the brush border of proximal tubular epithelial cells, and commonly referred to as fraction 1A or FxlA, develop a lesion that is pathologically indistinguishable from membranous nephropathy in man. Finely granular deposits of IgG and complement are present in all glomeruli, and by electron microscopy the deposits form exclusively on the subepithelial surface of the capillary wall, often in filtration slit pores (14). An identical lesion can be produced quite rapidly by the passive injection of rats with heterologous antibody to brush border antigen, the so-called passive Heymann nephritis, or PHN, model (15). The conventional explanation for the development of subepithelial immune deposits in the Heymann models has been that the antibody combines with a circulating renal tubular antigen that is present in the plasma of the rat to form a circulating immune complex that is then filtered out by the glomerulus which acts only as an innocent by-stander in this process (16).

In 1976 Dr. Vernier presented a paper at the American Society of Nephrology meetings in Washington D.C. describing work done in Dr. Phillip Hoedemaeker's laboratory in the Netherlands which represented the first step in demonstrating that the subepithelial immune deposits in this model probably do not represent circulating complex trapping but instead illustrate a second mechanism of glomerular immune deposit formation in which free antibody binds to an antigen already present in the glomerular capillary wall resulting in local, or *in situ*, complex formation (17). These workers used an *ex vivo* perfusion system, originally designed by Dr. John Hoyer, in which the left kidney is clamped off from the circulation and is then perfused through a needle inserted into the aorta. A hole in the renal vein allows perfusate to drain without entering the systemic circulation. When blood-free rat kidneys were perfused with rabbit antibody to rat tubular antigen and then studied by an immunoperoxidase technique, antibody deposits were identified at several sites in the capillary wall including the subepithelial space (18). Based on these and related findings, these workers proposed that the subepithelial deposits in the Heymann models of membranous nephropathy resulted from antibody binding

to a fixed glomerular antigen, presumably one which was cross-reactive
with tubular brush border (17, 18).

Work which was on-going in our laboratory at the same time produced
similar results using a somewhat different system. In our experiments a
rat kidney was isolated *in vitro* and perfused at $37^{\circ}C$ by a pulsatile perfusion pump at physiologic pressures with an oxygenated perfusate which
contains only albumin in a physiologic bicarbonate buffer. In this system
the kidney can be maintained functionally and morphologically intact for
about 2 hours *in vitro*. The system was also modified so that renal venous
effluent would not recirculate, thus producing a single-pass system in
which there was no possibility of tubular antigens escaping into the perfusate to form circulating immune complexes (19). Our experiment was to
perfuse isolated normal rat kidneys with either normal sheep IgG or with
sheep antibody to the rat tubular antigen used to produce subepithelial
deposits in the intact animal. Perfusion for up to two hours with normal
sheep IgG produced no non-specific binding of non-antibody IgG. However,
when kidneys were perfused for only ten minutes with antibody IgG the
development of diffuse, discontinuous subepithelial deposits could be seen
by routine immunofluorescence along the glomerular capillary walls. By
two hours we produced a membranous glomerular lesion essentially indistinguishable from that produced in the whole animal, although there were no
circulating immune complexes in this system. Electron microscopy of these
kdineys confirmed that the deposits, like those in the intact animal,
were primarily in filtration slit pores and in the subepithelial space
(19). In collaboration with Drs. T. James Neale and Curtis Wilson in La
Jolla, California we have recently obtained similar results in the isolated
perfused kidney using radiolabelled rat antibody eluted from the kidneys
of rats with Heymann nephritis (20). The isolated perfused kidney studies
are not the only evidence for a fixed antigen in this model. If radiolabelled IgG antibody eluted from Heymann rat kidneys is incubated with
isolated rat glomeruli there is also a definite binding of eluted antibody
to glomeruli *in vitro* compared to acid-treated control IgG (21).

The recognition that subepithelial immune deposits in the Heymann
nephritis models can result from *in situ* immune deposit formation due to
the binding of free antibody to a fixed glomerular antigen has enabled
several other studies to be carried out to characterize the factors which
regulate this new process of glomerular immune deposit formation.

Dr. David Salant, in our laboratory, has recently defined the kinetics of immune deposit formation in experimental membranous nephropathy using radiolabelled antibody and measuring antibody deposition in glomeruli at various times after intravenous antibody administration (22). These data illustrate that there is a very slow progressive accumulation of antibody in glomerular deposits despite the rapid decline in serum levels of circulating antibody. Only after five days of on-going deposit formation has enough antibody localized in glomeruli to finally cause an increase in urine protein excretion (22). This rather indolent course of antibody deposition in subepithelial immune deposits and slow development of glomerular injury is in marked contrast to either anti-GBM antibody disease or pre-formed immune complex infusion where maximum amounts of glomerular deposits are seen within hours. These data suggest that depositon of circulating antibody to form subepithelial immune deposits is restricted by some factors. Knowing some of the properties which regulate the ability of macromolecules to penetrate the glomerular basement membrane, and the fact that these deposits form exclusively on the subepithelial side of the capillary wall, we postulated that deposit formation in membranous nephropathy may be affected by both size and charge-selective properties of the glomerular filtration barrier (23). Dr. Salant and Dr. Michael Madaio, in our laboratory, have now demonstrated that both of these factors are, in fact, critical in determining the rate and quantity of antibody binding to form subepithelial deposits.

If antibody to rat tubular antigen is digested to form 3 reagents: intact IgG weighing 160,000, divalent $F(ab')_2$ weighing 96,000 and univalent Fab' weighing 48,000, and these 3 reagents are then administered in varying doses to rats and blood levels and glomerular deposition measured at 24 hours the following data are obtained. First of all, the amount of glomerular antibody deposition is directly related to blood level of antibody for all three reagents (24). At any given blood level of antibody, glomerular deposit formation occurs more readily with the $F(ab')_2$ fragment then with whole IgG and more readily still with the univalent Fab' fragment (24). In other words, at any given blood level, the smaller the antibody the more readily it forms deposits in the subepithelial space. The ability of the univalent Fab antibody fragments to form subepithelial deposits virtually excludes a role for circulating immune complexes in this process since univalent antibodies are not capable of immune complex lattice formation (24).

Charge is also an important determinant of the ability of antibody to form subepithelial immune deposits. In another study, done largely by Dr. Michael Madaio in our laboratory, antibody was eluted from kidneys of rats with Heymann nephritis, the IgG fraction was isolated and seperated into cationic and anionic sub-groups, both sub-groups were shown to have equivalent antibody content by *in vitro* binding studies, and equal amounts of the two antibodies were then re-administered to rats and glomerular antibody binding measured 24 hours later (25). The results demonstrated that at any given blood level of antibody the glomerular binding of the cationic subclass at 24 hours exceeded that of the anionic subclass by a factor of anywhere from 3.5 to over 5, and this difference was sustained over a 5 day period (25).

While the passive Heymann nephritis model has been of enormous use in characterizing the process of *in situ* subepithelial immune deposit formation, let me emphasize that the concept of glomerular immune deposits forming locally rather then representing circulating complex trapping is not limited to subepithelial deposits nor is it restricted to fixed antigens. In 1973 Dr. Michael Mauer and his colleagues at the University of Minnesota, did a study in which heat-aggregated human IgG was administered to rabbits and was trapped in the glomerular mesangium (26). Incidently, this study demonstrates the validity of the concept that mesangial deposits may represent circulating complex trapping. Kidneys containing this planted exogenous antigen were then transplanted into normal rabbits to eliminate the possibility of circulating antigen. The recipient rabbits were then injected with antibody to human IgG. The result was local immune deposit formation within the mesangium, complement activation and a striking focal proliferative glomerulonephritis (26). In addition to demonstrating that glomerulonephritis can be induced by local deposit formation in the mesangium, I would particularly call your attention to the severity of the histologic lesion which was demonstrated. When mesangial deposits are produced by circulating complex trapping there is generally little or no accompanying inflammatory response, an observation which I think may provide a clue to the relative importance of these two mechanisms in human disease.

With regard to subendothelial deposits, in 1978 Golbus and Wilson injected rabbits with the plant lectin concanavalin A which binds avidly through receptor proteins to the mannose and glucose present in basement membrane glycoproteins (27). Following injection, the Con A bound to the glomerular capillary wall. When rabbit antibody to Con A was administered, *in situ* deposit formation occurred, and a proliferative glomerulonephritis was produced (27). In this model *in situ* deposit formation appeared to occur primarily on the subendothelial surface of the capillary wall.

The latter two studies illustrate two mechanisms by which exogenous antigens may be localized in the glomerulus, that is through mesangial uptake of antigen or by direct binding of antigen to basement membrane glycoprotein. To return to the subepithelial deposits of membranous nephropathy again it is now clear, as it almost has to be if one is to invoke the *in situ* mechanism in human disease, that exogenous as well as fixed antigens are also capable of initiating *in situ* deposit formation. The study which demonstrates this most clearly was again carried out in the laboratory of Dr. Hoedemaeker (28). Using the *ex vivo* perfusion system described previously and working with the standard BSA-anti-BSA system used to induce the serum sickness models, these investigators did two studies. First, they made pre-formed BSA-anti-BSA immune complexes and perfused them directly into the renal artery, a study which has been done many times before. Secondly, they carried out a series of perfusions in which the kidney was perfused for approximately thirty seconds with BSA alone, followed by perfusion with saline to remove circulating BSA, and then perfused with anti-BSA, followed again by a saline flush. This cycle was repeated five times so the kidney was exposed alternately to antigen and then to antibody but never to both at the same time. As has been found by many investigators before them, perfusion with preformed immune complexes produced only a few mesangial deposits. However, alternate perfusions with antigen followed by antibody resulted in definite granular deposit formation along the capillary wall. By electron microscopy these deposits were localized in the subepithelial space (28).

While the mechanism which leads to the retention of free BSA in the subepithelial space is not yet clear, it is apparent that there must be available circulating unbound antigen, or antigen excess, for this process to proceed. This accords with a number of observations regarding the immunologic environment in which subepithelial deposits develop in both experimental and clinical membranous nephropathy. The available data suggests that it may well be the presence of free antigen, rather than the relative size of any circulating immune complexes that may be present, which accounts for subepithelial immune deposit formation in the following situations: in the acute serum sickness rabbits with a poor antibody response, in chronic serum sickness rabbits maintained in antigen excess, or in animals that produce only low avidity antibodies. It is also conceivable that this inability to clear free circulating antigen accounts for the association between the presence of very low levels of non-precipitating anti-DNA antibody in some patients with systemic lupus and the tendency of such patients to develop a membranous nephropathy which has been reported by Friend et al (29), or the apparently diminished capacity to produce IgG, associated with a suppressor monocyte, which has now been described in idiopathic membranous nephropathy by Dr. Ooi and his associates (30).

With regard to how free antigen becomes localized in the subepithelial space, there is now considerable evidence from more recent studies of the mechanisms of glomerular permeability that various free antigens with the appropriate biophysical properties may localize in a subepithelial distribution for totally non-immunologic reasons. For instance, if one looks at the glomerular transport of ferritin, a large molecule with a molecular weight of about 500,000, anionic ferritin is confined entirely to the capillary lumen (31). As the isoelectric point of the molecule, and thereby its net positive charge, increases, it exhibits greater penetration through the glomerular basement membrane. Cationic ferritin, with a pI of 9-10, localizes along the subepithelial surface and in filtration slit pores in a distribution very similar to that of the deposits in membranous nephropathy (31). An analogous phenomenon is observed when kidneys are perfused first with the polcation protamine and then with heparin, a sequence which results in the formation of protamine-heparin complexes which are localized in a subepithelial distribution on a totally non-immunologic basis (32). These complexes result from the initial interaction between the cationic protamine and negatively charged structures in the glomerular capillary wall followed by complex formation with heparin. If an antibody response were to develop against either component of this complex one would develop subepithelial immune deposits and a membranous nephropathy.

The situations in which *in situ* immune deposit formation is now known to be involved in producing renal injury are classified in Table I.

Table I. Mechanisms of *In Situ* Immune Deposit Formation

FIXED (ENDOGENOUS) ANTIGENS

> Tubular brush border antigen (Heymann nephritis)
>
> GBM and TBM antigens
>
> Epithelial cell antigen in rabbits
>
> ? Mesangial antigens
>
> Tamm-Horsfall protein (interstitial nephritis)

PLANTED (EXOGENOUS) ANTIGENS

> Antigen uptake by mesangium
>
> Antigen-glycoprotein binding
>
> Antigen (IgG) binding to capillary wall
>
> > Autologous phase of nephrotoxic nephritis
> >
> > Autologous phase of passive Heymann nephritis
>
> Antigen interaction with glomerular charged structures
>
> > Protamine-heparin
> >
> > ? BSA, ? DNA
>
> Antigen concentration by glomerular filtration

Granular immune deposits may result from antibody binding to either fixed endogenous antigens or planted exogenous antigens. With respect to the Heymann models in rats, it must be apparent that the mechanism of granular deposit formation in these models is no different from that of linear deposit formation in anti-GBM or TBM disease. Thus, it is important that we now recognize that discontinuity or granularity of immune deposits may not represent a different mechanism of deposit formation as previously believed but can be due to differences in either the distribution of antigen or variations in antibody access to it, particularly at more distal sites in the capillary wall. Antibodies have also been shown to bind in a granular pattern to an epithelial cell antigen in rabbits by Wilson (33), and probably to mesangial antigens in other models (34). It should also be noted that a similar mechanism involving Tamm-Horsfall protein has been implicated in the pathogenesis of interstitial nephritis by Dr. John Hoyer (35). No fixed antigens have yet been positively identified in association with granular deposits in human renal disease. As our knowledge of glomerular antigens continues to expand, however, it seems highly likely that a role for fixed antigens will be defined in man, and this possibility will be addressed by Dr. Fish in the paper which follows.

With respect to planted exogenous antigens at least four different processes have now been identified which may result in glomerular antigen trapping (Table I). These include mesangial uptake of antigen, antigen binding to GBM glycoprotein, antigen in the form of immunoglobulin binding immunologically to fixed glomerular antigens as in the so-called autologous phases of nephrotoxic nephritis or passive Heymann nephritis, and charge interaction between antigen and charged components of the glomerular filter as in the protamine-heparin studies. Finally, the distribution of deposits in filtration slit pores in membranous nephropathy suggests that the filtration process must play some role in the glomerular localization of some antigens. None of these processes really adequately explain the observations reported with BSA, however, and it seems certain that other mechanisms will be added to this list in the future.

In addition to these new insights into how granular immune deposit formation occurs and the factors which regulate it, it has also recently become clear that the mechanisms by which immune complex deposits cause glomerular injury differ from the complement-neutrophil dependent mechanism which has traditionally been held to be operative in the pathogenesis of immune complex disease. With respect to the acute serum sickness model of immune complex nephritis, in which mesangial and subendothelial deposits usually predominate, a study from Dr. Curtis Wilson's laboratory shows quite clearly that proteinuria in acute serum sickness is mediated almost exclusively by macrophages and does not involve either complement or neutrophils (36).

With respect to the subepithelial deposits in membranous nephropathy, the mediation of glomerular injury also involves an apparently new and previously unrecognized mechanism. Again, using the passive Heymann nephritis model of membranous nephropathy, if one compares glomerular antibody deposition at 5 days and urine protein excretion in normal rats and rats depleted of complement components C3-C9 by daily administration of cobra venom factor, we have shown that one can totally abolish proteinuria by complement depletion, although this maneuver has no effect at all on the amount of antibody deposited (37). Thus, despite the totally non-inflammatory glomerular lesion in membranous nephropathy, proteinuria in this model is highly complement dependent. However, if one does a similar

study in which one group of rats is depleted of neutrophils with specific
anti-rat neutrophil serum and the other group is not, neutrophil depletion
has no effect on proteinuria (37). Thus proteinuria in this model is
complement-dependent but neutrophil-independent, a finding which represents
a new and potentially important role for the complement system in mediating glomerular injury. We now suspect this phenomenom may represent a
membranolytic mechanism in the glomerulus, perhaps analagous to complement-
dependent lysis of antibody coated red blood cells.

In conclusion, it is now clear that mesangial and subendothelial deposits may result from either circulating complex trapping or *in situ*
complex formation. While there is no way at the present time to assess
the relative importance of these two mechanisms in human renal disease,
I would remind you again that experimentally glomerular trapping of pre-
formed immune complexes does not produce much glomerular injury while
local complex formation is associated with inflammatory lesions much like
those seen in man.

With respect to subepithelial deposits I believe we must remain open
to the possibility that certain very low avidity or highly positively
charged immune complexes may localize at this site. However, most evidence
now favors an *in situ* mechanism for the formation of these deposits which
may involve either fixed endogenous antigens or planted exogenous ones.
Finally, in two standard models of immune complex nephritis, two new mechanisms by which these granular deposits cause tissue injury have now been
identified. In acute serum sickness the principal mediator appears to be
macrophages. In experimental membranous nephropathy complement has been
shown to cause proteinuria by a direct membranolytic effect rather than
by an inflammatory process.

Clearly there is much still to be learned about this most common of
the immunologic mechanisms of glomerular disease. Hopefully the impetus
generated by these recent advances will not be lost, and progress in the
future will continue at the rate it has in the past few years.

REFERENCES

1. Merrill, J.P.: Glomerulonephritis, NEJM 290:257-266, 1974.
2. Couser, W.G. and Salant, D.J.: *In situ* complex formation and glomerular injury. Kidney Int. 17:1-13, 1980.

3. Germuth, F.G., Jr., Rodriguez, E.: Immunopathology of the renal glomerulus: Immune complex deposit and anti-basement membrane disease. Boston, Little Brown and Co. 1973.
4. Dixon, F.J., Vazquez, J.J. Weigel, W.O., Cochrane, C.J.: Pathogenesis of serum sickness. Arch. Pathol. 68:18-28, 1958.
5. Dixon, F.J., Feldman, J.D. Vazquez, J.J.: Experimental glomerulo-nephritis: The pathogenesis of a laboratory model resembling the spectrum of human glomerulonephritis. J. Exp. Med. 113:899-920, 1961.
6. Pincus, T., Haberkern, R., Christian, C.L.: Experimental chronic glomerulitis. J. Exp. Med. 127:819-831, 1968,
7. Okumura K., Kondo, Y., Tada, T.: Studies of passive serum sickness I. The glomerular fine structure of serum sickness nephritis induced by pre-formed antigen-antibody complexes in the mouse. Lab. Invest. 24:283-391, 1971.
8. Koyama, A., Niwa, Y., Shigematsu, H., Taniguchi, M., Tada, T.: Studies on passive serum sickness. II. Factors determining the local-ization of antigen antibody complexes in the murine renal glomerulus. Lab. Invest. 38:253-262, 1978.
9. Ward, H.J., Kamil, E.S., Cohen, A.H., Border, W.A.: Role of electrical charge in the pathogenesis of experimental membranous nephropathy. Abstracts of the American Society of Nephrology, 1980.
10. Hebert, L.A., Allheiser, C.L., Koethe, S.M.: Some hemodynamic deter-minants of immune complex trapping by the kidney. Kidney Int. 14:452-465, 1978.
11. Haakenstad, A.O., Mannik, M.: Saturation of the reticuloendothelial system with soluble immune complexes. J. Immunol. 112:1939-1948, 1974.
12. Cochrane, C.G.: Mechanisms involved in the deposition of immune com-plexes in tissues. J. Exp. Med. 134:79s-89s, 1971.
13. Germuth, F.G.Jr., Rodriguez, E., Lorelle, C.A., Trump, E.I., Milano, L.L., Wise, O.: Passive immune complex glomerulonephritis in mice, models for various lesions found in human disease. II. Low avidity complexes and diffuse proliferative glomerulonephritis with subepi-thelial deposits. Lab. Invest. 41:366-371, 1979.
14. Couser, W.G., Stilmant, M.M., Darby, C.: Autologous immune complex nephropathy: I. Sequential study of immune complex deposition, ultra-structural changes, proteinuria and alterations in glomerular sialo-protein. Lab. Invest. 34:23-30, 1976.
15. Barabas, A.Z., Lannigan, R.: Induction of an autologous immune-complex glomerulonephritis in the rat by intravenous injection of heterologous anti-rat kidney tubular antibody: I. Production of chronic progressive immune complex glomerulonephritis. Brit. J. Exp. Pathol. 55:47-55, 1974.
16. Edgington, T.S., Glassock, R.J., Dixon, F.J.: Autologous immune com-plex pathogenesis of experimental allergic glomerulonephritis. Science 155:1432-1434, 1967.
17. Van Damme, B., Fleuren, G.J., Bakker, W.W., Hoedemaeker, P.J., and Vernier, R.L.: Fixed glomerular antigens in the pathogenesis of heterologous immune complex glomerulonephritis. Kidney Int. 10:551, 1976.
18. Van Damme, B.J.C., Fleuren, G.J., Bakker, W.W., Vernier, R.L., Hoedemaeker, P.J.: Experimental glomerulonephritis in the rat induced by antibodies directed against tubular antigens: IV. Fixed glomerular antigens in the pathogenesis of heterologous immune complex glomerulo-nephritis. Lab. Invest. 38:502-510, 1978.
19. Couser, W.G., Steinmuller, D.R., Stilmant, M.M., Salant, D.J., Lowenstein L.M.: Glomerulonephritis in the isolated perfused rat kidney. J. Clin. Invest. 62:1275-1287, 1978.

20. Neal, T.J., Wilson, C.B., Couser, W.G., Salant, D.J.: Personal communication.
21. Madaio, M.P., Salant, D.J., Stilmant, M.M., Darby, C., Capparell, N., Couser, W.G.: Comparative study of subepithelial immune deposit formation in active and passive Heymann nephritis. Abstracts of the American Society of Nephrology, 1980.
22. Salant, D.J., Darby, C., Couser, W.G.: Experimental membranous glomerulonephritis in rats. Quantitative studies of glomerular immune deposit formation in isolated glomeruli and whole animals. J. Clin. Invest. 66:71-81, 1980.
23. Venkatachalam, M.A., Rennke, H.G.: The structural and molecular basis of glomerular filtration. Circ. Res. 43:337-347, 1978.
24. Salant, D.J., Capparell, N., Darby, C., Stilmant, M.M., Couser, W.G.: Effect of antibody size on subepithelial immune deposit formation. Kidney Int. 16:801, 1979.
25. Madaio, M.P., Salant, D.J., Couser, W.G., Darby, C., Capparell, N.: Influence of antibody charge and concentration on subepithelial immune deposit formation. Abstracts of the American Society of Nephrology, 1980.
26. Mauer, S.M., Sutherland, D.E.R., Howard, R.J., Fish, A.J., Najarian, J.S., Michael, A.F.: The glomerular mesangium: III. Acute immune mesangial injury: A new model of glomerulonephritis. J. Exp. Med. 137:553-570, 1973.
27. Golbus, S., Wilson, C.B.: Experimental glomerulonephritis induced by *in situ* formation of immune complexes in glomerular capillary wall. Kidney Int. 16:148-157, 1979.
28. Fleuren, G., Grond, J., Hoedemaeker, P.J.: *In situ* formation of subepithelial glomerular immune complexes in passive serum sickness. Kidney Int. 17:631-637, 1980.
29. Friend, P.S., Kim, Y., Michael, A.F., Donadio, J.V.: Pathogenesis of membranous nephropathy in systemic lupus erythematosis: Possible role of non-precipitating DNA antibody. Brit. Med. J. 1:25, 1977.
30. Ooi, B.S., Ooi, Y.M., Hsu, A., Hurtubise, P.E.: Diminished synthesis of immunoglobulin by peripheral lymphocytes of patients with idiopathic membranous glomerulonephropathy. J. Clin. Invest. 65:789-797, 1980.
31. Rennke, H.G., Cotran, R.S., Venkatachalam, M.A.: Role of molecular charge in glomerular permeability. Tracer studies with cationized ferritins. J. Cell Biol. 67:638-645, 1975.
32. Seiler, M.W., Rennke, H.G., Venkatachalam, M.A., Cotran, R.S.: Pathogenesis of polycation-induced alteration ("fusion") of glomerular epithelium. Lab. Invest. 36:48-58, 1977.
33. Neale, T.J., Wilson, C.B.: Non-GBM glomerular antigen in spontaneous nephritis in rabbits. Kidney Int. 14:715, 1978.
34. Seelig, H.P., Seelig, R., Roth, E: Antibodies reacting with the glomerular mesangium. Isolation and immunopathology. Virchows Arch (Pathol Anat) 306:313-330, 1975.
35. Hoyer, J.R.: Tubulointerstitial immune complex nephritis in rats immunized with Tamm-Horsfall protein. Kidney Int. 17:284-292, 1980.
36. Wilson, C.B., Holdsworth, S.R., Neale, T.J.: Abrogation of immune glomerulonephritis in rabbits by anti-macrophage serum. Abstracts of the American Society of Nephrology, 1980.
37. Salant, D.J., Belok, S., Madaio, M.P., Couser, W.G.: A new role for complement in experimental membranous nephropathy in rats. J. Clin. Invest. 66:Dec., 1980.

CELL-MEDIATED MECHANISMS IN RENAL DISEASE

B. S. OOI

This communication focuses on three renal disorders in which
there may be evidence of cell-mediated mechanisms: (a) lipoid
nephrosis, (b) acute interstitial nephritis, (c) idiopathic
membranous nephropathy.

Lipoid Nephrosis

Shalhoub (1) first proposed that lipoid nephrosis may be a
disorder of T cell function in which a clone of T cells produces
lymphokine(s) toxic to the glomerular basement membrane.
Evidence for lymphocyte-associated mechanisms in this disorder
has been obtained, including: (a) elaboration of leukocyte
migration factor when lymphocytes of patients with lipoid
nephrosis were cultured with kidney antigen (2); (b) cell-
mediated lymphocytoxicity exhibited by lymphocytes to cultured
renal epithelial cells (3); (c) presence of "cold" lymphocytotoxins in the serum of such patients suggesting the presence
of a foreign clone of lymphocytes (4); and (d) tentative
identification of a vascular permeability factor produced by
lymphocytes cultured with Concanavalin-A (5,6). This factor
has been characterized as being a molecular weight of 12,000
daltons, sediment coefficient of 1.8S and pI of 6.4.

However, none of these phenomena are specific to lipoid
nephrosis, and have been found in relation to other types
of renal disease; furthermore, a direct relationship between
these phenomena and the pathophysiology of the disease has not
been established.

Acute Interstitial Nephritis

Drug-induced acute interstitial nephritis in patients serves

as a model for discussion. The disorder is characterized
histologically by pronounced infiltration of the tubulointerstitial structure with mononuclear cells and eosinophils. The
presence of this cellular infiltrate has prompted studies of
cell-mediated mechanisms in the disorder. While no reliable
animal model of drug-induced tubulointerstitial nephritis has
been reported, models for the induction of tubulointerstitial
nephritis have been developed:

(a) a model in which the principal mechanism is delayed
hypersensitivity. Animals were immunized with bovine gamma
globulin by methods known to favor delayed hypersensitivity (7).
The antigen was then injected directly into the subcortical
areas of the kidney. An intense mononuclear infiltrate developed
in the injected areas. This reaction was shown to be due to
delayed hypersensitivity, since transfer of the disease could
be accomplished only by cell transfer and not by serum.

(b) tubulointerstitial nephritis produced by immunizing
animals with tubular basement antigens (3,9,10,11). This model
has relevance to the human illness, since circulating anti-TBM
antibody can be demonstrated in some patients with drug-induced
interstitial nephritis (12,13). The animal model can be transferred by serum alone (9), but requires the presence of bone
marrow cells in the recipient for the complete histologic
expression of disease (10). This led to recent studies by
Neilson and Phillips (11) who showed that the lymphocytes of
animals immunized by tubular basement membrane antigens
developed cytotoxic capacities against cultured kidney cells;
sequential observations showed concordance between maximum
in vitro cytotoxicity and in vivo histologic nephritis. However, transfer of the disease by cells has not to date been
reported.

Idiopathic Membranous Nephropathy

Studies in our laboratory (14) have recently shown evidence
for monocyte modulation of the immune response in patients with
membranous nephropathy. The rationale for the studies stems
from observations in animal models of chronic serum sickness
nephritis which have suggested that animals exhibiting a poor

antibody response to the antigen develop membranous lesions. To test this hypothesis, we examined the ability of lymphocytes isolated from 11 patients with this disorder to produce immuno-globulin (Ig)G and IgM on stimulation with a polyclonal B-cell activator, pokeweed mitogen. The peripheral blood lymphocytes (2×10^6 cells) from 24 normal individuals had geometric mean production rates of 1,779 ng for IgG, and 2,940 ng for IgM after 7 days of culture in the presence of pokeweed mitogen. By contrast, under identical conditions, lymphocytes from the 11 patients with membranous nephropathy produced significantly lower quantities of both immunoglobulins, with geometric mean concentrations of 511 ng for IgG and 439 ng for IgM. When lymphocytes from patients with membranous nephropathy were co-cultured with normal lymphocytes, the production of immuno-globulin by normal lymphocytes was depressed by 22-82%, sug-gesting that a population of suppressor cells was responsible for this disturbance in B-cell function. By co-culturing normal lymphocytes with patient lymphocytes depleted of either T cells or monocytes, the suppressor cell was identified as a monocyte.

These studies suggest that analogous to the animal model of chronic serum sickness nephritis, patients with idiopathic membranous nephropathy may have a defective antibody response -- this defect being mediated by monocyte suppressor cells. Such a defect would allow the formation of soluble immune complexes in large antigen excess leading to small sized immune complexes localized in the subepithelial position in the glomerulus. The reduced antibody concentrations would also result in only small amounts of immune complexes being formed, which would explain the relative absence of these complexes in the circulation (15); it would also account for the slow deterioration in renal function observed in these patients.

REFERENCES
1. Shalhoub RJ. 1974. Pathogenesis of lipoid nephrosis: A disorder of T cell function. Lancet 2:556

2. Mallick NP, Williams RJ, McFarlane H, Taylor B, and Williams G. 1972. Cell mediated immunity in nephrotic syndrome. Lancet 1:507

3. Eyres KE, Mallick NP, Taylor G. 1976. Evidence for cell-mediated immunity to renal antigens in minimal change nephrotic syndrome. Lancet 1:1158

4. Ooi BS, Orlina A, and Masaitis L. 1974. Lymphocytotoxins in renal disease. Lancet 2:1348

5. Lagrue G, Branellec BA, Blanc C. 1978. A vascular permeability factor in lymphocyte culture supernatants from patients with nephrotic syndrome. II. Pharmacological and physico-chemical properties. Biomedicine 23:73

6. Sobel AT, Branellec AJ, Blanc CJ, and Lagrue GA. 1977. Physicochemical characterization of a vascular permeability factor produced by Con A-stimulated human lymphocytes. J. Immunol. 119:1230

7. Van Zwieten MJ, Leber PD, Bhan AK, and McCluskey RT. 1977. Experimental cell-mediated interstitial nephritis induced with exogenous antigens. J. Immunol. 118:589

8. Steblay RW, and Rudofsky UH. 1971. Renal tubular disease and autoantibodies against tubular basement membrane induced in guinea pigs. J. Immunol. 107:589

9. Steblay RW, Rudofsky UH. 1973. Transfer of experimental autoimmune renal cortical tubular and interstitial disease in guinea pigs by serum. Science 180:966

10. Rudofsky UH, Pollara B. 1976. Studies on the pathogenesis of experimental autoimmune renal tubulointerstitial disease in guinea pigs. II. Passive transfer of renal lesions by antitubular basement membrane autoantibody and non-immune bone marrow cells to leukocyte-depleted recipients. Clin. Immunol. Immunopathol. 6:107

11. Neilson EG, and Phillips SM. 1979. Cell-mediated immunity in interstitial nephritis. J. Immunol. 123:2381

12. Border WA, Lehman DH, Egan JD, Sass HJ, Glode JE, and Wilson CB. 1974. Anti-tubular basement-membrane antibodies in methicillin-associated interstitial nephritis. N. Engl. J. Med. 291:381

13. Ooi BS, Ooi YM, Mohini RL, Pollak VE. 1978. Humoral mechanisms in drug induced acute interstitial nephritis. Clin. Immunol. Immunopathol. 10:330

14. Ooi BS, Ooi YM, Hsu A, and Hurtubise PE. 1980. Diminished synthesis of immunoglobulin by peripheral lymphocytes of patients with idiopathic membranous glomerulonephropathy. J. Clin. Invest. 65:789

15. Ooi YM, Ooi BS, and Pollak VE. 1977. Relationship of levels of circulating immune complexes to histologic patterns of nephritis: a comparative study of membranous glomerulonephropathy and diffuse proliferative glomerulo-nephritis. J. Lab. Clin. Med. 90:891

THE USE OF ISOLATED TUBULES IN THE STUDY OF REGULATION OF CELL VOLUME

M.A. LINSHAW AND J.J. GRANTHAM

INTRODUCTION

Renal tubule cells are capable of transporting large quantities of water
and solute across their plasma membrane and yet they maintain a remarkably
constant ionic composition and cellular volume. It is generally held that
volume and ionic composition of kidney tubule cells are regulated by a cation
pump. Under normal conditions, intracellular nondiffusible substances such
as protein exert a colloid osmotic pressure which promotes the continual
diffusion of water into the cell. A cation pump extrudes sodium from the
cell and prevents cell swelling. When cation transport is blocked by ouabain,
an inhibitor of membrane $Na^{+}+K^{+}$ ATPase (2), cell swelling occurs. One would
expect that if the ouabain sensitive pump were the only determinant of cell
size, ouabain should cause enormous cellular swelling. In fact, however,
renal tubule cells in ouabain swell to only a limited degree (1,7) indicating
that some system resistant to the effect of ouabain contributes to the
control of cell size. Some years ago, Kleinzeller (4) suggested that the
ouabain insensitive volume control system resided in the plasma membrane
which under certain experimental conditions could increase its rigidity,
develop a transmembrane hydrostatic pressure and offset the pressure created
by intracellular colloid. However, this theory has not been widely accepted
because the plasma membrane of a variety of mammalian cells including renal
tubule cells is highly deformable (3). It had also been previously suggested
that the relatively rigid tubule basement membrane might influence cell size
(1,7). Alternatively, Whittembury and his co-workers (11, 12) postulated
that cell volume was controlled by a ouabain resistant electrogenic sodium
pump, a notion derived primarily from studies of slices of kidney cortex
in which metabolism was blocked by chilling to $0^{\circ}C$ in anaerobic medium.
Under these conditions, the slices swelled by taking up water and saline.
Upon rewarming to room temperature in an aerobic medium, the slices regulated

their volume by extruding water and salt. If ouabain were added to the
slices during the chilled incubation period, the tissue when rewarmed still
extruded salt and water suggesting that volume regulation occurred even in
the presence of ouabain. However, when other metabolic inhibitors such as
2-4 dinitrophenol (DNP) were added to the bathing medium, the tissue upon
rewarming was unable to extrude saline and remained considerably swollen.
These studies were interpreted to indicate that cell volume was not regulated
by the ouabain sensitive Na-K exchange pump, but rather by a different
sodium pump not blocked by ouabain but nevertheless requiring cellular
metabolism for its operation. However, Mills and co-workers (9) raised
questions about the interpretation of data from ouabain treated slices of
kidney cortex. These investigators found that ouabain binding to $Na^+ + K^+$
ATPase occurred principally when there was actual movement of sodium ion
across the membrane. Since passive solute movement is considerably decreased
at temperatures around $0-4^\circ C$, the temperature used in Whittembury's studies,
the decreased sodium flux at this low temperature might have precluded
sufficient ouabain binding to completely block the ouabain sensitive pump.

Over the past several years, we have concentrated our research efforts on
clarifying the role of passive forces in the overall regulation of cell size.

METHODS

Rabbit proximal tubules from the outer cortex were isolated by microdissection and the ends tightly crimped between two pipets (Figure 1).

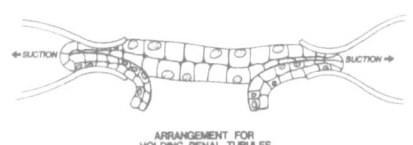

ARRANGEMENT FOR
HOLDING RENAL TUBULES

FIGURE 1. Arrangement for holding
nonperfused tubules. (From Am. J.
Physiol. 233:F325, 1977, reproduced
by permission).

Using an inverted microscope and high powered magnification tubule volume
was assessed visually by measuring tubule diameter with an image splitting
micrometer. The tubules were incubated at $37^\circ C$ in a balanced electrolyte
solution containing 6 gm% protein. Since the tubule ends were tightly
crimped, fluid did not enter the lumen. Since the lumen remained collapsed
during the experiment, fluid entered the cells primarily across the basolateral membrane. Cell volume was estimated from the formula $\pi r^2 l$, r being
the radius of the tubule and l a constant length. By obtaining frequent
measurements of cell diameter (volume) over a given time frame, we could

quantitate the rate of fluid entry across the basolateral membrane. This
preparation allowed us to study a single layer of renal epithelial cells
and assure a more efficient exposure of cell surfaces to the bathing medium
than might occur in a slice of cortex.

RESULTS AND DISCUSSION

Our initial studies clearly confirmed that the classical ouabain sensitive
Na-K pump was important in the regulation of cell size (Figure 2).

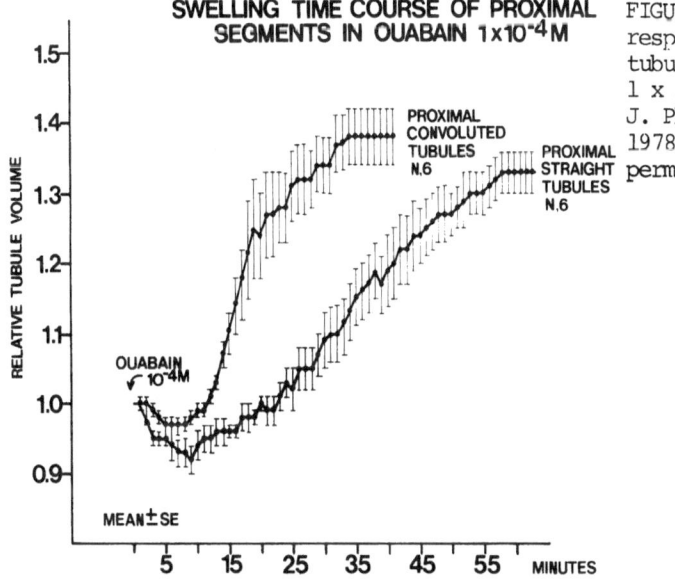

FIGURE 2. Swelling response of proximal tubules in ouabain 1×10^{-4}M. (From Am. J. Physiol. 235:F480, 1978, reproduced by permission).

In 10^{-4}M ouabain proximal convoluted and straight tubules swelled predictably
to a steady state about 35-40% above the control level. We did not know
why cell swelling leveled off at that point. The ouabain sensitive pump
may have been incompletely blocked. However, when we performed ouabain dose
response curves, we found that the 10^{-4}M concentration was sufficient to
evoke a maximal swelling response in proximal tubules (Figure 3). The dose
response was similar for proximal convoluted and straight tubules. It
seemed plausible that a ouabain resistant sodium pump might further regulate
volume and prevent enormous swelling in ouabain. However, when we added
metabolic inhibitors known to eliminate cell volume regulation such as DNP,
we found that tubules in ouabain, DNP or ouabain + DNP all swelled to the
same extent (Figure 4), although tubules in DNP began to swell earlier.
In further experiments when we removed all the energy substrate from the

58

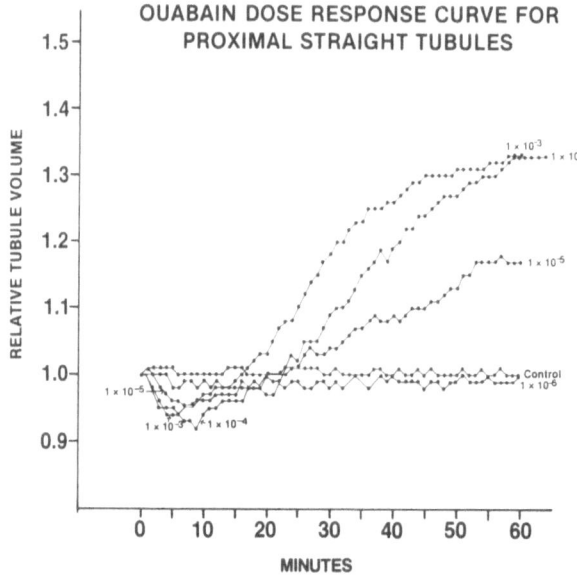

FIGURE 3. Swelling response of proximal straight tubules in different concentrations of ouabain (mM/L). Note that 10^{-4}M ouabain induced a maximal response. (From Am. J. Physiol. 235:F480, 1978, reproduced by permission).

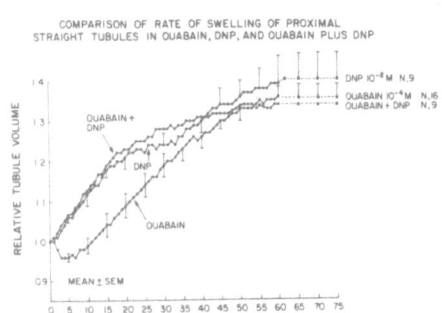

FIGURE 4. Response of proximal tubules to ouabain and DNP. Note that maximal cell swelling was similar in ouabain and DNP. (From Am. J. Physiol. 239, 1980, In Press, reproduced by permission).

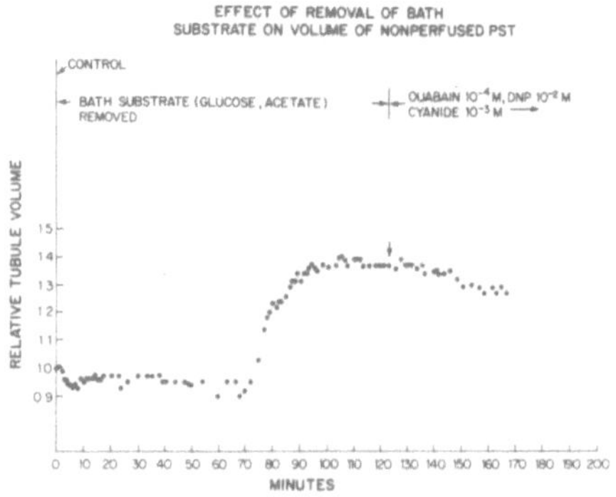

FIGURE 5. Swelling response of a single nonperfused proximal straight tubule following removal of bath substrate. Maximal tubule swelling though delayed was similar to swelling in ouabain. Note lack of further effect of metabolic inhibitors. (From Am. J. Physiol. 239, 1980, In Press, reproduced by permission).

bathing medium, tubules maintained their volume until their endogenous energy supply was gone and then swelled, but again to the same degree as tubules in ouabain - about 35-40% above control (Figure 5). The subsequent

addition of ouabain, cyanide and DNP caused no further swelling. These
findings seemed strong evidence that cell size in ouabain was not limited
by an energy dependent sodium pump.

It had been previously suggested that the tough elastic tubule basement
membrane might appear to constrain cell size by developing a transmembrane
hydrostatic pressure as the tubule swelled (1). When we removed the
basement membrane with collagenase from our ouabain treated tubules, the
tubule swelled enormously, developed huge surface blebs (Figure 6) and
eventually disaggregated. It is of course possible that collagenase removed

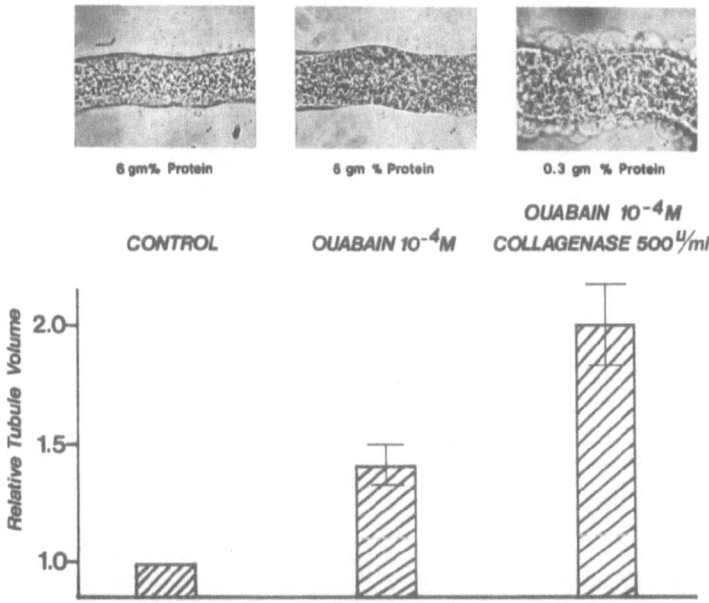

FIGURE 6. Effect of ouabain and collagenase on cell volume of proximal
straight tubules. Cell volume increased to steady state 40% above control
in ouabain, and increased much more in ouabain + collagenase. Note swollen
tubule in ouabain appears intact. Tubule in collagenase developed extensive
surface blebs which eventually burst. Values are MEAN ± SE. N,11. (From
Am. J. Physiol. 233:F325, 1977, reproduced by permission).

pump protein from the plasma membrane allowing for further cell swelling.
However, when tubules were incubated in collagenase and not ouabain so that
their basement membranes were removed but their transport mechanisms were
intact the cells swelled only slightly (6, 7). Furthermore, increasing the
concentration of collagenase from 10 to 1,000 units per ml did not cause
a corresponding increase in cell size (8). One would expect that if

60

collagenase were removing pump protein, higher concentrations of collagenase should cause progressively greater degrees of cell swelling.

We were also reminded that the peritubular capillaries are perfused with blood which might affect cell size by counterbalancing the osmotic pressure of intracellular colloid. Indeed, bath protein had a considerable effect on cell size (Figure 7). Note the reversible decrease in tubule diameter upon addition of hyperoncotic protein and increase in tubule diameter upon protein removal. This effect could be translated to collagenase treated tubules as

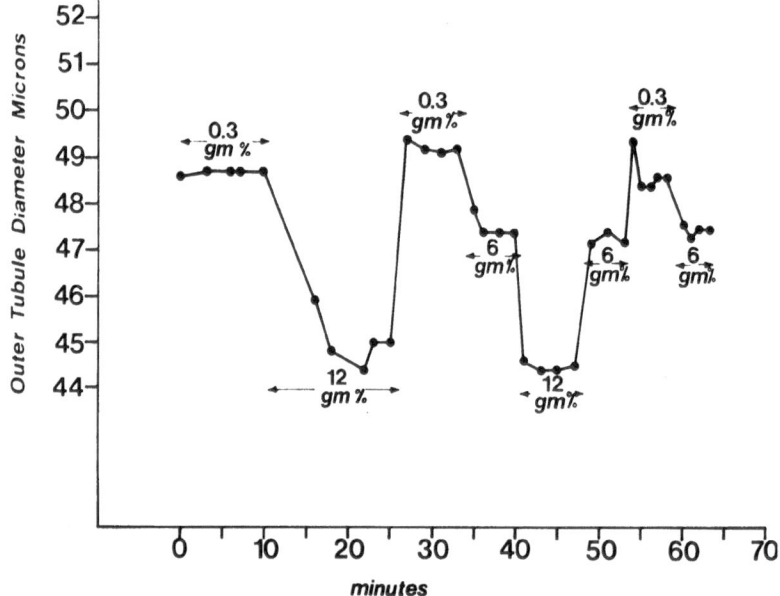

FIGURE 7. Effect of peritubular protein (albumin) concentration on outer diameter of a single nonperfused ouabain treated proximal straight tubule. Basement membrane was intact. Note reversible changes in diameter as protein concentration was varied. (From Am. J. Physiol. 233:F325, 1977, reproduced by permission).

well (Figure 8). In collagenase alone, relative volume of these tubules increased only slightly. However, after ouabain was added, swelling was extensive in the absence of protein, modest in the presence of 6 gm% protein and tubules could be shrunk below the control level and swelling minimized in hyperoncotic protein. These experiments taken together showed that proximal tubules maintained their volume primarily by the action of the ouabain sensitive classical Na-K pump. When that pump was inhibited either by ouabain, DNP, cyanide or by removing energy supplies, cell size was controlled to a major extent by external protein (colloid osmotic force)

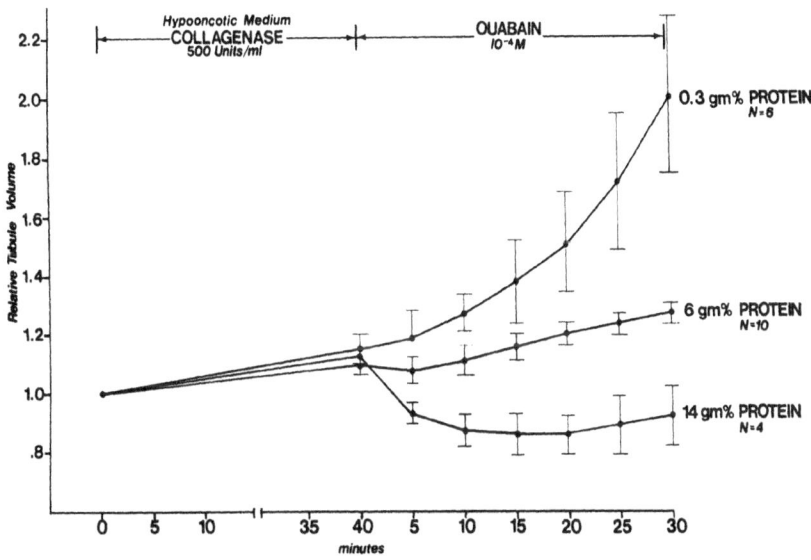

FIGURE 8. Effect of bath protein on cell volume. Nonperfused proximal straight tubules were first treated with collagenase to remove basement membrane. Swelling was slight. After cation transport was blocked by ouabain, cell swelling varied depending on the bath albumin concentration. Values are MEAN ± SE. (From Am. J. Physiol. 233:F325, 1977, reproduced by permission).

and the elastic constraint of the tubule basement membrane (hydrostatic force).

We have used this technique to evaluate relative peritubular membrane permeability of different proximal tubular segments. We had observed that in ouabain, proximal convoluted tubules swelled more rapidly that did proximal straight tubules (Figure 2). In an effort to define if there were a difference in the permeability of the respective basolateral membranes to salt, we compared the rate of cell swelling in ouabain to their respective basolateral membrane surface areas. We found that proximal convoluted tubules had a faster rate of swelling in ouabain and a greater basolateral membrane surface area than proximal straight tubules. However, the ratio of the rate of swelling to the surface area was nearly identical in both segments (6). Therefore, differences in rates of swelling among proximal segments are probably not related to intrinsic differences in peritubular membrane permeability.

We have made similar observations on neonatal rabbit tubules. Neonatal tubules in ouabain swell predictably about 40% above control and show the same qualitative response when protein is removed or collagenase added to the bathing medium. The neonatal tubules do swell somewhat more slowly than adult tubules. We also performed a cell volume experiment on a human proximal tubule several years ago. This tubule behaved as did our rabbit tubules and supports the notion that our observations made on rabbit tubules are broadly applicable to the human condition (10).

This project was supported in part by Public Health Service Grants AM 13476 (J.J. Grantham) and AM 25748 (M.A. Linshaw).

REFERENCES

1. Dellasega M and Grantham JJ. Regulation of renal tubule cell volume in hypotonic medium. Am. J. Physiol. 224:1288-1294, 1973.
2. Glynn IM and Karlish SJD. The sodium pump. Ann. Rev. Physiol. 37:13-55, 1975.
3. Grantham JJ. Vasopressin: effect on deformity of urinary surface of collecting duct cells. Science 168:1093-1095, 1970.
4. Kleinzeller A. Cellular transport of water in metabolic pathways. In: Metabolic Transport(3rd ed.) Edited by LE Hokin. New York: Academic Press, 1972, vol. 6, p 91-131.
5. Linshaw MA. Effect of metabolic inhibitors on renal tubule cell volume. Am. J. Physiol. 239, 1980, In Press.
6. Linshaw MA and Stapleton FB. Effect of ouabain and colloid osmotic pressure on renal tubule cell volume. Am. J. Physiol. 235 (Renal Fluid Electrolyte Physiol. 4):F480-F491, 1978.
7. Linshaw MA, Stapleton FB, Cuppage FE and Grantham JJ. Effect of basement membrane and colloid osmotic pressure on renal tubule cell volume. Am. J. Physiol. 233 (Renal Fluid Electrolyte Physiol. 2):F325-F332, 1977.
8. Linshaw MA and Grantham JJ. Effect of collagenase and ouabain on renal cell volume in hypotonic media. Am. J. Physiol. 238 (Renal Fluid Electrolyte Physiol. 7):F491-F498, 1980.
9. Mills JW, Dayer JM, MacKnight ADC and Ausiello DA. Ouabain binding to epithelial cells (LLc-PKI) in culture. Kidney Internat. 14:770, 1978 (Abstract).
10. Stapleton FB and Linshaw MA. Regulation of cell volume in a human proximal straight tubule. Renal Physiol. 1:334-337, 1978.
11. Whittembury G. Sodium extrusion and potassium uptake in guinea pig kidney cortex slices. J. Gen. Physiol. 48:699-717, 1965.
12. Whittembury G and Proverbio F. Two modes of sodium extrusion in cells from guinea pig kidney cortex slices. Pfluegers Arch. 316:1-25, 1970.

ROLE OF Na ENTRY IN THE REGULATION OF PROLIFERATION OF CULTURED FIBROBLASTS:
EFFECT OF VASOPRESSIN

S.A. MENDOZA

INTRODUCTION

This study reports the measurement of monovalent ion fluxes and content
in cultured cells. The study is based on the fact that normal, untransformed
fibroblasts reduce their rate of entry into the S (DNA synthesizing) phase
of the cell cycle and accumulate in a viable quiescent state (G_0/G_1) when
the content of   growth factors in the medium becomes limiting. Addition
of fresh serum or growth factors to such quiescent cells stimulates a complex
array of biochemical events leading to DNA synthesis and cell division (1,2).
Recently, a variety of information has led to the suggestion that the uptake
of sodium plays an important role in the regulation of cell proliferation (3).
Serum, the most widely used stimulator of cell proliferation, rapidly
increases sodium entry into quiescent cells (4) and stimulates the sodium
potassium pump (5). A variety of other growth factors including platelet
derived growth factor (6) and fibroblast derived growth factor (7) also
increase sodium entry and/or activity of the sodium potassium pump. The
synthesis of DNA is dependent upon the concentration of sodium in the
extracellular medium (4). The proliferative response to serum is strikingly
inhibited by ouabain, an inhibitor of the sodium potassium pump (5), and
by amiloride, an inhibitor of sodium entry into the cells (3). In certain
transformed cells, the entry of sodium and the activity of the sodium
potassium pump greatly exceeds that found in the nontransformed parent
cells (3,6). Since cell proliferation and sodium transport seemed to be
related, the mitogenic effect of a variety of substances which stimulate
sodium transport in other systems was tested. Rozengurt and coworkers
found that the neurohypophyseal peptide hormone, vasopressin, is strongly
mitogenic for Swiss 3T3 cells (8). The effect of vasopressin on monovalent
ion fluxes in quiescent Swiss 3T3 cells was then studied. This work was
performed in the laboratory of Dr. Enrique Rozengurt at the Imperial

Cancer Research Fund Laboratories in London, England during my recent sabbatical leave. This study has been reported in more complete form (9).

MATERIALS AND METHODS

Swiss 3T3 cells (10) were maintained in 90 mm Nunc Petri dishes in Dulbecco's modified Eagle's medium (DME), 10% fetal bovine serum, 100 unit/ml penicillin and 100 µg/ml streptomycin in a humidified atmosphere of 10% CO_2 and 90% air at $37^{o}C$. The cells were subcultured to 30 mm, 50 mm, or 90 mm Nunc Petri dishes with medium containing 10% fetal bovine serum. The medium was changed two days after plating and studies were performed on quiescent confluent dishes 4-7 days later. The cultures were shown to be quiescent by autoradiography after 48 hours with ^{3}H-thymidine as previously described (5). Intracellular Na and K content and the uptake of ^{86}Rb (a K tracer) were measured via a modification of previously reported methods (4,5). At the beginning of each experiment, the media from quiescent cultures in 50 mm dishes was replaced with experimental media. After a variable preincubation period, 50 µl of ^{86}Rb (Amersham/Searle) containing $2-3 \times 10^{6}$ dpm were added. When the uptake period was complete, the dishes were washed rapidly 6 times with 0.1 M $MgCl_2$ at $4^{o}C$. The dishes were allowed to drain a few minutes to ensure the compelte removal of the final $MgCl_2$ wash. When the dishes were dry, 1 ml of 15 mM LiCl containing 1% toluene was added to each dish. This solution was tested directly in the flame photometer to measure intracellular sodium and potassium. An aliquot of the solution was transferred to the liquid scintillation counter to measure Cerenkov radiation. Ouabain sensitive ^{86}Rb uptake was calculated by subtracting the ^{86}Rb uptake in the presence of 1 mM ouabain from ^{86}Rb uptake in the absence of the inhibitor. The uptake of ^{22}Na was measured by the method of Smith and Rozengurt (4). The media from quiescent cultures were replaced with modified DME in which sodium chloride was replaced by choline chloride to increase the specific activity of ^{22}Na. In addition, the Na-K pump was inhibited by lowering the concentration of KCl to 0.5 mM and by adding 1 mM ouabain. Twenty minutes after the addition of this medium, 50 µl of ^{22}NaCl containing $1-2 \times 10^{6}$ dpm were added. Three minutes later, dishes were washed as described above. When the dishes were dry, 1.5 ml of 15 mM LiCl containing 1% toluene was added to each dish, the solution aspirated and radioactivity assayed in a gamma spectrometer.

Cell electrolyte content, ^{86}Rb uptake and ^{22}Na uptake are expressed
as a function of total cell protein (11). Statistical analysis was performed
using the paired or unpaired t test as appropriate. The data presented
are the means$\overset{+}{-}$ the standard error of two or more identically treated
cultures and are typical of experiments each done several times. Synthetic
arginine vasopressin was obtained from Sigma.

RESULTS AND DISCUSSION

Vasopressin stimulated ^{86}Rb uptake in quiescent Swiss 3T3 cells.
Vasopressin did not affect ^{86}Rb uptake in the presence of ouabain. This
indicated that vasopressin stimulated ^{86}Rb uptake was mediated by the Na-K
pump. The magnitude of the stimulation of ouabain sensitive ^{86}Rb uptake
produced by 10 ng/ml of vasopressin varied but averaged 59$\overset{+}{-}$ 5% in 43
independent experiments. Ouabain sensitive ^{86}Rb uptake in the absence
and presence of vasopressin was linear for at least 40 minutes after the
addition of the isotope. In contrast, vasopressin had no effect on ^{86}Rb
efflux from cells pre-loaded with the isotope. (Figure 1)

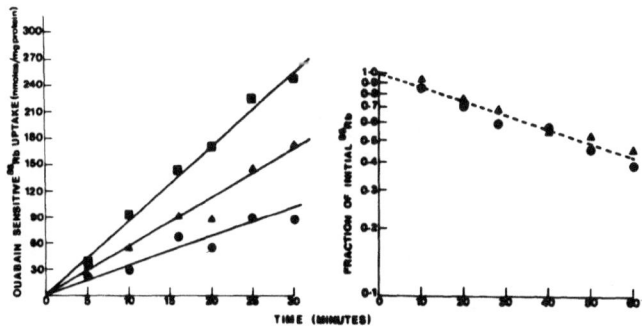

66

FIGURE 1. <u>Left panel</u>: Time-course of ouabain-sensitive ^{86}Rb$^+$ uptake in the absence or in the presence of vasopressin or serum. Quiescent cultures of Swiss 3T3 cells grown in 30 mm dishes were incubated in DME (O), DME + 10% fetal bovine serum (■) or DME + 10 ng/ml arginine vasopressin (▲). After 20 minutes of incubation, ^{86}Rb$^+$ was added to the dishes and the uptake was terminated at the indicated times. All other experimental details were as described in Materials and Methods. <u>Right panel</u>: Time-course of ^{86}Rb$^+$ exit in the absence or in the presence of vasopressin. Quiescent cultures of 3T3 cells were loaded with ^{86}Rb$^+$ by adding 10^6 dpm of the isotope directly to the medium (2 ml) for 4 hours. Then, the cultures were rapidly washed three times with pre-warmed DME and incubated at 37° in 2 ml of DME (●) or DME containing 10 ng/ml arginine-vasopressin (▲). At the times indicated, remaining internal ^{86}Rb$^+$ was measured as described in Materials and Methods. The radioactivity still present in the cells at each time is expressed as a fraction of that present at the end of the loading period. This corresponded to 9747 cpm per dish; each dish contained 92 µg of protein.

When vasopressin and ^{86}Rb were added simultaneously, the stimulation of uptake by the hormone occurred rapidly. (Figure 2) As early as one minute after the addition of the hormone and isotope, total ^{86}Rb uptake was higher in vasopressin treated cultures than in control cultures. Similar differences were noted in ouabain sensitive ^{86}Rb uptake. Consistent with the speed of the hormonal effect on the stimulation of ^{86}Rb uptake, cyclohexamide was ineffective in inhibiting this response.

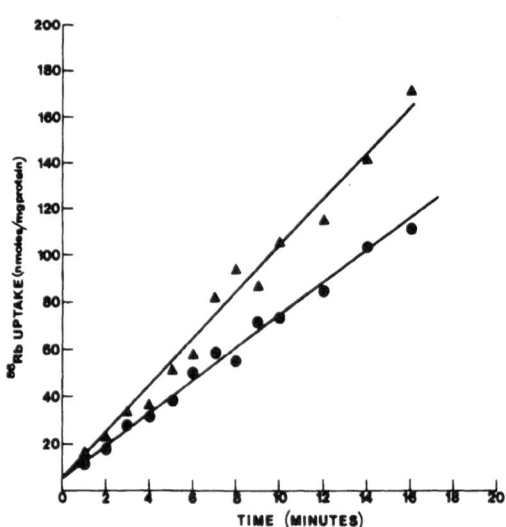

FIGURE 2. Kinetics of stimulation by vasopressin of ^{86}Rb$^+$ uptake in quiescent 3T3 cells. The growth medium of quiescent cultures of Swiss 3T3 cells was replaced by DME (●) or DME containing 10 ng/ml vasopressin (▲). Both media contain 3.5x10^6 dpm of ^{86}Rb$^+$ per ml. The cultures were incubated for different periods of time as indicated.

Vasopressin stimulated ^{86}Rb uptake in a concentration dependent manner. (Figure 3) Oxytocin also stimulated the Na-K pump but at significantly higher concentrations than vasopressin. The difference in the sensitivity to the two peptides was similar to that seen for the mitogenic effects of vasopressin and oxytocin. Furthermore, the concentrations of vasopressin which stimulated ^{86}Rb uptake (1-100 ng/ml) were the same as the concentrations which stimulated DNA synthesis (8).

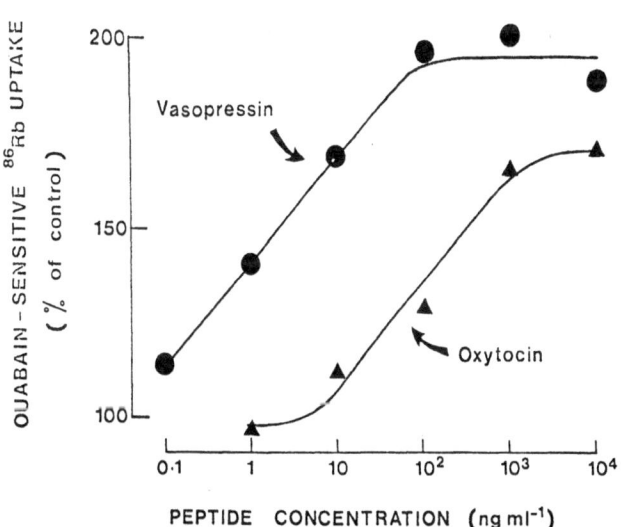

FIGURE 3. Effect of different concentrations of arginine vasopressin or oxytocin on ouabain-sensitive ^{86}Rb uptake by Swiss 3T3 cells. Quiescent cultures of Swiss 3T3 cells grown in 30 mm dishes were incubated in DME or in DME containing different concentrations of vasopressin or oxytocin either in the presence or in the absence of 1 mM ouabain. Each value represents the average of 2-4 cultures treated identically and is expressed as percentage of the ^{86}Rb uptake obtained in cultures treated with DME alone (2,772 ± 267 cpm/dish; mean ± S.E., n=6).

The rate of ^{86}Rb uptake was dependent upon the concentration of potassium in the medium both in the absence and presence of vasopressin. (Figure 4) The hormone had no effect on the apparent affinity of the Na-K pump for potassium. The maximum velocity (V_{max}) increased from 8 to 13 nmoles/mg protein/min. The apparent K_m for potassium was 1.3 mM in both the absence and presence of vasopressin, agreeing closely with previously reported values in Swiss 3T3 cells (5). The stimualtion of ^{86}Rb uptake by vasopressin was not dependent upon the presence of calcium in the medium and did not appear to be mediated by cyclic AMP (data not shown).

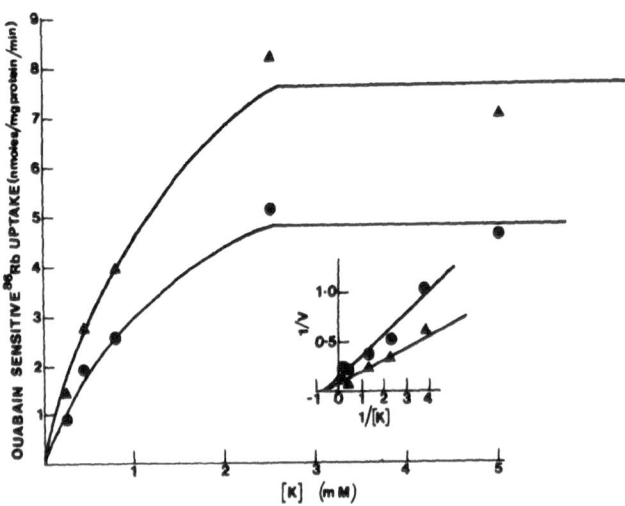

FIGURE 4. Rate of ouabain-sensitive ^{86}Rb$^+$ uptake as a function of K$^+$ concentration in the absence (●) or presence of 10 ng/ml vasopressin (▲). Quiescent cultures of Swiss 3T3 cells were rapidly washed three times with pre-warmed KCl-free medium and then incubated with medium containing different concentrations of K$^+$ (checked by flame photometry) in the absence or presence of 1 mM ouabain and, in each case, with or without 10 ng/ml vasopressin. After 20 minutes, the cultures were labeled with ^{86}Rb$^+$ for an additional 10 minutes, during which uptake was linear with time. All other experimental details were as described under Materials and Methods.

When the concentration of sodium in the medium was lowered by the isotonic replacement of NaCl by choline Cl, ^{86}Rb uptake fell. Addition of vasopressin shifted the sodium dependence of the Na-K pump. Half maximal activity of the Na-K pump occurred at 40 mM Na in the absence of vasopressin and 20 mM Na in the presence of the hormone. Vasopressin caused a nine fold stimulation in ^{86}Rb uptake when external Na concentration was ·20·mM. (Figure 5)

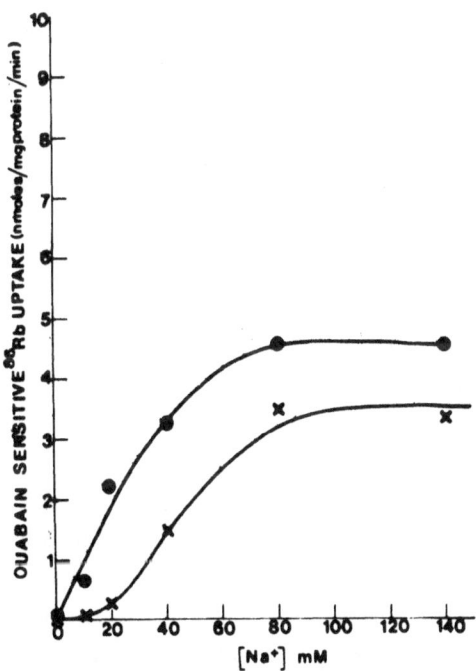

FIGURE 5. Dependence of ouabain-sensitive ^{86}Rb$^+$ uptake on Na$^+$ concentration in the absence (X) or in the presence (●) of 10 ng/ml vasopressin. Quiescent cultures of 3T3 cells were washed three times with pre-warmed DME from which the NaCl and NaHCO$_3$ were omitted and replaced by 140 mM choline Cl and 20 mM Tris-Hepes (pH 7.3). The cultures were incubated with this medium but containing different concentrations of Na; NaCl was. replaced by equimolar choline Cl.

These findings were suggestive of the possibility that vasopressin stimulated the sodium-potassium pump by increasing sodium entry into the cells. This hypothesis was tested by measuring ^{22}Na uptake. There was a marked stimulation of ^{22}Na uptake by vasopressin. This stimulation of ^{22}Na uptake was also present when amino acids were removed from the medium (data not shown).

Vasopressin altered intracellular electrolyte content in a manner similar to the effects of serum on quiescent 3T3 cells (6). In the presence of the Na-K pump inhibitor ouabain, vasopressin caused a statistically significant increase in intracellular Na content without affecting intracellular potassium. In the absence of the pump inhibitor, intracellular sodium was changed little but intracellular potassium increased significantly. These results are interpreted as follows: the initial effect of vasopressin on monovalent ion fluxes was stimulation of sodium entry into the cells. Since the activity of the Na-K pump is strongly dependent on intracellular Na concentration (4), the increase in Na entry resulted in a stimulation of the Na-K pump. Vasopressin-mediated stimulation of the Na-K pump resulted in a stimulation of ouabain sensitive ^{86}Rb uptake as well as an increase in intracellular potassium with little or no change in intracellular sodium. When ouabain was present, ^{22}Na uptake was increased but there was no stimulation of the Na-K pump by vasopressin. Intracellular potassium was unchanged but intracellular Na rose dramatically.

Three independent lines of evidence indicated that the initial effect of vasopressin was an increase of Na entry into the cells. First, the changes in electrolyte composition in the presence of ouabain were most compatible with the theory that the hormone is increasing Na entry rather than stimulating the pump directly. Second, when the pump was inhibited both by lowering potassium in the medium and by the addition of ouabain, ^{22}Na entry into the cells was markedly stimulated by vasopressin. Third, the Na dependence of the activity of Na-K pump was markedly shifted by the addition of vasopressin.

Several recent studies have reached conclusions in other cell culture systems similar to those which we have reported in Swiss 3T3 cells. It has been reported in neuroblastoma-glioma hybrid cells that an increase in intracellular Na was associated with stimulation of the Na-K pump and a marked increase in membrane potential difference (12). In addition, it has been shown that the addition of serum to quiescent neuroblastoma cells causes a rapid increase in Na permeability (13).. Phytohemagglutinin or Concanavalin A stimulated lymphocytes show a rapid increase in Na permeability and Na-K pump activity (14). Entry of Na into the isolated guinea pig atrium is a primary determinant of ouabain sensitive ^{86}Rb uptake (15). Epel has shown an influx of Na ions into the cells occurs rapidly following fertilization of sea urchin eggs (16). Leffert and Koch have suggested that Na entry into liver is one of the earliest, if not the earliest, event in the stimulation of liver regeneration (17).

In addition to the regulation of the activity of the Na-K pump, changes in Na entry into cells could affect cell metabolism in a variety of different ways. First, cytoplasmic Na may play a role in the release of mitochondrial calcium (18,19). Cytosolic calcium has been implicated in the control of cell proliferation and in the control of various enzymatic activities (20-24). Another possible regulatory effect of changes in Na entry is in the control of intracellular pH. Sodium-hydrogen exchange has been recorded in membrane vesicles from a variety of cell types (25,26) and it is possible that an increase in intracellular pH could occur simultaneously with the increase in Na entry which we have measured. It is known that proliferation of a variety of cell types is very sensitive to small changes in extracellular pH (27,28). In addition, an increase in Na entry with the concomitant Na-K pump activation could cause either depolarization or hyperpolarization of the cell membrane depending on the relative magnitude of the increased Na conductance and the electrogenicity of the pump. Changes in cell membrane potential would affect a variety of cellular transport processes. Thus, the increase of Na entry into the cells could trigger a series of ionic movements with changes in membrane potential and cytosolic Na, K, H and Ca concentrations and these in turn could each produce major changes in cellular metabolism and ultimately cell proliferation. At the present time, there is no information incompatible with this hypothesis although it certainly requires a considerable amount of further verification.

At the present time in our laboratory, we are doing experiments similar to those just described using renal epithelial cells rather than fibroblasts. Epithelial cells in culture have been shown to form a monolayer with tight junctions and lateral intracellular spaces. These monolayers are capable of oriented active transport, response to hormones and generation of a transmembrane potential difference (29-31). The possible role of ion fluxes in the proliferation of these cells which have a separate transepithelial ion transport system has not been studied previously.

REFERENCES

1. Todaro G, Matsuya Y, Bloom S, Robbins A, Green H. 1967. Stimulation of RNA synthesis and cell division in resting cells by a factor present in serum. In: Growth Regulating Substances for Animal Cells in Culture. V. Defendi and M. Stoker, eds, Wistar Institute Press. Philadelphia. Monograph Number 7, p.87.
2. Holley RW. 1975. Control of growth of mammalian cells in cell culture. Nature (London) 258:487.
3. Rozengurt E, Mendoza S. 1980. Monovalent ion fluxes and the control of cell proliferation in cultured fibroblasts. Ann.N.Y.Acad.Sci. 339:175.
4. Smith JB, Rozengurt E. 1978. Serum stimulates the Na^+-K^+ pump in quiescent fibroblasts by increasing Na^+ entry. Proc.Natl.Acad.Sci. USA 75:5560.
5. Rozengurt E, Heppel LA. 1975. Serum rapidly stimulates ouabain-sensitive $^{86}Rb^+$ influx in quiescent 3T3 cells. Proc.Natl.Acad.Sci. USA 72:4492.
6. Mendoza SA, Wigglesworth NM, Pohjanpelto P, Rozengurt E. 1980. Na entry and Na-K pump activity in murine, hamster,and human cells - effect of monensin,serum,platelet extract and viral transformation. J.Cell Physiol. 103:17.
7. Bourne HR, Rozengurt E. 1976. An 18,000 molecular weight polypeptide induces early events and stimulates DNA synthesis in cultured cells. Proc.Natl.Acad.Sci. USA 73:4555.
8. Rozengurt E, Legg A, Pettican P. 1979. Vasopressin stimulation of mouse 3T3 cell growth. Proc.Natl.Acad.Sci. USA 76:1284.
9. Mendoza SA, Wigglesworth NM, Rozengurt E. 1980. Vasopressin rapidly stimulates Na entry and Na-K pump activity in quiescent cultures of mouse 3T3 cells. J.Cell Physiol. (in press)
10. Todaro GJ, Green H. 1963. Quantitative studies of the growth of mouse embryo cells in culture and their development into established lines. J.Cell Biol. 17:299.
11. Lowry OH, Rosebrough NJ, Farr AL, Randall RJ. 1951. Protein measurement with the Folin phenol reagent. J.Biol.Chem. 193:265.
12. Lichtshtein D, Dunlop K, Kaback HR, Blume AJ. 1979. Mechanism of monensin-induced hyperpolarization of neuroblasmona-glioma hybrid. NG 108-15. Proc.Natl.Acad.Sci. USA 76:2580.
13. Moolenaar WH, de Laat SW, van der Saag PT. 1979. Serum triggers a sequence of rapid ionic conductance changes in quiescent neuroblastoma cells. Nature (London) 279:721.
14. Kaplan JG, Owens T. 1980. Activation of lymphocytes of man and mouse: monovalent cation fluxes. Ann.N.Y.Acad.Sci. 339:191.
15. Yamamoto S, Akera T, Brody TM. 1979. Sodium influx rate and ouabain-sensitive rubidium uptake in isolated guinea pig atria. Biochim. Biophys.Acta 555:270.
16. Epel D. 1980. Ionic triggers in the fertilization of sea urchin eggs. Ann.N.Y.Acad.Sci. 339:74.

17. Leffert HL, Koch KS. 1980. Ionic events at the membrane initiate rat liver regeneration. Ann.N.Y.Acad.Sci. 339:201.

18. Carafoli E, Crompton M. 1978. The regulation of intracellular calcium. Current Topics in Membranes and Transport. 10:151.

19. Haworth RA, Hunter DR, Berkoff HA. 1980. Na$^+$ releases Ca^{++} from liver, kidney and lung mitochondria. FEBS Letters 110:216.

20. Balk SD, Whitfield JF, Youdale T, Braun AC. 1973. Roles of calcium, serum, plasma and folic acid in the control of proliferation of normal and Rous Sarcoma virus-infected chicken fibroblasts. Proc.Natl.Acad. Sci. USA 70:675.

21. Maino VC, Green NM, Crumpton MJ. 1974. The role of calcium ions in initiating transformation of lymphocytes. Nature (London) 251:324.

22. Hazelton B, Mitchell B, Tupper J. 1979. Calcium, magnesium, and growth control in the WI-38 human fibroblast cell. J.Cell.Biol.83:487.

23. Schneider JA, Diamond I, Rozengurt E. 1978. Glycolysis in quiescent cultures of 3T3 cells: Addition of serum, epidermal growth factor, and insulin increases the activity of phosphofructokinase in a protein synthesis-independent manner. J.Biol.Chem.253:872.

24. Cheung WY. 1980. Calmodulin plays a pivotal role in cellular regulation. Science 207:19.

25. Christensen HN. 1975. Biological Transport. WA Benjamin Inc. Reading, Massachusetts.

26. Murer H, Hopfer U, Kinne R. 1976. Sodium/proton antiport in brush-border-membrane vesicles isolated from rat small intestine and kidney. Biochem. J. 154:587.

27. Eagle H. 1973. The effect of environmental pH on the growth of normal and malignant cells. J.Cell.Physiol. 82:1.

28. Rubin H. 1971. pH and population density in the regulation of animal cell multiplication. J.Cell.Biol. 51:686.

29. Misfeldt DS, Hamamoto ST, Pitelka DR. 1976. Transepithelial transport in cell culture. Proc.Natl.Acad.Sci. USA 73:1212.

30. Cereijido M, Robbins ES, Dolan WJ, Rotunno CA, Sabatini DD. 1978. Polarized monolayers formed by epithelial cells on a permeable and translucent support. J.Cell.Biol. 77:853.

31. Goldring SR, Dayer J-M, Ausiello DA, Krane SM. 1978. A cell strain cultured from porcine kidney increases cyclic AMP content upon exposure to calcitonin or vasopressin. Biochem.Biophys.Res.Comm. 83:434.

32. Handler JS, Steele RE, Sahib MK, Wade JB, Preston AS, Lawson NL, Johnson JP. 1979. Toad urinary bladder epithelial cells in culture: maintenance of epithelial structure, sodium transport and response to hormones. Proc.Natl.Acad.Sci. USA 76:4151.

33. Rindler MJ, Chuman LM, Shaffer L, Saier MH,Jr. 1979. Retention of differentiated properties in an established dog kidney epithelial cell line (MDCK). J.Cell.Biol.81:635.

Acknowledgements: During the course of this work, the author was a Senior International Fellow of the Fogarty International Center, United States Public Health Service. The author is extremely grateful to Dr. Enrique Rozengurt in whose laboratory this work was done and without whose guidance the work would have been impossible. The excellent technical assistance of Noel M. Wigglesworth is greatly appreciated.

MICROPUNCTURE IN DEVELOPMENTAL RENAL PHYSIOLOGY

A. SPITZER

The prevailing trend in biology, as well in other fields of human endeavor is to study smaller and smaller components in greater and greater detail. This continuous process is punctuated by technicological breakthroughs which result in a burst of activity and new knowledge. Such a step forward was achieved when Alfred Newton Richards and his collaborators provided the means of studying the function of single nephrons in vivo by micropuncture techniques (1,2). It is here, at the University of Pennsylvania, that this pioneering work has been done, and this is, therefore, the most appropriate place to acknowledge that all we know in renal physiology has either been proved or confirmed by renal micropuncture.

The technique, greatly improved and extended over the years, consists of three basic approaches for the study of glomerular function and of three basic approaches for the study of tubular function (Fig. 1). Description of the process of glomerular ultrafiltration requires quantitation of colloid-osmotic and hydrostatic forces. The colloid osmotic pressures can be assessed by collecting blood from the systemic circulation and from the stellate vessels - the latter reflecting the changes in blood composition that have occurred during filtration. The

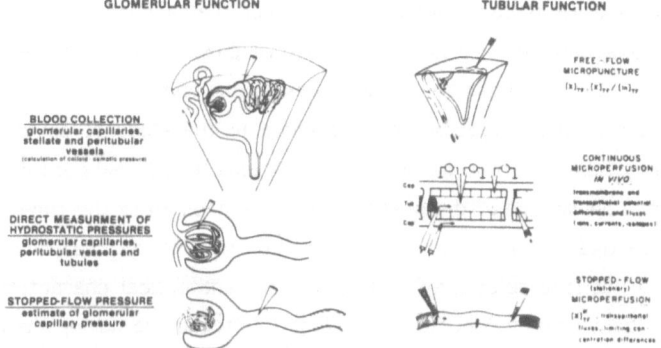

FIGURE 1: Schematic representation of micropuncture techniques for measurements of glomerular and tubular function.

measurement of glomerular capillary hydrostatic pressure necessary for the assessment of glomerular function, can be done directly in animals which possess glomeruli on the surface, such as the Munich-Wistar rat, or indirectly by the stop-flow technique. This latter approach is based on the assumption that blockage of the tubule with viscous oil allows filtration to continue until the pressure in the segment of the tubule located above the obstruction reaches a level similar to that in the glomerular capillary. Good correlations between direct and indirect measurements performed in the same animals have been reported (3). As this presentation proceeds it will become apparent that all these methods have been applied successfully to the study of glomerular dynamics during development.

The most commonly used technique for the study of tubular function is the free flow collection. This requires the identification on the surface of the kidney of the tubular segment to be studied, and a complete, timed collection of tubular fluid as it reaches the impelling micropipette. This method has been used extensively to determine sites of concentration gradients and the transport of solutes and water. The stop flow stationery microperfusion consists in the injection in the tubule of a solution of known amount and composition. This permits expression of transport processes in terms of tubular length exposed per unit time. In addition, limiting concentration differences can be measured when initially electrolyte free test solutions are used. This information can be used to assess pump and leak properties of various tubular segments. Continuous microperfusion of the tubule, either alone or in conjunction with perfusion of peritubular capillaries, provides an even greater range of freedom in altering the composition of both the tubular and peritubular environments. This approach has permitted to measure transmembrane and transepithelial potential differences, and fluxes of ions, currents and isotopes across various segments of the nephron. Only free flow collections have been used in developing animals.

Application of the micropuncture technique to the study of developmental renal physiology has been late to come. It took exactly 50 years from the time Richards started his voyage of discovery through the nephron to the time that this method of investigation has been applied to the study of the maturing animal. One reason for this long delay may be found in the anatomical characteristics of the immature kidney which preclude the use of this technique during the newborn period in most mammalian species (Fig. 2). The laboratory animals customarily used for micropuncture, namely the rat and the dog, have no discernible superficial nephrons at birth. Two to three weeks of extrauterine life have to pass in these species before nephrogenesis is completed and the superficial nephrons become amenable to sampling. An exception to this rule is the guinea pig, which, like the human, is born with a full complement of functioning nephrons and, as a consequence, can be subjected to micropuncture experiments from the very first day of extrauterine life.

Using this animal model we have been able to demonstrate that the process of morphological differentiation, which starts from the center of the kidney and proceeds toward the periphery, is parallelled by a similar pattern of functional development (4). A schematic representation of our findings (Fig. 3) highlights the fact that during the first two weeks of life of a guinea pig there is little change in the SNGFR of the superficial nephrons, while the total kidney GFR rises. During a subsequent period of development, the increase in total kidney GFR occurs in conjunction with a sharp increase in superficial SNGFR. Quantitative analysis of the data (Table I) indicates that a 3-fold increase in deep nephron GFR should occur during the initial period of postnatal development and that the 20-fold increase in superficial SNGFR, observed during the second period of postnatal maturation is sufficient to account for the overall increase in GFR. A similar pattern of postnatal development is evident in the data of Horster and Valtin (5), obtained in the dog, and that of Aperia and Herin (6), that of Dlouha (7), and that of deRouffignac and Monnens (8), obtained in the rat.

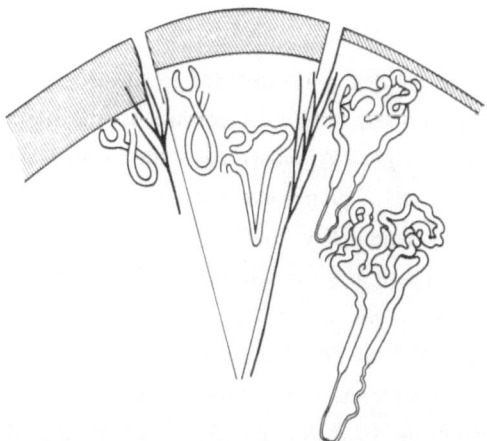

FIGURE 2: Schematic representation of the morphological changes occurring in the kidney during development. Modified from Speller, A.M. and Moffat, D.B.: J. Anat. 123: 487, 1977).

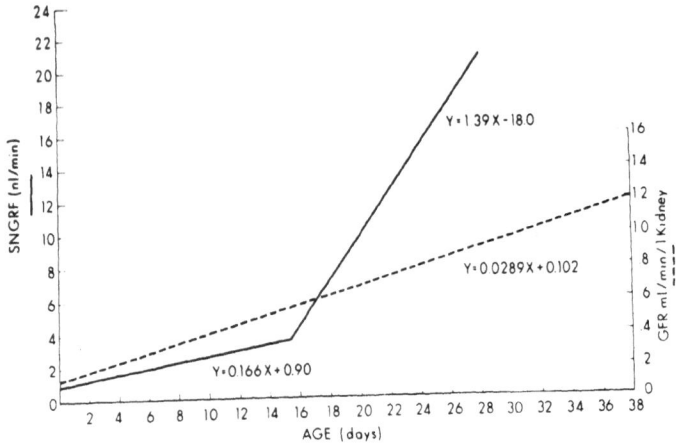

FIGURE 3: Schematic representation of the changes' in SNGFR (continuous line) and total kidney GFR (dashed line) in the developing guinea pig.

Table I
Measured Values of Superficial Nephron GFR (nl/min)
and Calculated Values of Deep Nephron GFR
in Guinea Pigs of Different Ages

Age (days)	Cortical (80%)	Juxtamedullary (20%)
1	0.9	17.2
15	4.1	43.2
30	19.3	42.1

Measurements of SNGFR are important to the investigation of the regulation of the filtration process itself. According to the mathematical model of Deen et al., (9) SNGFR = $\Delta P \times K_f$ where ΔP = the mean transcapillary hydraulic pressure difference, and K_f = glomerular ultrafiltration coefficient which in turn is a function of k = permeability coefficient and S = capillary surface area. Measurements of hydrostatic pressures in the tubule and the glomerular capillary, combined with measurements of colloid osmotic pressure of the glomerular capillary blood, have led to the quantification of the various terms of this equation in developing animals. Our study in guinea pigs (10), documented an increase in the effective filtration pressure (ΔP) at the afferent end of the glomerular capillary of about 2.5 fold between the age of 1 and 40 days, a period of time during which GFR increases by about 25 fold. Consistent with these data are the observations made by Ichikawa, et al. (11), and by Tucker and Blantz (12) in the rat. The inescapable conclusion is that the increase in SNGFR, and consequently in total kidney GFR, during maturation is mainly a function of the increase in Kf. Since we have detected very little change in the permeability of the glomerular capillary during development (an increase of approximately 1.4 fold) (13), it became apparent that the increase in glomerular capillary surface area is the most prominent factor. That this is indeed the case was confirmed by us in studies in which the neutron activation of a rubber compound injected in the renal microvasculature was used to demonstrate an 8 fold increase in the glomerular capillary surface area of the dog between the ages of 1 and 6 weeks (14).

Knowing the rate of glomerular filtration in single nephrons is also crucial to the determination of absolute rates of reabsorption or secretion by the renal tubules. For instance, assessment of factors involved in the control of sodium reabsorption depends on knowing the rate at which sodium enters and leaves the tubule. The relationship between GFR and tubular reabsorption during development has been a matter of continued interest and controversy. Morphological investigations performed by microdissection and functional studies performed by clearance techniques have indicated the existence of a glomerular-tubular imbalance in early life. According to this theory, the capacity for tubular reabsorption is smaller than the ability to form an ultrafiltrate of plasma, resulting in low rates of fractional reabsorption and high rates of fractional excretion. Although recent studies demonstrate that previous investigations were flawed by the lack of consideration given to the effect of changes in extracellular fluid volume on tubular reabsorption, the issue is far from being resolved. Measurements performed by Brandis and myself in the guinea pig (4) (Fig. 4) and those performed by Horster and Valtin in the puppy (5) indicate a constancy of the TF/P inulin ratio during development. It should be pointed out however, that these studies

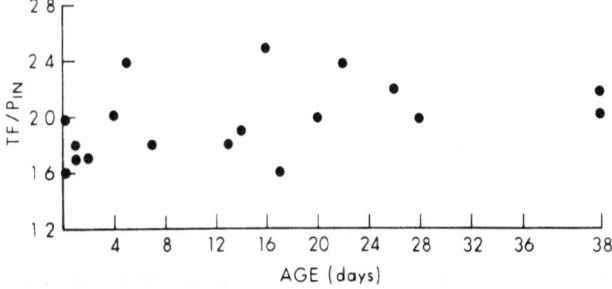

FIGURE 4: Fractional reabsorption of fluid by the proximal convoluted tubule of the developing guinea pig.

were done under hydropenic conditions. It is possible that the changes in fractional reabsorption in the expanded state are of a different magnitude in the newborn than in the adult animal and that the disturbance in the glomerular tubular balance is greater in the former than in the latter. Measurements performed by Schoeneman and myself (15) by the recollection technique, in guinea pigs subjected to volume expansion with an isoncotic albumin solution equal to 5% of body weight failed to reveal age related differences in fractional reabsorption of fluid (Fig. 5). However, when Zink and Horster measured proximal tubular fluid reabsorption in 2 and 4 week old rats, which were the progeny of mothers subjected to a high sodium intake, they noticed a graded incrase in proximal net fluid transport relative to the filtered load: the fractional reabsorption in the proximal tubules of the younger animals was only 72% of that observed in the older ones (16).

The inconsistency of these findings may be related to differences in the experimental conditions or in the developmental stage but they also can be due to the technical difficulties and possible pitfalls associated with these measurements. Potential sources of artifactual results (Table II) include variations of intratubular pressure at the collection site, collection from more than one tubule, the retrograde flow of tubular fluid during sampling, and the effect of repeated sampling at the same site. Some of these problems are of particular concern in the study of immature animals; the small diameters of the tubules makes

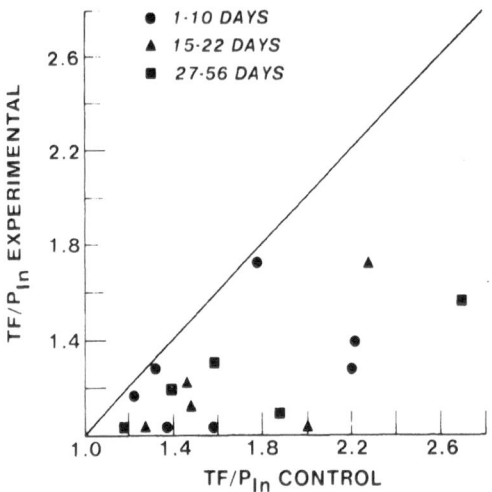

Figure 5: Measurements of proximal fluid reabsorption by the recollection technique in guinea pigs of various ages before (control) and after volume expansion (experimental).

Table II
SOURCES OF ARTIFACTUAL RESULTS
IN MICROPUNCTURE

Variations in intratubular pressure
Collection from more than one tubule
Retrograde flow
Leakage of tubular fluid

inadvertant puncture of a second nephron below the kidney surface much more likely than in the adult animal and the small rate of tubular fluid flow may result more often in suction and reduction in intratubular pressure.

Despite the lingering controversy regarding proximal tubular reabsorption of salt and fluid, we all agree that the retention of sodium intrinsic to the process of growth is made possible by enhanced reabsorption at tubular sites located beyond the proximal tubule (17). Fig. 6 taken from work performed with Schoeneman (18), portrays the behavior of the proximal tubule and that of the rest of the nephron (distal nephron) both under conditions of hydropenia and volume expansion with an isoncotic albumin solution equal to 5% of body weight. Please note that the general pattern is a decreased dependence on distal sodium reabsorption for the maintenance of external balance. That the thick ascending limb of the loop of Henle is not responsible for the enhanced sodium reabsorption observed during growth has been demonstrated by Zink and Horster (16). These investigators provided evidence that the absolute reabsorption of fluid in the loop of Henle increase by about 3 fold between 12 and 35 days of the life of the rat. Simultaneously, the osmolarity of early distal fluid decreased significantly, from 284 ± 19.8 to 180.9 ± 18.2 ml/L during the same period of observation. These findings demonstrate that the ability of the loop of Henle to generate a hypotonic fluid, and thus to increase the tonicity of the surrounding interstitium, is attained only gradually during ontogeny. The study also indicates that the loop of Henle is not the site which accounts for the retention of sodium in early postnatal life. As reported elsewhere at this meeting, Aperia and Elinder (19) have investigated one group of rats around 24 days of age and another one around 40 days of age, both during hydropenia and volume expansion. They found that both the delivery of sodium from the ascending loop of Henle and the reabsorption along the distal convoluted tubule were higher in the younger than in the older animals. While the first of these findings is mainly confirmatory of the work performed by Zink and Horster (16), the second finding strongly suggests that the distal convoluted tubule contributes to the retention of sodium observed in the newborn. It is our contention that the enhanced absorptive capacity of the distal convoluted tubule is related to the high levels of aldosterone prevailing during early postnatal life (18).

Thus, during the span of only 9 years, an impressive amount of information has been unravelled applying micropuncture techniques to the study of the developing nephron: 1) we have demonstrated that the centrifugal pattern which characterizes the morphologic and functional development of the kidney continues after birth, even in those animal species which are born with a full complement of nephrons, 2) we have described the factors which underly the increase in GFR with age, 3) established that the relative inability of the newborn to dispose of a sodium load in order to grow, far from reflecting an "immaturity" of the transporting process, represents an adaptive mechanism which allows the growing subject to maintain a positive sodium balance, 4) have been able to localize this phenomenon to the distal convoluted tubule, the site of aldosterone action. These accomplishments become more impressive in view of the fact that the world literature on micropuncture in developing animals is limited to some 15 publications generated by four laboratories.

The large potential that micropuncture holds is yet to be fulfilled in our field of science. Whether we consider the process of glomerular filtration and the factors that control it, or the tubular reabsorption of substances such as calcium,

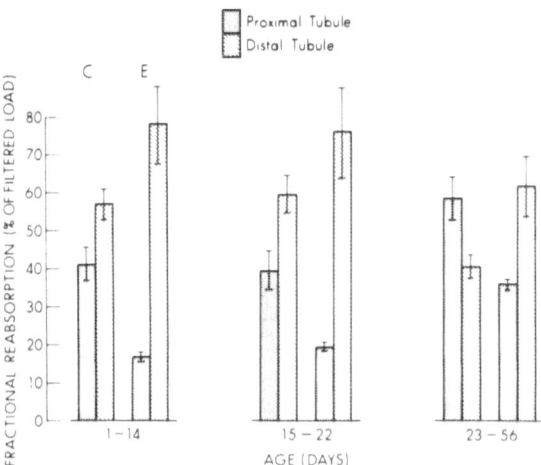

Figure 6: Functional reabsorption of sodium in the proximal and distal nephron of the guinea pig at various ages under control (C) and experimental (E) conditions (acute loading with an isoncotic albumin solution equal to 5% of body weight).

phosphate and bicarbonate, the renal handling of potassium, the electrical forces involved in the transport of these various solutes, or the handling of urea and its role in limiting the ability of the newborn to concentrate the urine, there is a considerable amount of information that can be gained in the growing animal by the use of micropuncture techniques. The description of these processes needs to be accomplished and accomplished fast if developmental renal physiology is to progress towards a new era of research, that of the intracellular mechanisms governing transport processes. This journey beyond cell boundaries is paramount not only to the understanding of physiological phenomena but also to the understanding of the disturbances that occur in disease states. It is not accidental that the two major weapons in our therapeutic armamentarium are transplantation and dialysis, both addressing the results rather than the intrinsic cause of kidney disease. The tools which permit us to cross the cell membrane barrier and thus get closer to the cellular events, are available and are being used successfully by investigators in the field of nephrology. Microvesicles of membrane fragments, electronprobe analysis, and nuclear magnetic resonance are only a few of the techniques which we will have to master and apply to the study of the developing kidney in order to obtain answers to our pressing questions.

REFERENCES:

1. Richards, A.N.: Kidney function. Harvey Lect. 16: 163, 1920.
2. Wearn, G.T. and Richards, A.N.: Observations on the composition of glomerular urine with particular reference to the problem of reabsorption in the renal tubule. Am. J. Physiol. 71: 209, 1924.
3. Allison, M.E.M., Lipsham, E.M. and Gottschalk, C.W.: Hydrostatic pressure in the rat kidney. Am. J. Physiol. 223: 975, 1972.
4. Spitzer, A. and Brandis, M.: Functional and morphological maturation of the superficial nephrons. Relationship to total kidney function. J. Clin. Invest. 53: 1, 1974.
5. Horster, M. and Valtin, H.: Postnatal development of renal function: micropuncture and clearance studies in the dog. J. Clin. Invest. 50: 779, 1971.
6. Aperia, A. and Herin, P.: Development of glomerular perfusion rate and nephron filtration rate in rats 17-60 days old. Am. J. Physiol. 228: 1319, 1975.
7. Dlouha, H.: A micropuncture study of the development of renal function in the young rat. Biol. Neonate 29: 117, 1976.
8. deRouffignac, C. and Monnens, L.: Functional and morphologic maturation of superficial and juxtamedullary nephrons in the rat. J. Physiol. (London) 262: 119, 1976.
9. Deen, W.M., Robertson, C.R. and Brenner, B.M.: A model of glomerular ultrafiltration in the rat. Am. J. Physiol. 223: 1178, 1972.
10. Spitzer, A. and Edelmann, C.M., Jr.: Maturational changes in the pressure gradients for glomerular filtration. Am. J. Physiol. 221: 1431, 1971.
11. Ichikawa, I., Maddox, D.A. and Brenner, B.M.: Maturational development of glomerular ultrafiltration in the rat. Am. J. Physiol. 236 (5): F465, 1979.
12. Tucker, B.J. and Blantz, R.C.: Factors determining superficial nephron filtration in the mature growing rat. Am. J. Physiol. 232(2): F97, 1977.
13. Goldsmith, D.I., Jodorkovsky, R.A., Kleeman, S.R., Sherwinter, J. and Spitzer, A.: Changes in glomerular capillary permeability to dextrans during development. Ped. Res. 13: 1126, 1979.
14. John, E., Goldsmith, D.I. and Spitzer, A.: Quantitative changes in canine glomerular vasculature during development: physiologic implications. Kidney Int. (in press).
15. Schoeneman, M. and Spitzer, A.: The effect of intravascular volume expansion on the proximal tubular reabsorption during development. Proc. Soc. Exp. Biol. Med. 165: 319, 1980.
16. Zink, H. and Horster, M.: Maturation of diluting capacity in loop of Henle of rat superficial nephrons. Am. J. Physiol. 233(6): F519, 1977.
17. Kleinman, L.I.: Renal sodium reabsorption during saline loading and distal blockade in newborn dog. Am. J. Physiol. 228: 1403, 1975.
18. Spitzer, A.: Renal Physiology and Functional Development. In Pediatric Kidney Disease, Vol. I, C.M. Edelmann, Jr., ed. Little, Brown and Co., Boston, 1978, p. 25.
19. Aperia, A. and Elinder, G.: Distal tubular reabsorption in the developing rat kidney. Am. J. Physiol. (in press).

THE CLINICAL FEATURES OF CHRONIC INTERSTITIAL NEPHRITIS

THOMAS G. MURRAY, M.D.

Today I would like to review with you the major clinical features of
chronic interstitial renal disease. In my opinion, the term chronic
interstitial disease should be applied to any structural renal disease
in which the renal failure is due to scarring and fibrosis of the tissues
surrounding the glomeruli rather than to direct glomerular damage. According
to this definition, any case of renal failure where the initial cortical
damage is to the interstitial tissue rather than to the glomeruli, is a
case of interstitial renal disease.

Of course, chronic interstitial renal disease is not a single entity
any more than primary glomerular disease is a single entity. Rather, it
is a final common pathway by which damage to one or more discrete areas of
the kidney is converted to diffuse renal scarring. The initial cause and
site of the damage can and does vary widely, but diffuse interstitial
scarring is a common feature. Chronic interstitial renal disease can be
initiated by papillary damage, tubular damage, or damage to the renal
vasculature as well as by direct damage to the interstitial tissue itself.

If interstitial renal disease is defined in this broad manner, there are -
in fact, only two major causes of chronic renal failure - primary glomerular
disease and interstitial renal disease. Most of the many etiologies of
chronic renal failure cause azotemia either by damaging the glomeruli
themselves or by causing scarring of the interstitial tissue in which the
glomeruli are "suspended".

Chronic interstitial renal disease is the same disease as that commonly
referred to as chronic pyelonephritis - or as chronic interstitial nephritis.
I prefer not to use these latter names because they imply something about
the etiology of this disease which is actually not known and in the case
of the term chronic pyelo, is probably wrong. Patients labeled as having
any of these diseases, all, in fact, have the same disease, as do many
patients who are said to have idiopathic renal failure. Chronic interstitial

disease is responsible for a substantial amount of all chronic renal failure. In adults, it is the cause of at least 50% of all azotemia. The proportion of childhood azotemia which is secondary to interstitial, as opposed to glomerular disease is, as far as I can tell, unknown.

An understanding of the clinical features of chronic interstitial renal disease is important for at least two reasons. The most important reason is that it allows you to arrive at the diagnosis of chronic interstitial renal disease in most patients even if renal tissue is not available. Most patients with chronic interstitial renal disease manifest clinical characteristics which, considered collectively, allow the diagnosis to be made.

Determining that a patient with renal failure has chronic interstitial renal disease is, in turn, important because in many cases this disease can be treated. The level of renal failure can be stabilized or even improved if the cause of the interstitial damage is identified and treated. Since it is virtually impossible to search in every patient for every possible cause of renal failure, it is essential that the list of potential etiologies which need to be seriously entertained, be narrowed as much as possible. Deciding - on the basis of clinical features or histologic data - that a patient has an interstitial disease permits you to narrow the list of potential etiologies from the long list of all causes of renal failure to the shorter, more managable, list of causes of interstitial disease.

A second benefit of determining that a patient has chronic interstitial renal disease is that it allows you to predict the course of the renal failure. Chronic interstitial renal disease, in general, progresses quite slowly and plans for the future therapy must take this fact into account.

The second reason that an understanding of the clinical features of chronic interstitial renal disease is important is that it allows you to anticipate some of the complications which are likely to occur in a patient with this disease. This anticipation in turn allows you to take preventative measures to avoid these complications or, failing this, to treat them before they cause significant morbidity.

The clinical features I will concentrate on today, are those which are a consequence of the chronic interstitial disease itself. These features are present in a large proportion of patients with interstitial renal disease whatever its etiology. They are the features which allow a diagnosis of chronic interstitial disease to be made and which cause predictable complications in patients with this disease. Little attention will be given to the clinical features of the individual diseases which serve as the causes of interstitial scarring since time does not permit their discussion.

Azotemia is present by definition in patients with chronic interstitial renal disease. Quite commonly, the azotemia is discovered accidentally or coincidentally. Often it is discovered during a routine examination or perhaps as part of the evaluation of a urinary tract infection or of hypertension; both of which are frequently early complications of chronic interstitial disease. In some patients, the azotemia is discovered when a second complication of the disease which is the cause of the interstitial disease develops. The passing of a kidney stone, or an attack of gout, are examples of such complications.

In a large number of patients with chronic interstitial disease, the renal failure is not noted until uremic symptoms develop. This happens much more commonly in patients with interstitial disease than it does in those with other forms of renal failure. The delayed discovery of the renal failure appears to be a consequence of the slow rate of progression and the lack of dramatic complications of this form of renal disease. It is not uncommon for ten or more years to elapse between the time renal function first declines and the time advanced renal failure develops. This slow rate of deterioration allows most patients to adapt to the presence of azotemia without a noticeable change in their state-of-well-being. Without a specific change in the way they feel, the patients do not seek medical assistance. In addition, no dramatic manifestations of the renal disease develop to give notice of its presence. Complications such as the nephrotic syndrome, gross hematuria, or malignant hypertension are not commonly seen in patients with chronic interstitial renal disease.

This leads us to the second category of features of chronic interstitial disease which are helpful in establishing its presence. Patients with interstitial disease do not have any of the so-called "pathognomonic" features of primary glomerular disease. They do not have red blood cell casts and they seldom have a very active urine sediment. In addition, they generally do not have heavy proteinuria and rarely, if ever, have the nephrotic syndrome.

Almost all patients with chronic interstitial disease have proteinuria. In the vast majority of patients, the level of protein excretion is less than

2.0 grams per day and rarely, if ever, is it more than 3.5 grams per day unless it is acutely increased by a superimposed process; such as accelerated hypertension or severe congestive heart failure. The protein which is excreted is principly albumin which suggests that a "glomerular" leak is its principal cause. The pathogenesis of the glomerular leak of protein is unclear.

If nephrotic range proteinuria co-exits with clinical features which suggest that an interstitial disease is present, the patient probably has either; one of the forms of primary glomerular disease which regularly has has a major amount of associated interstitial damage(for example, focal glomerular sclerosis or membrano-proliferative glomerulonephritis), or has an interstitial disease which has been complicated by the development of a glomerular disease. Reflux nephropathy is the major cause of this latter combination.

Evidence of interstitial inflammation and/or interstitial scarring is also useful in establishing the presence of chronic interstitial disease. Evidence of active interstitial inflammation would, if it were present, be found in the urinalysis. Only rarely is such evidence found in patients with chronic interstitial disease. This apparently reflects the fact that much of the active renal inflammation which was initially present, has by the time the renal disease is discovered, been replaced by interstitial fibrosis and scarring. The urinalysis in chronic interstitial renal disease is often notable only for its benignity. A moderate amount of sterine pyuria is a frequent finding and microscopic hematuria is often present. Only rarely are cellular casts present. Superimposed acute urinary tract disease is, of course, quite common in patients with chronic interstitial disease and when present, may dramatically change the urinalysis. Occasionally, etiologic information can be gleaned from the urinalysis - as well - most often, if calcium, uric acid, or cysteine cyrstals are seen.

Signs of interstitial scarring are present far more often than are signs of interstitial inflammation. Evidence of scarring is obtained from radio-logic examination of the kidneys. In most patients with chronic interstitial renal disease, the kidneys are small. In some, they are already markedly shrunken when the level of azotemia is only modest. Such dramatic shrinkage is highly suggestive that an interstitial disease is responsible for the azotemia, but it is relatively uncommon. More commonly, the kidneys, although small are no smaller than those which might be seen in primary

glomerular disease. The intravenous pyelogram is more often helpful.
Calyceal abnormalities(such as clubbing or blunting), and cortical scars
are commonly present in patients with chronic interstitial disease but are
not seen in cases of primary glomerular disease. Thus, when such findings
are present, they are very helpful diagnostically. Unfortunately, not all
patients with interstitial disease have these abnormalities. Information
concerning the etiology of the interstitial disease may also be obtained
from the intravenous pyelogram. For example, hydronephrosis, or renal
calcification may be seen.

The next group of clinical features we will discuss are also useful in
determining whether a patient with azotemia has chronic interstitial renal
disease. They are grouped together because they may share a common pathophysiologic basis - they may each develop as a consequence of a deficiency
of a hormone produced in the kidney - probably in the renal interstitium.
One explanation for the earlier onset and/or the increased severity of these
clinical complications in patients with interstitial renal disease would be
that the hormonal deficiency develops earlier in a disease which damages
the interstitium before it damages the glomeruli. There is at least one
equally tenable explanation for the increased importance of these complications
in patients with interstitial disease. It is possible that the long duration
of the period of azotemia in the typical patient with chronic interstitial
disease increases the chance that any given complication of chronic renal
failure will eventually occur or become severe enough to cause the patient
difficulty. In this case, the hormonal deficiency would not have to be
quantitatively more severe in interstitial disease than in glomerular disease,
it would simply be present for a longer period of time.

Anemia is an almost universal complication of chronic renal failure and
a decreased production of erythropoietin is its principal cause. There is
a widely held clinical opinion that patients with chronic interstitial disease
have a more severe degree of anemia at any given level of azotemia than do
patients with glomerular disease. There does not appear to be any data
supporting this contention; although I share the feeling that it is true.
There are no studies which compare the erythropoietin levels of patients
with interstitial disease to those of patients with a similar degree of
glomerular disease.

Complications related to disordered calcium metabolism are, on the other
hand, clearly more common and often more severe in patients with chronic

interstitial disease than they are in patients with other types of chronic
renal failure. Symptomatic renal osteodystrophy, severe hypocalcemia, and
non-skeletal manifestations of hyperparathyroidism or of Vitamin D deficiency
all occur much more commonly, and often develop much earlier in patients with
interstitial disease. At some point in the course of chronic renal failure
of any cause, the production of 1,25 dihydroxy vitamin D is decreased as a
result of a decrease in the activity of the enzyme responsible for 1 hydroxylation of 25 hydroxy Vitamin D. It has not been demonstrated that 1,25
dihydroxy Vitamin D production is decreased earlier, or to a greater degree,
in chronic interstitial renal disease, although it is logical to assume that
this might be the case. It is also conceivable that the increased frequency
of complications related to abnormal calcium homeostasis in patients with
chronic interstitial disease is simply a consequence of the prolonged duration
of their renal failure. Abnormalities of calcium metabolism which were
quantitatively the same in interstitial disease as in other forms of renal
failure could, as a result of their prolonged presence, result in more severe
consequences.

Hypertension is a common complication of chronic interstitial disease and
unlike the hypertension that occurs in primary glomerular disease, it is
usually not a consequence of subtle volume expansion. Whether it is caused
by a decrease in the production of an,as yet,unidentified vasodepressive
hormone is completely unknown.

Hyperkalemia normally does not complicate chronic renal failure until
very severe - essentially end-stage renal failure is present. In a small
percentage of patients with chronic interstitial disease, hyperkalemia which
is not due to severe renal failure occurs. In the majority of these cases,
the cause of the hyperkalemia is a decreased production of renin. The
resulting syndrome - hyporeninemic hyopaldosteronism - will be discussed
below.

A final set of clinical features which can aid in the diagnosis of chronic
interstitial renal disease, are those which are a consequence of abnormal
tubular function. All patients with chronic renal disease - whatever its
cause - have abnormalities of tubular function. In patients with chronic
interstitial disease, these abnormalities develop earlier and are more
severe than they are in patients with primary glomerular disease. The
increased severity of the tubular abnormalities, combined with the longer
period of time they are present, make it much more likely that they will

cause clinical complications in patients with interstitial disease than in those with other types of renal failure.

For example, although an inability to lower the urinary excretion of sodium in response to decreased sodium intake or volume depletion complicates all forms of chronic renal failure, it is more pronounced in cases of chronic interstitial disease. As a consequence, volume depletion and its attendant clinical complications occur much more commonly in patients with interstitial disease.

Urinary sodium losses can be so high in chronic interstitial disease that volume depletion develops despite the ingestion of a normal or even a high sodium intake. Fortunately, such severe salt wasting is a rare complication of chronic interstitial disease - it occurs in only a small proportion of patients with medullary cystic disease or obstructive nephropathy. The typical patient with interstitial disease can maintain a normal extracellular fluid volume as long as sodium intake is normal. If the intake of sodium is decreased, or if the non-renal losses of sodium containing fluid is increased, however, volume depletion develops as a consequence of continued urinary sodium losses. Because this defect in sodium conservation is present over a prolonged period of time in patients with interstitial disease, volume depletion is likely to be a clinical problem on one or more occasions in such patients.

An inability to conserve water as a result of a defect in urinary concentrating ability is also a feature of all forms of chronic renal failure. The defect in urinary concentrating ability develops earlier and is more severe in patients with chronic interstitial disease. A small number of patients with interstitial disease have frank nephrogenic diabetes insipidus; most, however, simply cannot concentrate their urine much above isotonic levels. Polyuria is, therefore, a common clinical feature of chronic interstitial disease.

A defect in the excretion of hydrogen ions also develops earlier in patients with chronic interstitial disease than it does in those with other forms of renal failure. The decreased ability to excrete the hydrogen ions is in most cases, a consequence of a decreased production and excretion of ammonia. In the face of decreased ammonia excretion, the daily load of acid cannot be excreted despite the presence of a low urine pH. Since the defect in hydrogen ion excretion develops before the glomerular filtration rate has fallen enough to cause the retention of organic anions, a hyperchloremic acidosis rather than an anion gap acidosis develops initially. Later as the GFR falls further, the hyperchloremic acidosis is replaced by the anion gap acidosis which is typical of advanced renal failure of any cause. Because hyperchloremic acidosis is much more common in chronic interstitial disease than it is in primary glomerular disease, its presence can aid in diagnosis of interstitial disease.

It should be mentioned that a small proportion of cases of chronic interstitial disease are complicated by the development of classical renal tubular acidosis and that patients with renal tubular acidosis who develop secondary renal failure develop an interstitial renal disease.

As mentioned previously, hyperkalemia usually does not complicate the course of renal disease until severe - essentially end-stage renal failure is present. The majority of patients with chronic interstitial renal disease are indistinguishable from those with renal failure of any other type in this regard - that is they do not develop early hyperkalemia. Some cases of chronic interstitial disease are, however, complicated by hyperkalemia which is not explained by the level of renal insufficiency. In these cases, hyperkalemia either occurs spontaneously, or more commonly, develops in response to a sudden increase in the load of potassium which must be excreted. The pathophysiologic explanation of the hyperkalemia in these patients is either hyporeninemic - hypoaldosteronism or tubular unresponsiveness to the action of aldosterone.

Hyporeninemic hypoaldosteronism is responsible for the majority of causes of early hyperkalemia. This syndrome is characterized by the presence of low levels of renin which cannot be increased by normal manuevers which stimulate its release. Aldosterone levels are low secondary to the low renin levels and potassium excretion is low because of the low aldosterone levels. This syndrome appears to occur more commonly in some types of chronic interstitial disease than in others. The majority of the reported cases have had diabetes mellitus; and a number have had lead, uric acid, or analgesic nephropathy.

Tubular unresponsiveness to aldosterone is the other cause of early hyperkalemia. It too occurs only in patients with chronic interstitial renal disease. Thus far, it has only been convincibly demonstrated in transplant rejection, lupus interstitial renal disease, and sickle cell nephropathy. In this syndrome, aldosterone levels are high, but potassium excretion is low.

Those are the clinical features of chronic interstitial renal disease. Ascertaining whether each is present or absent in a patient with chronic renal failure will allow you to determine, in most cases, whether an interstitial disease is responsible for the azotemia.

If the patient has an interstitial disease, the next step is to determine its etiology. Although there are many causes of chronic interstitial renal disease, the majority of causes are secondary to one of a fairly small number of causes. Anatomic abnormalities - including reflux - are responsible for the vast majority of cases. This is especially true in children and young adults. Prolonged analgesic use and nephrosclerosis are important causes of interstitial renal disease in the adult, but probably uncommon causes in children. The deposition of calcium salts, uric acid, or cysteine in the tubules and interstitium can lead to chronic interstitial scarring. The relationship of stone forming disease and sickle cell disease to chronic interstitial disease is well-known to all of you.

Medullary cystic disease, although given a name of its own, actually causes renal failure through a process of interstitial scarring. Heavy metal toxicity can cause chronic interstitial disease; the most common example of this type of disease is lead nephropathy. Radiation nephropathy has fortunately become relatively rare due to the use of new shielding techniques. It is still a problem in some individuals who receive large doses of radiation to areas close to the kidneys. The best examples of immunologically induced interstitial disease are acute interstitial nephritis and transplant rejection. Immunologic events are, however, almost certainly involved at some stage in the pathogenesis of all types of chronic interstitial disease.

As I'm sure most of you are aware, the role of bacterial infection in the pathogenesis of chronic renal failure is unsettled. A thorough discussion of the controversy surrounding this issue is certainly beyond the scope of this presentation. It is sufficient to say that bacterial infection alone is rarely, if ever, the cause of renal failure. In every case of interstitial renal disease, even if infection is present, other possible causes of the renal failure should be thoroughly investigated.

The cause of some cases of interstitial disease remain obscure despite an exhaustive search. Perhaps 5% of cases must currently be considered idiopathic.

Once the etiology of the interstitial disease has been identified, it should, if possible, be removed or treated. The level of renal failure can, in many patients, be stabilized or in some, improved by treatment of the cause. If these efforts are not successful, one must be content with treating the patient as his/her renal failure progresses. In this task, knowledge that the patient has an interstitial disease permits you to predict that certain complications are likely to occur and to be alert to their development. Recurrent volume depletion, long-standing metabolic acidosis, and renal osteodystrophy are three types of complications whose effects on the patient can be minimized by proper treatment.

Thus, to offer the best diagnostic and therapeutic help to the patient with azotemia, it is necessary to be aware of the clinical features of interstitial renal disease.

PATHOLOGY OF INTERSTITIAL NEPHRITIS

ELFENBEIN, I. BRUCE

In this review will be presented a working definition of the pathologic changes that constitute interstitial nephritis, a classification of morphologic types, descriptions of the histologic features of the types, a discussion of the various causes of interstitial nephritis and some discussion of the problems in the morphologic diagnosis of interstitial nephritis.

Why is there a need to develop a working definition of "interstitial nephritis"? Shouldn't "interstitial nephritis" be considered to be "inflammation in the interstitium of the kidney"? The first table shows that inflammation within the interstitium of the kidney is found to accompany most primary vascular diseases and most glomerular diseases. Inflammatory reactions in the interstitium are also a prominent morphologic component of the changes observed in acute renal failure be it either true morphologic "acute tubular necrosis" or the more common "tubulo-interstitial nephropathy" without obvious tubular cell death. It would seem, therefore, that the simple presence of inflammatory cell exudates and edema and/or fibrosis in the renal interstitium does not define a morphologic condition that should be called interstitial nephritis.

Table 1. Non-Interstitial Diseases in Which Interstitial Inflammation May Be a Major Component

VASCULAR DISEASES
Ischemic
Vasculitides
Infarcts
GLOMERULAR DISEASES
Primary Glomerulonephritides
Systemic Glomerulonephritides

Table 1. Non-Interstitial Diseases in Which Interstitial Inflammation
May Be a Major Component (continued)

ACUTE RENAL FAILURE
Acute Tubular Necrosis (with tubular cell necrosis)
Tubulo-interstitial Nephropathy (ATN without tubular cell necrosis)

Our working definition of interstitial nephritis is two-fold: First, there is a range of tubular damage and interstitial inflammatory cell infiltrates with either edema or fibrosis or both; second, there is relative or absolute preservation of the morphologic integrity of the glomeruli and blood vessels. As a corollary, the amount of tubular and interstitial damage must be greater than the glomerular and vascular damage in order to establish the diagnosis of interstitial nephritis. There is an overlap at one end of the spectrum between the morphologic changes of acute renal failure (tubulo-interstitial nephropathy) and those of acute interstitial nephritis.

Morphologically, interstitial nephritis can be classified in each of two ways. The anatomic distribution of lesions forms the basis for the first classification. Lesions can be characterized as either diffuse or widespread vs. localized. See Table 2. The second basis of classification is on the apparent age of the lesions: i.e., acute vs. chronic vs. mixed forms.

Table 2. Anatomic Classification of Interstitial Nephritis

DIFFUSE OR WIDESPREAD	LOCALIZED
1. Uniform or widespread and repetitive lesions	1. Localized lesions (often at renal poles) with large zones of spared parenchyma
2. Infiltrates and/or fibrosis without destroying gross architecture	2. Infiltrates and/or fibrosis with distortion of gross architecture

In localized forms of interstitial nephritis one or more different regions of a kidney may be involved. This is often associated with distortion of the architectural pattern of the involved region, particularly in the chronic type of localized interstitial nephritis. The vast majority of cases of localized interstitial nephritis are due either to infection or changes secondary to vesicoureteral reflux with or without infection. Because of sampling error it is possible that representative lesions in the localized forms of interstitial nephritis may not be present in biopsy specimens.

The diffuse or widespread type of interstitial nephritis is characterized by either relatively uniform involvement of the cortex and adjacent medulla or repetitive involvement of similar zones throughout the entire kidney. An example of the latter is the perivenous localization of inflammatory cell reaction in mild forms of rejection reaction. Generally, the uniform or repetitive pattern of involvement is not associated with distortions of the architectural pattern of the kidney.

The apparent age of interstitial lesions may be classified into acute vs. chronic types. The most significant difference between these two types is the presence of interstitial fibrosis in the chronic type and interstitial edema without fibrosis in the acute type. Table 3 summarizes the cellular characteristics of the inflammatory cell reactions. The heterogenous nature of the inflammatory cellular reaction seen in the acute type may be determined either by the etiology of the disease or by the timing of the biopsy in relation to the biology of the disease. Neutrophils and eosinophils will predominate very early in the acute type. Lymphocytes and plasma cells will predominate when cell mediated immune reactions are the mechanism and also in the later phases of the acute reaction. Neutrophils, especially, and also eosinophils will not be present in chronic interstitial nephritis. Classification into acute or chronic types has major prognostic significance. Generally, the loss of renal function that results from chronic interstitial nephritis cannot be reversed even if the cause is removed. The best that can be expected is stabilization of function at approximately the level of loss at diagnosis. On the other hand, in acute interstitial nephritis the loss of function is potentially totally reversible.

Table 3. Pathology of Interstitial Nephritis

ACUTE INTERSTITIUM	CHRONIC INTERSTITIUM
1. Edema	1. Fibrosis
2. Inflammatory infiltrates	2. Inflammatory infiltrates
a. Neutrophils	a. Lymphocytes
b. Eosinophils	b. Plasma cells
c. Lymphocytes	c. Macrophages
d. Plasma cells	
e. Macrophages	
TUBULES	TUBULES
1. Degeneration	1. Atrophy
2. Necrosis	2. Disappearance
GLOMERULI	GLOMERULI
1. No change	1. Relative preservation
2. Periglomerular inflammation	2. Periglomerular fibrosis
	3. Atrophy and hyalinization
BLOOD VESSELS	BLOOD VESSELS
1. No change	1. Probable arteriosclerotic changes

THE ETIOLOGIES OF INTERSTITIAL NEPHRITIS

There are a wide variety of causes of interstitial nephritis. Table 4 attempts to create an outline of the various causes and to place them in the context of the gross morphology: i.e., diffuse or widespread vs. localized interstitial nephritis. Of necessity radiation nephritis and obstructive uropathy may appear under both headings. Whether radiation nephritis is diffuse or localized depends on whether or not part or all of the kidneys are exposed to the ionizing radiation. Obstructive uropathy may be bilateral and relatively equal in severity or unilateral and even segmentally localized.

Table 4. Causes of Interstitial Nephritis

DIFFUSE OR WIDESPREAD	LOCALIZED
1. TOXIC direct tubular toxins	INFECTION
2. HYPERSENSITIVITY reactions to drugs	REFLUX NEPHROPATHY with or without infection
3. METABOLIC hypercalcemia, hypokalemia, gout	RADIATION
4. IMMUNOLOGIC rejection, SLE	OBSTRUCTIVE
5. ENVIRONMENTAL Balkan nephropathy	NEOPLASMS direct infiltration vascular involvement
6. HEREDITARY Alport's, medullary cystic disease, medullary sponge kidney	
7. OBSTRUCTIVE	
8. RADIATION	

In many situations a careful history and physical examination will elicit the cause of the interstitial nephritis. Careful correlation of history, physical examination and laboratory studies is of great importance because most of the morphologic findings of interstitial nephritis are non-specific. Furthermore, in order to make some anatomic diagnoses such as urate nephropathy, the diagnosis must be suspected in advance and tissue must be fixed in absolute alcohol rather than the usual fixatives. On the other hand, some diseases may be diagnosed or suggested by specific histopathologic features. Examples of the latter include: massive oxalate crystal deposition (crystals polarize) in oxalate nephropathy; calcified casts and calcified tubular cells and tubular basement membranes in hypercalcemic nephropathy; large clear vacuoles in proximal and occasionally distal tubular cells in hypokalemic nephropathy; eosinophilic intranuclear inclusions in tubule cells in lead nephropathy; large intranuclear inclusions with halos in cytomegalic virus infection; multinucleation of glomerular epithelial cells and peculiar inclusion bodies in cystinosis; tophi with urate crystals and giant cell reaction in gout; specific neoplastic infiltrates particularly of leukemias and lymphoproliferative diseases; interstitial foam cells in association with irregular glomerular lesions histologically and lamellation of GBM by

electron microscopy in Alport's hereditary nephritis; non-caseating granu-
lomas in the active phase of sarcoidosis; specific membranous inclusions in
tubular cells in toxic reactions to the aminoglycoside antibiotics; ectasia
of medullary collecting ducts in medullary sponge kidney; cysts in lower
cortex and upper medulla with cortical atrophy in medullary cystic disease;
marked glomerular hypertrophy in oligomeganephronia; yellow autofluorescence
of renal tubules in tetracycline toxicity.

In some cases there may be a differential diagnosis between "acute
tubular necrosis" and hepatorenal syndrome. Most patients with hepatorenal
syndrome, but not those with ATN, have hypertrophy of the juxtaglomerular
apparatus. They also have more calcium casts and are more likely to have
bile stained oxalate crystals.

There has been a rising incidence of patients with one primary renal
disease acquiring a superimposed interstitial nephritis. In most instances
the interstitial nephritis is drug related. Many of the patients biopsied
for steroid-dependent lipoid nephrosis and who have also received Lasix
have shown scattered tubular calcifications with an adjacent low grade interstitial inflammatory cell reaction. This may be due to the hypercalcuric
effects of the Lasix. This can cause confusion with the diagnosis of focal
segmental sclerosis by causing tubular atrophy. A smaller group of patients
with nephrotic syndrome and treatment with both lasix and one of the synthetic penicillins have developed overt acute renal insufficiency and even
acute renal failure. Biopsies of these patients have shown a non-specific
diffuse interstitial nephritis superimposed on the underlying glomerular
disease.

In transplanted patients the problem of the cause of renal insufficiency
will arise with increasing frequency. Recently, one such patient treated
with a synthetic penicillin, lasix, and suspected of having cytomegalic
virus infection or enhancement of rejection was biopsied. In these instances if specific findings such as intranuclear viral inclusions cannot
be demonstrated, a specific diagnosis of the cause of the interstitial
nephritis cannot be made and the best solution is to remove all potentially
causative agents and follow the patient closely. The most obvious problem
in transplanted patients may be the differential diagnosis between rejection and "acute tubular necrosis". If acute tubulo-interstitial nephropathy is the cause, it will be manifested morphologically by dilatation of

cortical tubules, flattening of the tubular epithelium, and a variety of tubular casts without inflammatory cells. Rejection is characterized by interstitial inflammation, particularly of plasma cells, lymphocytes, and immunoblasts, tubular cell swelling with or without infiltration by lymphocytes. Both conditions will have interstitial edema.

Interstitial inflammation may be a prominent feature in the kidney biopsies of some patients with systemic lupus erythematosus. Rarely, it has been the major feature. Most commonly the interstitial inflammation in SLE is associated with the more severe forms of glomerular injury with either or both diffuse proliferative glomerular lesions or crescents. In these cases the predominant cell type is the plasma cells. Many of these cases the immunofluorescence will also show granular IgG deposits along the tubular basement membranes. If interstitial inflammation is a prominent histologic feature in SLE patients with membranous glomerulonephritis, a superimposed, non-SLE related, condition should be suspected.

In summary, a working definition of interstitial nephritis has been presented: interstitial inflammation and/or fibrosis and tubular damage with relative preservation of glomeruli and blood vessels. It has been divided into diffuse/widespread or localized forms; and into acute or chronic forms (with resultant prognostic significance). The histologic characteristics have been described. In most instances the histology of interstitial nephritis is not specific for its etiology. A partial list of discriminating features to diagnose specific etiologies has been given. Interstitial nephritis has been recognized as being superimposed on other underlying renal diseases. It is likely in the future with newer therapeutic modalities that this will become a greater problem in the diagnosis and treatment of patients with renal disease.

HENOCH-SCHÖNLEIN PURPURA : A PROBLEM OR NOT?

R. H. R. WHITE

I am not sure what sort of response the Chairman of this Symposium expected to the question posed in the title which he gave me; the short answer is 'yes and no'! It is well recognised that the only significant mortality associated with Henoch-Schönlein (HS) purpura today is the outcome of serious renal involvement; I propose to review some of recently published data concerning the renal prognosis, as well as presenting some new findings.

Contributions to the literature during the past decade give the impression that the condition is more common in Europe and Japan than in America, and this is also reflected by the numbers of patients entered into a therapeutic trial conducted by the International Study of Kidney Disease in Children (ISKDC) by January, 1980 (Table 1).

Table 1. Geographical distribution of HS Nephritis (ISKDC, January, 1980)

Zone	Centres	Patients
United Kingdom	3	35
Rest of Europe	4	18
North America	6	20
Mexico	1	1

The incidence of renal involvement in HSP is difficult to assess; it depends on the population studied and the criteria used to define renal involvement. Some recent studies (1-3) give a range of 41-60.5% renal involvement using acceptable criteria. However, it is pertinent that Greifer et al. (4) and Meadow et al. (5) independently observed mild focal glomerulonephritis in biopsy specimens obtained from children without clinical evidence of nephritis, so the true incidence may be somewhat higher.

There is a small but significant death rate from renal failure; 3-7.7% of children entering dialysis programmes in Europe (6,7) were suffering from HSP. Counahan et al. (8) reported that 14% of a group of 88 children followed up for a mean of 10 years had died or were in chronic renal failure (CRF), while a further 10% had active disease. However, their patients were mostly selected on the basis of comparatively severe illness clinically, and the mortality rate is an over-estimate. In a large Japanese series (3), 123 (60.6%) out of 203 children with HSP showed renal involvement and the estimated death rate of the latter (allowing for 10 children lost to follow-up) was 8.9%.

Prediction of the outcome has been the focus of a good deal of attention in the past decade. Good prognostic criteria are needed because treatment with cytotoxic drugs is, at best, of dubious value (5,7,8), and it is therefore desirable to elaborate a means of detecting those patients who are most greatly at risk, and in whom exposure to the potential hazards of these drugs is justified. For several years the ISKDC has been conducting a controlled trial in which a 6 weeks' course of cyclophosphamide is compared with supportive treatment only. However, the number of patients who have satisfied the trial criteria and have completed 2 years' follow-up is yet too small to yield meaningful results.

A clinical presentation with a mixed nephritic-nephrotic pattern has for many years been recognised as denoting a poor prognosis (5,7,8), and this is further substantiated in a new study recently completed at the Birmingham Children's Hospital by Drs. Yoshikawa, Cameron and myself (9). Even so, 47-54% of these patients were either in complete remission or had only minor urinary abnormalities an average of 6-10 years after onset (9,8). Counahan et al. (8) extended the minimum observation period of the patients originally reported by Meadow et al. (5) from 2 to 6½ years and noted that the proportion of patients who had either died, were in CRF, or showed active disease had increased from 20-24%. A disturbing feature was that 4 children with a non-nephritic clinical presentation were doing badly; one had died, one was on regular dialysis and two were in early CRF. Thus the clinical presentation is not a very good discriminator of prognosis.

The involvement of a high percentage of glomeruli with epithelial

104

crescents is claimed by a number of authors (2,7,8,9) to denote a bad prognosis. However, Counahan et al. (8) drew attention to the problems of defining crescents and quantitating them with reasonable accuracy. The figure illustrates how histological sections at different levels in individual glomeruli may under- or overestimate both the size of crescents and the number of glomeruli affected. Even when allowance is made for this, it should be realised that the number of patients with more than 75% of affected glomeruli is small:- 6% (8), 11% (9) and 21% (7) in three recent series in which patients were already selected for biopsy because of their clinical severity. The group of patients in whom prognostication is particularly hazardous are those with 50-75% crescentic glomeruli, of whom approximately 60% appear to do well (8,9).

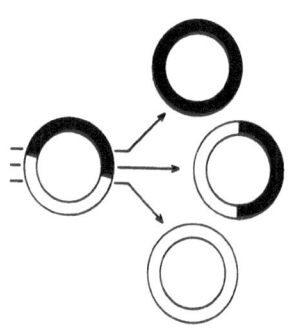

EPITHELIAL CRESCENTS
Distribution according to level of section

The immunofluorescence pattern of HS nephritis is predominantly diffuse mesangial IgA, often with lesser deposits of other immunoglobulins and complement components, especially C3. Capillary wall deposits are sometimes observed, especially in those cases with extensive crescent formation (7).

A number of workers have reported the electron microscopic (EM) changes in HS nephritis but with little or no comment on their prognostic significance (10). Electron-dense deposits are predominantly mesangial but are also seen in subendothelial and subepithelial locations, the latter somewhat less frequently (7,9,11-14). Our own data, which has been submitted elsewhere for publication in detail (9), shows some interesting correlations between certain ultrastructural abnormalities and the prognosis. After a mean observation period of 6 years the clinical status of each patient was classified according to the system used by Counahan et al. (8):

State A - Normal: physical examination (including blood pressure), urine and GFR all normal;
State B - Minor urinary abnormalities: normal physical examination and GFR, with microscopic haematuria or proteinuria < 40 mg/h/m^2 (< 1.0 g/24h);
State C - Active renal disease: proteinuria > 40 mg/h/m^2 (> 1 g/24h) or hypertension (diastolic BP persistently > 90 mmHg) or both, with GFR > 60 ml/min/1.73m^2.

State D - Renal insufficiency: active renal disease but with GFR
< 60 ml/min/1.73m² (including dialysis and transplantation) or
deceased.

Table 2 shows the results in 50 children with adequate EM tissue
available for examination. It can be seen that all 6 children in state D
and 3 out of 5 in state C showed subepithelial deposits associated with

Table 2. relationship between location of deposits on EM and outcome (9).

		Follow-up status			
Location of deposits	n	A	B	C	D
None	1		1		
Mesangial only	16	9	6	1	
Mesangial + subendothelial	17	12	4	1	
Mesangial + subepithelial	1	1			
All 3 locations	15	3	3	3	6

subendothelial and mesangial deposits. Heaton et al. (14) noted that
subepithelial deposits were generally seen where the light microscopy
changes were more severe, although they did not discuss the relationship
to outcome.

Finally - and surprisingly - we observed clusters of 'lead shot'
microparticles in the lamina densa or mesangial matrix in 16 out of 35 EM
specimens examined; they were present in 9 out of 10 children in states
C and D at follow-up (Table 3). These are probably paracrystalline

Table 3. Prognostic significance of 'lead shot' microparticles (9).

'Lead shot'		Follow-up status			
microparticles	n	A	B	C	D
Present	16	5	2	4	5
Absent	19	7	11	1	

structures of protein origin, perhaps resulting from glomerular injury
or immune complex deposition (15), and we have observed them in a variety
of other nephropathies.

In summary, more than half of all children suffering from HSP will
have renal involvement and, although up to half of these will exhibit a

seemingly severe clinical presentation, less than 10% of affected children
will have their lives threatened. Predicting this last group is of
considerable importance because there is little evidence that treatment
favourably influences the outcome in the remainder. The clinical presentatic
alone is a poor discriminator of outcome although an acute nephritic onset
is an indication for renal biopsy. In order to increase the precision of
prognostication, both light and electronmicroscopy should be performed.

REFERENCES

1. Hurley, R.M. & Drummond, K.N. Anaphylactoid purpura nephritis:
   clinicopathological correlations. J. Pediat., 81: 904, 1972.
2. Koskimies, O., Rapola, J., Savilahti, E. & Vilska, J. Renal involvement:
   Schönlein-Henoch purpura. Acta. Paediatr. Scand., 63: 357, 1974.
3. Kobayashi, O., Wada, H., Okawa, K. & Takeyama, I. Schönlein-Henoch's
   syndrome in children. In Contr. Nephrol., vol. 4, (ed. G.M. Berlyne
   & S. Giavonetti); Karger, Basel, 1977, p48.
4. Greifer, I., Bernstein, J., Kikkawa, Y. & Edelmann, C. Histologic
   evidence of nephritis in patients with Schönlein-Henoch syndrome
   without clinical evidence of renal disease. Abstract, 3rd International
   Congress of Nephrology, Washington, 1966, p.203.
5. Meadow, S.R., Glasgow, E.F., White, R.H.R., Moncrieff, M.W.,
   Cameron, J.S. & Ogg, C.S. Schönlein-Henoch nephritis. Quart. J.
   Med., 41: 241, 1972.
6. Chantler, C., Donckerwolcke, R.A., Brunner, F.P., Brynger, H.A.O.,
   Gurland, H.G., Hathway, R.A., Jacobs, C., Selwood, N.H. & Wing, A.J.
   Combined report on regular dialysis and transplantation of children in
   Europe, 1977. In Proc. E.D.T.A. (ed. B.H.B. Robinson & J.B. Hawkins);
   Pitman, London, p.77.
7. Levy, M., Broyer, M., Arsan, A., Levy-Bentolila, D. & Habib, R.
   Anaphylactoid purpura nephritis in childhood: natural history and
   immunopathology. Adv. Nephrol., 6: 183, 1976.
8. Counahan, R., Winterborn, M.H., White, R.H.R., Heaton, J.M.,
   Meadow, S.R., Bluett, N.H., Swetschin, H., Cameron, J.S. & Chantler, C.
   Prognosis of Henoch-Schönlein nephritis in children. Brit. med. J.,
   2: 11, 1977.
9. Yoshikawa, N., White, R.H.R. & Cameron, A.H. Prognostic significance
   of the glomerular changes in Henoch-Schönlein nephritis. Submitted to
   Clinical Nephrology, 1980.
10. Meadow, S.R. The prognosis of Henoch-Schönlein nephritis. Clin.
    Nephrol., 9: 87, 1978.
11. Urizar, R.E., Michael, A., Sisson, S. & Vernier, R.L. Anaphylactoid
    purpura: II. Immunofluorescence and electron microscopic studies of
    the glomerular lesions. Lab. Invest. 19: 437, 1968.
12. Brun, C., Bryld, C., Fenger, L. & Jorgensen, F. Glomerular lesions
    in adults with the Schönlein-Henoch syndrome. Acta Pathol. Microbiol.
    Scand., 7: 569, 1971.
13. Striker, G.E., Quadracci, L.J., Larter, W., Hickman, R.O., Kelly, M.R.
    & Schaller, J. The nephritis of Henoch-Schönlein purpura. In
    Glomerulonephritis (ed. P. Kincaid-Smith, T.H. Mathew & E.L. Becker);
    Wiley, New York, 1973, p.1105.

14. Heaton, J.M., Turner, D.R. & Cameron, J.S. Localization of glomerular deposits' in Henoch-Schönlein nephritis. Histopathology, 1: 93, 1977.
15. Cameron, A.H. & Standring, D. Ultrastructure of unusual protein aggregates on the glomerular basement membrane. Abstract, Fourth International Symposium of Pediatric Nephrology, Helsinki, 1977, p.96.

MEMBRANOPROLIFERATIVE GLOMERULONEPHRITIS: CLASSIFICATION AND TREATMENT

CLARK D. WEST, M.D.

1. INTRODUCTION

Considerable experience has been gained with membranoproliferative glomerulonephritis since it was first recognized in 1965 (1). It has been shown to consist of three diseases which have many factors in common but differ in glomerular morphology at the ultrastructural level. Little is known about differences in their pathogenesis.

The following discusses the distinguishing features of these three diseases, then indicates what is known of their pathogenesis and finally, discusses the results of treatment.

2. CLASSIFICATION

The three diseases do not differ clinically. Presentation may be by the chance finding of proteinuria and hematuria or by advent of asymptomatic gross hematuria, of a nephrotic syndrome or of an acute nephritic syndrome. In many, the acute symptoms, if present, subside and for long periods the patients exhibit only microhematuria and proteinuria and have normal renal function. Eventually, however, function deteriorates and end-stage disease is usually preceded by 18 to 24 months of increasing azotemia, nephrotic syndrome and hypertension.

The distinguishing features of these three diseases lie in their glomerular morphology and, as will be noted later, in the response of glomerular morphology to treatment. Differences in morphology are summarized in Table 1. Type I, which is most frequently encountered, has subendothelial and mesangial deposits and the basement membrane is intact. The mesangial deposits seem to be capable of producing a most severe inflammatory reaction in that the glomerulus is extremely proliferative, resulting in marked mesangial interposition, great thickening of the capillary walls, and glomerular enlargement.

Table 1. Frequency and distinguishing features of glomerular
morphology in the three types of MPGN

	Incidence	Glomerular deposits	Basement membrane	Mesangial cellularity
Type I	50%	Subendothelial Mesangial	Intact	++++
Type II	20%	Mesangial Subepithelial occasionally	Intramembr. "deposit"	+ - ++
Type III	30%	Subendothelial Subepithelial Mesangial	Disrupted, frayed, replicated	+ - +++

Type II is characterized by mesangial and occasionally subepithelial
deposits and by densification of the lamina densa of the glomerular
basement membrane, giving the appearance of an intramembranous deposit.
This densification is responsible for the designation "dense deposit
disease". The densification does not appear to do harm; the glomeruli of
renal transplants in patients with this disease frequently develop the
same basement membrane abnormality but often have no signs of glomerulonephritis (2). The dense basement membrane may represent a unique
degenerative change; we have seen a similar abnormality in the basement
membranes of patients with idiopathic rapidly progressive glomerulonephritis (3). The mesangial deposits do not produce as severe an inflammatory reaction as they do in Type I and the glomerulus is less proliferative than in Type I.

Among the questions that arise concerning this disease are the origin
of the basement membrane abnormality, the reasons for the association of
the disease with partial lipodystrophy and for the frequent presence of
C3 nephritic factor. The C3 nephritic factor is found occasionally also
in patients with Type I, with lupus and with post-streptococcal
glomerulonephritis, but is most frequent in Type II. We have not found
it in any of 17 patients with Type III.

Type III MPGN is noteworthy for the markedly altered glomerular
basement membrane which is best appreciated in silver impregnated
specimens (4). There are subendothelial, subepithelial and mesangial
deposits. The basement membrane appears to respond to the deposits in
that it tends to replicate and surround them much as it does in membranous nephropathy but in a more disordered fashion. The result is a
basement membrane which appears frayed, laminated and fenestrated. These
changes, in our experience, are permanent. On the other hand, the

mesangial deposits often do not produce as severe an inflammatory
reaction as occur in the other two forms. In fact, the proliferation
varies widely in extent; the glomeruli of some patients are minimally
proliferative and resemble those seen in membranous nephropathy.

3. PATHOGENESIS

Although MPGN apparently results from glomerular deposition of
complement reactive material, details of the pathogenesis are lacking.
Others have detected immune complexes in the circulation but no attempt
has been made to correlate them with the clinical course. Dr. Charles A.
Davis, in our laboratory, correlated clinical course with the levels of
complexes detected by the solid phase Clq method (5). Since, in this
method, the complexes are ultimately detected by their ability to react
with radiolabeled IgG, they, by definition, must contain IgG as well as
be reactive with Clq.

The results for specimens obtained when the patient was first seen
are shown in Fig. 1. For contrast, the results in a series of patients

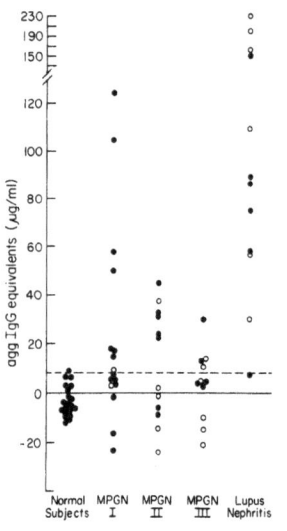

FIGURE 1. Levels of circulating
complexes in patients with MPGN and
SLE expressed as aggregated IgG
equivalents. The closed circles
indicate specimens obtained shortly
after diagnosis before prednisone
therapy started and the open circles,
specimens obtained a short time after
therapy started.

with lupus nephritis are also shown. It is apparent that complexes are
present in all three Types. They tend to be somewhat more abundant in
Type I but this was not statistically significant. In none of the

diseases were they as abundant as in lupus nephritis.

The correlation between levels of the complexes and clinical course was the opposite of that which might be predicted. Thus, as seen in Table 2, complexes were present in 100% of the patients whose disease was judged mild in that they had minimal or no proteinuria and hematuria. To the contrary, complexes were infrequently found in those whose disease had progressed to renal insufficiency or would develop renal

Table 2. Correlation between clinical status and presence of circulating immune complexes in 39 patients with MPGN

Clinical Status	Complexes present/ total patients	percent
Mild or "silent" glomerulonephritis	6/6	100
Typical MPGN without renal insufficiency	11/23	48
Renal insufficiency present or imminent	1/10	10

insufficiency in a few months. Patients between these extremes had complexes detectable with a frequency of about 50%. These results might indicate that the complexes detected are not nephritogenic; they may be by-products of an immune response and not harmful to the host. If the complexes measured are nephritogenic, the glomerular insult must occur early in the disease and, at that time, the subsequent course programmed to evolve in the absence of circulating complexes.

We tend to feel that the complexes measured are not nephritogenic but that complexes containing immunoglobulin are, on the other hand, responsible for the pathogenesis of Type I but may not be for the pathogenesis of Types II and III. That the complexes measured are not nephritogenic is evidenced by the fact that in the face of the continuing presence of complexes over periods of up to 11 years, several patients showed no signs and symptoms of progressive nephritis and, indeed, glomerular morphology may greatly improve despite high levels of complexes.

Evidence that immunoglobulin containing complexes are, on the other hand, responsible for Type I disease is the fact that (a) IgG determinants are usually found in the glomerular deposits (6) (b) that the disease responds well to therapy with corticosteroid as does lupus and (c) that glomerular morphology resembles closely that which can be seen in nephritides which are undoubtedly of immune complex origin. A prime example of the latter is the nephritis of chronic bacteremia in which morphology identical to idiopathic Type I may be seen (7,8).

That immunoglobulin containing complexes are not responsible for Types II and III is suggested by the lack of IgG in the glomerular deposits (6,9). Whereas this may be due to covering of Ig determinants by complement or to rapid loss of Ig integrity, it seems equally possible that some form of non-Ig containing complement reactive material is depositing.

Regardless of the pathogenic significance of the complexes detected by the solid phase Clq method, the observations indicate that their measurement is of little diagnostic or prognostic value and has no advantage over measurements of serum complement levels in following the response to therapy.

4. THERAPY

The actuarial survival of renal function in 37 patients treated with high dose long term alternate day prednisone can be compared with the survival of untreated patients in Fig. 2. The abscissa indicates the total duration of the disease. The dashed lines give the survival of three series of patients who had no treatment or were treated sporadical-ly. One is the series reported by Davis, et al. (10), another, the 105 patients reported in 1973 by Habib, et al. (11) and the third is our own experience with 17 patients who had no treatment (12). The survival of our 37 treated patients is significantly better than that in the other three series. Of the 37, three have developed ESRD in the 16 year period. All three had had their disease for 4 to 8 years before treat-ment started and renal biopsy at the start of therapy indicated severe glomerular involvement. Our impression is that treatment would have been successful in these children if it had been started earlier.

There are differences in the response of the three types to treatment and, in fact, this is one of the prime reasons for distinguishing types. We feel that all three diseases can be rendered inactive by this form of therapy, using as criteria for inactivity the disappearance of hematuria and normalization of the complement profile. However, when the disease is inactive, proteinuria often continues unabated and hypertension may remain a problem. Type I disease responds well to treatment if it is

initiated early. Deposits disappear and proliferation greatly diminishes. When therapy is initiated late, progression may be halted but
hypoproteinemia, nephrotic syndrome and hypertension often persist.

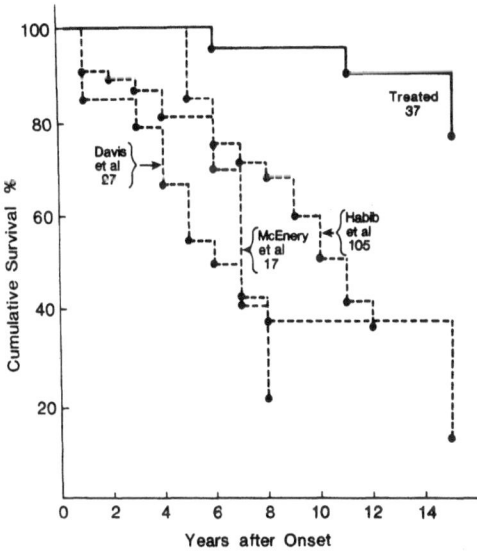

FIGURE 2. Actuarial
survival of renal
function for patients
with MPGN who were
untreated or treated
sporadically (dashed
lines) and for those
treated for 1.5 years or
more with an alternate
day prednisone regimen
(solid line). The number
of patients in each
series is indicated.

Treatment in Type II disease has also been successful although our
experience is not large (12). Of 7 patients treated for 3 years or
longer, one has developed ESRD and one is lost to follow-up. The remaining 5 are doing well after being treated for an average of 8 years. Two
of these have delivered healthy infants without complications. The
abnormality in the basement membrane persists but overall glomerular
morphology improves.

The response of the glomerular morphology of Type III to treatment
is, on the other hand, minimal. As can be seen from the data in Table 3
(12), most of the patients with Type I or Type II disease had a marked or
at least moderate increase in the number of open capillary lumens 2 years
after the start of treatment whereas this evidence of improvement was not
seen in those with Type III. Perhaps related to this is the observation
that there was no loss of capillary wall deposits whereas in Type I,
these deposits frequently disappeared. Despite the persistence of very
abnormal morphology in Type III, treatment seems to be of value; 9 of the

10 we have treated for an average of 5 years have evidenced no progression.

Table 3. Changes in glomerular morphology after 2 years of treatment according to type of MPGN.

	Type I n = 12 per cent	Type II n = 5 per cent	Type III n = 6 per cent
Number of open capillary lumens:			
Marked increase	75	60	0
Mod. to slight increase	17	20	0
No increase	8	0	100
Loss of capillary wall deposits	83	0	0

We feel it is important for successful therapy to use high doses of prednisone initially. The maximum for children over 40 kg is 80 mg q.o.d. and for children less than 40 kg, the dose is at least 2 mg/kg. This dose is continued for one year and then can be reduced if the complement profile becomes normal and the hematuria has diminished or disappeared. It may take more than a year for the disease to become inactive by these criteria and in many children, high doses have been maintained for 3 or more years. Subsequently, the dose has been slowly diminished so that patients treated for 5 or 10 years may be taking only 20 mg q.o.d. We have on occasion seen, after several years of treatment, the complement profile again become abnormal or hematuria develop. When the alternate day dose is increased, these abnormalities disappear.

Anecdotal observations have given evidence that prednisone given daily should not precede the alternate day regimen. Several patients given prednisone daily in divided dose for several weeks have shown irreversible deterioration.

The high dose alternate day therapy has not produced alarming side effects. Many of the children gain weight, develop slight moon facies and growth in height may be transiently slowed (12). However, height velocity returns to normal when the dose is reduced. The regimen has not produced striae, cataracts or osteoporosis and it does not greatly augment blood pressure in those already hypertensive.

It should be pointed out that the dose of prednisone used on alternate days in the treatment protocol for MPGN in the International

Study was 3/4 of that which was used in our patients. The results of the
International Study would suggest that the lower dosage significantly
reduces the effectiveness of the regimen. It also should be noted that
it is not optimum to treat these patients according to a strict protocol
since the duration of high dose treatment is not fixed but dependent on
the response of the patient.

REFERENCES

1. West, C.D., McAdams, A.J., McConville, J.M., Davis, N.C. and
    Holland, N.H.: Hypocomplementemic and normocomplementemic persis-
    tent (chronic) glomerulonephritis: clinical and pathologic charac-
    teristics. J. Pediatr. 67:1089-1112, 1965.
2. Turner, D.R., Cameron, J.S., Bewick, M., et al.: Transplantation in
    mesangiocapillary glomerulonephritis with intramembranous dense
    "deposits": Recurrence of disease. Kidney Int. 9:439-448, 1976.
3. Davis, C.A., McEnery, P.T., Maby, S., McAdams, A.J. and West, C.D.:
    Observations on the evolution of idiopathic rapidly progressive
    glomerulonephritis. Clin Nephrol. 9:91-101, 1978.
4. Strife, C.F., McEnery, P.T., McAdams, A.J. and West, C.D.: Mem-
    branoproliferative glomerulonephritis with disruption of the glomer-
    ular basement membrane. Clin Nephrol 7:65-72, 1977.
5. Davis, C.A., Marder, H. and West, C.D.: Circulating immune com-
    plexes in membranoproliferative glomerulonephritis. J Pediat Neph &
    Urol. In press.
6. Ooi, Y.M., Vallota, E.H. and West, C.D.: Classical complement
    pathway activation in membranoproliferative glomerulonephritis.
    Kidney Int. 9:46-53, 1976.
7. Strife, C.F., McDonald, B.M., Ruley, E.J., McAdams, A.J. and West,
    C.D.: Shunt nephritis: The nature of the serum cryoglobulins and
    their relation to the complement profile. J. Pediatr. 88:403-413,
    1976.
8. Michael, A.F., Herdman, R.C., Fish. A.J., Pickering, R.J. and
    Vernier, R.L.: Chronic membranoproliferative glomerulonephritis
    with hypocomplementemia. Transplant Proc. 1:925, 1969.
9. Habib, R., Gubler, M-C, Loirat, C., Ben-Maiz, H and Levy, M.: Dense
    deposit disease: A variant of membranoproliferative glomeruloneph-
    ritis. Kidney Int. 7:204-215, 1975.
10. Davis, A.E., Schneeberger, E.E., Grupe, W.E. and McCluskey, R.T.:
    Membranoproliferative glomerulonephritis (MPGN Type I) and dense
    deposit disease (DDD) in children. Clin. Nephrol. 9:184-193, 1978.
11. Habib, R., Kleinknecht, C., Gubler, M-C, and Levy, M.: Idiopathic
    membranoproliferative glomerulonephritis in children. Report of 105
    cases. Clin. Nephrol. 1:194-214, 1973.
12. McEnery, P.T., McAdams, A.J., and West, C.D.: Membranoproliferative
    glomerulonephritis: Improved survival with alternate day prednisone
    therapy. Clin. Nephrol. 13:117-124, 1980.

PLASMA CATECHOLAMINES IN NORMOTENSIVE CHILDREN AND IN CHILDREN WITH ESSENTIAL HYPERTENSION

J.G. MONGEAU, A. DAVIGNON, A. LAMARRE and J. DE CHAMPLAIN*

1. INTRODUCTION

In the last decade, the availability of highly sensitive radioenzymatic techniques has permitted the accurate and reproducible measurement of circulating catecholamines in human plasma. Under standardized protocols, it has been possible to use those measures as a valid index of sympathetic activity in man.

The purpose of the present study was to evaluate supine and standing plasma catecholamines (CA) and norepinephrine (NE) levels in children suffering from essential hypertension. These observations were correlated with cardiovascular parameters to determine whether a state of sympathetic hyperactivity could play a role in the development of essential hypertension early in life in a subgroup of patients.

2. DEFINITIONS AND METHODS

The hypertensive subjects were chosen according to the following criteria: thirty-eight (38) children, aged 5 to 20, were selected on the basis that their blood pressure was found above two standard deviations of the normal values for French Canadian children (1) after measurement on at least three different occasions. Physical examination and a serie of biochemical and radiological analysis were carried out on each patient to eliminate any primary disease that could be responsible for their hypertension. The measurement of plasma catecholamines was done on an outpatient basis and under strictly standardized conditions for all subjects. Plasma CA and NE levels were determined after resting in the supine position for 30 minutes and after standing for 10 minutes. Each hypertensive child was paired with a normotensive control of the same sex, age and approximately the same height and weight. Both were tested on the same day, under the same experimental

* Dept of Pediatrics, Ste-Justine Hospital and Dept of Pediatrics and Physiology, Université de Montréal, Montréal, Canada

protocol.

Plasma CA were determined using the radiometric enzymatic technique of Coyle and Henry, as modified by de Champlain et al (2,3). Plasma NE was determined by the radioenzymatic assay described by Henry et al (4).

Hypertensive children were classified into two categories: the systolic hypertensive (SH) and the systolic and diastolic hypertensive (SDH). At the beginning of our study, the SH children were divided in two subgroups: the children in whom the systolic blood pressure was 2 standard deviations above normal at the time catecholamines were determined, and the children in whom systolic blood pressure was statistically higher than their controls, but was between one and two standard deviations above normal at the time catecholamines were determined. Since it was found that CA and NE levels did not differ in these two subgroups, all these patients were included in the group of SH children.

3. RESULTS

CA and NE levels in patients and controls are shown in Table 1.

Table 1. Plasma catecholamines (CA) and norepinephrine (NE) in children suffering from essential hypertension and their controls.

	Age in years	B.P. mm Hg	SUPINE		STANDING	
			CA pg/ml	NE pg/ml	CA pg/ml	NE pg/ml
Controls n = 31	15	110/72	353 (± 19)	200 (± 15)	563 (± 30)	394 (± 26)
Systolic HTA n = 30	15	130/77	431* (± 29)	243 (± 28)	701** (± 41)	482* (± 32)
Systolic and diastolic HTA n = 8	12	137/92	464 (± 61)	199 (± 64)	688 (± 115)	375 (± 47)

(±) SEM
*   p < 0.05
** p < 0.01   vs control values

Hypertensive children tended to have higher CA and NE values than their own controls. In supine position the mean CA values were 353 pg/ml for controls, 431 pg/ml for SH children, and 464 pg/ml for SDH children. After standing for 10 minutes, the values of CA were 563, 701 and 688 pg/ml respectively. These results suggest that children with SH demonstrate a greater sympathetic reactivity to postural changes as reflected by the marked increase in CA (from 431 to 701 pg/ml i.e. 65%).

NE values in supine position were approximately the same for controls and SDH children, 200 and 199 pg/ml whereas children with SH have a mean NE value of 243 pg/ml. The fact that SDH childrenhave high CA values and normal NE values suggest that, in this group of children, epinephrine levels are probably greater. In standing position, NE levels showed the same pattern as in supine position: 394 and 375 pg/ml respectively for controls and SDH children, but SH children were characterized by a higher values of 482 pg/ml.

The distribution of CA and NE values found in each group of children was relatively scattered. In order to better evaluate individuals in each group, the percentage of distributions of values above one standard deviation from the mean normal values were calculated for each group of children, and are shown in Table 2.

Table 2. Percentage of plasma catecholamines (CA) and norepinephrine (NE) values above one standard deviation from the mean normal values.

	SUPINE		STANDING	
	High CA > 461 pg/ml	High NE > 284 pg/ml	High CA > 726 pg/ml	High NE > 533 pg/ml
Controls n = 31	13%	16%	14%	7%
Systolic HTA n = 30	33%	29%	46%	41%
Systolic and diastolic HTA n = 8	50%	29%	14%	14%

It becomes obvious that a greater proportion of hypertensive children (SH or
SDH) have elevated plasma CA and NE levels than controls. Moreover, the percentage of elevated values is markedly greater in children with SH than in
any other group in the standing position.

In order to assess the significance of plasma catecholamines as an index
of sympathetic activity, these levels were correlated with hemodynamic parameters calculated from echocardiography. Patients with CA values higher than
500 pg/ml were defined as hyperadrenergic and patients with values under
500 pg/ml as normoadrenergic.

Table 3. Cardiovascular parameters in normotensive (control) and hypertensive
normoadrenergic (CA < 500 pg/ml) and hyperadrenergic (CA > 500 pg/ml) children

	Controls	Normoadrenergic HTA	Hyperadrenergic HTA
n	31	28	12
Plasma CA (pg/ml)	403	350	639*
B.P. (mm Hg)	110/72	129/79**	136/83**
Heart Rate (B /min)	76	81	90**
Cardiac Index (1/m2)	2.89	3.27	3.66*
Aortic PEP (msec)	85.8	85.2	81.6

*   p < 0.05
** p < 0.01

As seen in Table 3, heart rate and cardiac index are significantly higher
in hyperadrenergic hypertensive than in normoadrenergic patients and normotensive controls. Moreover, the pre-ejection period (PEP) tended to be shorter

in hyperadrenergic hypertensive children compared to the other two groups.
These findings suggest hyperkinetic cardiac functions in hyperadrenergic
hypertensive patients.

Finally, because plasma CA may be influenced by physical fitness, physical working capacity (PWC) was assessed in all children.

Table 4. Percentile of the physical working capacity (PWC) in normotensive
and hypertensive children (HT)

	Controls n = 28	Normoadrenergic Ht n = 20	Hyperadrenergic Ht n = 10
PWC centile	76.6	53.3*	58.5*
		55*	

* $p < 0.01$

PWC results are shown in Table 4 as percentiles of normal for age and sex.
It is interesting to find that hypertensive children have significantly lower
PWC than their controls. This difference is not secondary to a difference in
body weight, since all children were paired with a control of the same body
size.

4. CONCLUSIONS

Values of circulating plasma catecholamines in normal children are slightly
higher than those measured in a group of normal adults by the same laboratory
using the same technique (5). As observed in adults with established or labile
essential hypertension, plasma catecholamines are elevated in an important subgroup of children with SH or SDH in supine position suggesting a higher basal
sympathetic tone. The higher CA and NE values observed in a subgroup of children with SH in the standing position also suggest that an increased sympathetic reactivity is present in these patients. Moreover, since high levels of
plasma catecholamines were found to be associated with hyperkinetic cardiac
functions reflected by an elevation of heart rate and cardiac index, it may be
postulated that although essential hypertension is probably the result of
combined multiple etiological factors, the sympathetic nervous system seems

nevertheless to play an important contributory role in the development of hypertension in a significant subgroup of hypertensive children.

5. ACKNOWLEDGEMENT

The Authors would like to express their gratitude to Ms Janine Lagarde, R.N., Lise Farley, R.T. for their most efficient technical assistance in the realization of these studies.

These studies were supported by grants from the Medical Research Council of Canada and from the Quebec Heart Foundation.

J. de Champlain is the holder of the J.C. Edward Professorship in Cardio-vascular Research at the Université de Montréal.

6. REFERENCES

1. Biron P, Mongeau JG, Bertrand D. 1976. Blood pressure values in 116 French Canadian children. CMA Journal, 114:432.
2. Coyle JT, Henry D. 1973. Catecholamines in fetal and newborn rat brain. J. Neurochem. 21:61-67.
3. de Champlain J, Farley L, Cousineau D, Van Ameringen MR. 1976. Circulating catecholamine levels in human and experimental hypertension. Circulation Research, 38:109-114.
4. Henry DP, Starman BS, Johnson DG, Wilhains RH. 1975. A sensitive radio-enzymatic assay for norepinephrine in tissues and plasma. Life Science, 16:375-384.
5. Cousineau D, Lapointe L, de Champlain J. 1978. Circulating catecholamines and systolic time intervals in normotensive and hypertensive patients with and without left ventricular hypertrophy. Amer. Heart J. 96:227-234.

URIC ACID REGULATION IN HYPERTENSIVE CHILDREN

JAMES W. PREBIS, M.D., ALAN B. GRUSKIN, M.D., H.JORGE BALUARTE AND
MARTIN S. POLINSKY, M.D. St. Christopher's Hospital for Children,
Philadelphia, PA.

The purpose of this presentation is threefold: 1) to review the normal
renal handling of uric acid in man; 2) to present our data on the subject of
hyperuricemia in hypertensive pediatric patients and 3) to discuss several
mechanisms which may be responsible for the production of hyperuricemia in our
hypertensive children.

Approximately 7-10% of the adult American population have elevated serum
uric acid levels. Of concern is the fact that hyperuricemia rarely occurs
alone but often appears as part of a clinical complex that may include obesity,
hypertension, hyperlipidemia, diabetes mellitus and atherosclerosis. Numerous
epidemiologic studies have documented that hyperuricemia occurs in 22 to 38% of
untreated hypertensive adults.[1,2,3] There are, however, no published studies
dealing with the subject of uric acid metabolism in hypertensive children. The
presence of hyperuricemia in hypertensive children would be of significant
clinical concern since numerous studies have demonstrated that hyperuricemia is
a cardiovascular risk factor.[4-11]

Hyperuricemia results from either an overproduction of uric acid or from a
decrease in its excretion from the body. There is little data to suggest that
hyperuricemia in hypertensive patients is secondary to an increase in uric acid
production. Thus, most studies have focused on possible abnormalities in uric
acid excretion. In normal individuals, approximately two-thirds of the daily
uric acid excretion occurs via the kidney with the remainder eliminated
through the gastrointestinal trace.[12] In 1961 Gutman and Yu proposed the classical three component system for the normal renal handling of uric acid.
Firstly, virtually all the serum uric acid is filtered at the glomerulus.
Secondly, 98 to 100% of the filtered urate is actively reabsorbed in the early
proximal tubule. Thirdly, a variable percentage of the filtered load is
actively secreted into the proximal tubular lumen.[13,14] Subsequent studies
have confirmed the validity of this three component model and they have also
identified a fourth component - a post secretory reabsorption of urate.[15,16]

The net interaction of these four renal mechanisms usually results in 6 to
10% of the filtered urate being excreted. Several important points should be
made concerning this model. Studies by Steele, Jenkins and Rieselbach indicate
that the transport capacity for the active proximal reabsorption of urate is
sufficiently large that the fractional reabsorption of urate remains at more

than 98% of the filtered load even at plasma urate concentrations exceeding 16 mg/dl.[17,18] In 1959, Gutman was able to demonstrate that the rate of urate secretion was a direct function of the plasma uric acid concentration i.e. the higher the plasma uric acid level the greater the rate of urate secretion.[19] These data demonstrated that there was "bi-directional transport" of uric acid since increases in plasma uric acid were associated with proportional increases in proximal tubular reabsorption and secretion of urate.

The most recent addition to our understanding of the renal handling of urate deals with the concept of post secretory reabsorption. Independent studies by Diamond and Steele[15,16] indicated that significant quantities of secreted urate were again reabsorbed back into the peritubular blood. This post secretory reabsorption occurs at a site distal to or coextensive with the urate secretory site. Animal studies would imply that the tubular maximum for this distal reabsorptive site is quite limited and may account for only 15% of the total urate reabsorbed. Yet this reabsorption would still have significant effects on the amount of secreted urate that was finally excreted. Since one hundred percent of plasma uric acid is filterable and virtually all filtered urate is then promptly reabsorbed, the amount of urate which is actually excreted must be controlled by alterations in the rate of secretion and post secretory reabsorption. I'll return to this concept later when I present our data on the renal handling of urate in hypertensive, hyperuricemic children.

In order to determine the degree to which hyperuricemia occurs in children and adolescents with essential hypertension, the following study was performed. Thirty-one hypertensive patients ranging in age from 3½ to 18 years were evaluated for their hypertension in the Clinical Research Center of St. Christopher's Hospital for Children. The diagnosis of hypertension was based on the presence of systolic and/or diastolic blood pressures consistently greater than the 95th percentile for age and sex according to the standards published by the National Heart, Lung and Blood Institute's Task Froce on Blood Pressure Control in Children.[20] All patients had a normal creatinine clearance and no child had received prior drug or dietary therapy before being evaluated. Serum uric acid levels and 24 hour urinary uric acid excretion rates were determined in each child during two different dietary regimens: first, while ingesting an unrestricted sodium intake; and second, after receiving a 200 mg sodium diet for three days. The purpose of placing the children on low sodium diets was to determine whether sodium restriction has any effect on uric acid metabolism in these hypertensive children.

The results of these tests were compared to previously established age-related values in healthy children and adults.[21] Hyperuricemia was defined as a serum uric acid value which exceeded the 95th percentile for age. Values above 7 mg/dl in males and 6 mg/dl in females were considered elevated in patients over 16 years of age. Thirteen of 31 or 42% of the children and adolescents with essential hypertension were hyperuricemic for age.

We next considered the possible physiologic mechanisms responsible for this hyperuricemia. As mentioned earlier, one mechanism known to produce hyperuricemia is a decrease in the renal excretion of urate. For this reason, we analyzed our data to determine whether there was a correlation between serum uric acid levels and the fractional excretion of urate. When the patient's serum uric acid level was compared with the fractional excretion of urate we found that there was a strong inverse correlation between the two factors, i.e. the lower the fractional excretion of urate the higher the serum uric acid concentration for both the normouricemic and hyperuricemic hypertensive children. These data, therefore, suggest that the hyperuricemia of these hypertensive children was in part due to a defect in the renal excretion of urate.

When these children were placed on a low sodium diet we found that 17/31 or 55% of the hypertensive subjects were hyperuricemic for age. When the patient's serum uric acid was compared to their fractional excretion of urate strong inverse correlation again existed between these two factors indicating that a decrease in the renal excretion of urate was at least partially responsible for the further increase in serum uric acid levels. In order to further explore the possible renal mechanisms underlying this hyperuricemia we used the Lasix stimulation test to compare the relative secretory function of the hyperuricemic vs normouricemic hypertensive patients. Of importance is the fact that the diuretic action of furosemide is due to the presence of this drug within the tubular lumen rather than in the peritubular blood. In addition, furosemide gains access to its site of action by secretion at the proximal tubule via the transport pathway for organic acids. The higher the concentration of Furosemide in the lumen of the tubule the greater the rate of sodium and chloride excretion.[22,23,24]

Since we knew that the organic acids furosemide and uric acid are both secreted by the proximal tubule although by different transport systems, we reasoned that if there is a decrease in the secretion of urate in the proximal tubule of the hypertensive, hyperuricemic patient there may also be a decrease in the secretion of furosemide which in turn would be reflected by a diminished rate of excretion for sodium, chloride, and urine.

Twenty-eight children with essential hypertension were evaluated. Thirteen were hyperuricemic and 15 were normouricemic. After breakfast, the patient was made NPO and blood was drawn for electrolytes, BUN and creatinine. After the patient voided, 1 mg/kg furosemide was administered orally. Hourly urine specimens were collected for five consecutive hours and measured for volume and electrolytes. At the completion of the urine collections blood was again drawn for electrolytes, BUN and creatinine.

The hyperuricemic patients excreted statistically less sodium during the first hour collection than the normouricemic children. Although the finding of a decreased sodium excretion in the hyperuricemic patients tended to persist throughout the remaining four collection periods, it approached but did not reach statistically significant proportions. The total five hour sodium excretion, however, was significantly lower by approximately 1/3, in the hyperuricemic patients. Identical patterns of excretion were observed for chloride and water.

These data permit several conclusions. Firstly, there is a statistically significant reduction in the diuretic response to furosemide in the hyperuremic children. Secondly, since the diuretic response to furosemide is directly related to its concentration in the renal tubule there must be a decreased secretion of this organic acid into the proximal tubule of the hyperuricemic children. Thirdly, this abnormality in the tubular organic acid transport of furosemide may reflect a similar defect in the transport of uric acid. We, therefore, feel it is reasonable to suggest that the decrease in uric acid excretion seen in hypertensive, hyperuricemic children is due to a reduction in uric acid secretion.

In summary: 1) hyperuricemia occurs with increased frequency in children with essential hypertension; 2) the ingestion of low sodium diet in hypertensive children results in an increased serum uric acid and diminished urate excretion; 3) a decrease in the renal excretion of urate is in part responsible for hyperuricemia of these children; 4) there appears to be a defect in the tubular secretion of urate in hypertensive hyperuricemic children and 5) insofar as hyperuricemia represents a cardiovascular risk factor, it is already operative in hypertensive children and adolescents.

REFERENCES

1. Maas, A.R.: The role of uric acid as a potential risk factor in hypertension, Smith Kline Corporation, 1978.
2. Cannon, P.J., Stason, W.B., DeMartini, F.E., Sommers, S.C. and Laragh,J.H.: Hyperuricemia in primary and renal hypertension. N. Engl.J.Med. 275:457, 1966.
3. Breckinridge, A.: Hypertension and hyperricemia. Lancet 1:15, 1966.
4. Newland, H.: Hyperuricemia in coronary, cerebral and peripheral artery disease:An explanation. Med.Hypoth. 1:152, 1975.
5. Bluhm, G.B. and Riddle, J.M.: Platelets and vascular disease in gout. Sem. Arth.Rheum. 2:355, 1973.
6. Gertler, M.M., Garn, S.M. and Levine, S.A.: Serum uric acid in relation to age and physique in health and in coronary heart disease. Ann.Int.Med. 34:1421, 1951.
7. Fessel, J.W., Siegelaub, A.B. and Johnson, E.S.: Correlates and consequences of asymptomatic hyperuricemia. Arch.Int.Med.132:44, 1973.
8. Persky, V.W., Dyer, A.R., Idris-Soven, E., Stamler, J., Shekelle, R.B., Schoenberger, J.A., Berkson, D.M. and Lindberg, H.A.: Uric acid:A risk factor for coronary heart disease? Circulation 59:969, 1979.

9. McEwin, R., McEwin, K. and Loudon, B.: Raised serum uric acid levels with myocardial infarction. Med.J.Aust. 1:530, 1974.

10. Fessel, J.W.: Hyperuricemia in health and disease. Rheum 1:275, 1972.

11. Stamler, J. et al: Relationship of multiple variables to blood pressure-findings from four Chicago epidemiologic studies, in Oglesby, P. (Ed): Epidemiology and Control of Hypertension. New York: Stratton, 307, 1975.

12. Sorenson, L.B. and Levison, D.J.: Origin and extrarenal elimination of uric acid in man, Nephrol 14:7, 1975.

13. Gutman, A.B. and Yu, R.F.: A three component system for the regulation of renal excretion of uric acid in man. Tr. Assoc. Am. Physicians 74:353,1961

14. Gutman, A.B.: Significance of the renal clearance of uric acid in normal and gouty man. Am.J.Med. 37:833, 1964.

15. Diamond, H.S. and Paolino, J.S.: Evidence for a postsecretory reabsorptive site for uric acid in man. J.Clin.Invest. 52:1491, 1973.

16. Steele, T.H. and Boner, G.: Origins of the uricosuric response. J.Clin. Invest. 52:1368, 1973.

17. Steele, T.H. and Rieselbach, R.E.: The renal mechanism for urate homeo stasis in normal man. Am.J.Med. 43:868, 1967.

18. Jenkins, P. and Rieselbach, R.E.: Unique characteristics of the mechanism for reabsorption of filtered versus secreted urate. Proc.Am.Soc.Clin. Invest. 66:36a, 1974.(Abstract).

19. Gutman, A.B., Yu, T.F. and Berger, L.: Tubular secretion of urate in man. J.Clin.Invest. 38:1778, 1959.

20. The National Heart, Lung and Blood Institute's Task Force on Blood Pressure Control in Children: Report of the Task Force on Blood Pressure Control in Children. Pediatrics Supplement 59(5):797, 1977.

21. Stapleton, F.B., Linshaw, M.A., Hassanein, K. and Gruskin, A.B.: Uric acid excretion in normal children. J.Pediatr. 92:911, 1978.

22. Deetjen, P.: Micropuncture studies on site and mode of diuretic action of furosemide. Ann.N.Y. Acad. Sci. 139:408, 1966.

23. Bowman, R.H.: Renal secretion of furosemide and its depression by albumin binding. Am.J.Physiol. 229(1):93, 1975.

24. Chennavasin, P., Seiwell, R., Brater, D.C. and Liang, W.M.: Pharmaco-dynamic analysis of the furosemide-probenecid interaction in man. Kidney Int. 16:187, 1979.

RENAL VEIN RENIN DETERMINATIONS IN EVALUATING HYPERTENSIVE CHILDREN

M.J. DILLON

1. INTRODUCTION

The determination of renal vein renin levels in identifying surgically curable forms of renal hypertension in adults is well established.[1,2] Since semi-micro methods for measuring plasma renin have become available these techniques have also been applied successfully to the investigation of children with various types of hypertensive renal disease.[3-5] Elevations of the renal venous plasma renin ratio between the affected kidney (R) and the contralateral or less affected kidney (Rc) has been used as an index of asymmetrical renin release and predictor of surgical relief of renal hypertension.[1,6] The plasma renin ratio between Rc and the inferior vena cava (P) has been suggested as an estimate of suppression of renin release from the contralateral kidney.[2]

Definition of a significant R/Rc ratio,i.e.,the minimum renal venous renin ratio clearly identifying pathological lateralization of renin release, was recently, based on empirical observations of operative success and varied considerably between different investigators.[6-10] The most widely accepted ratio has been 1.5[5,11] but ratios from 1.3 to 2.5 have been reported.[2,6-8,10] Less information is available about the Rc/P ratio inspite of Stockigt et al's suggestion that an Rc/P of <1.3 indicated contralateral negative feed back inhibition of renin release and was associated with a favourable response to surgical treatment of renal hypertension.

Renal vein renin measurements have not been undertaken systematically in normotensive adults although there have been a few reports of plasma renin ratios in adult patients with essential hypertension and apparantly normal kidneys.[12,13] In terms of paediatric patients there was also no data available until last year when Gerdts et al[14] reported their findings in normotensive children without kidney lesions. What is more, in pathological situations, although some reports indicated that these measurements aided assessment of childhood renal hypertension[5,15-17] there were others which cast doubt on their value.[3]

In view of this it was considered appropriate to review the experience of renal vein renin measurements at the Hospital for Sick Children, London, in terms of establishing a reference range for renal venous renin ratios in children and the use of the technique in assessing children with various pathological states associated with hypertension.

2.   PATIENTS AND METHODS

151 renal vein renin studies on 144 children were undertaken during a 5 year period. 49 studies were on normotensive children, free of renal disease, who were undergoing cardiac catheterization to elucidate their congenital heart lesions. The purpose of this study was to establish a reference range and the findings have been reported in more detail elsewhere.[14] The childrens' ages ranged from 1 - 16 years with a mean of 6.3 years. For them criteria for inclusion in the study were: a lack of history of renal disease, absence of heart failure, normal blood pressure, normal renal function and normal urinalysis.

The remaining 102 studies on 95 children were undertaken in the course of investigation of their sustained hypertension. 50 of these patients were included in an earlier report.[5] Their ages ranged from 8 months - 18 years with a mean of 4.9 years. 34 patients had renovascular disease (18 unilateral, 16 bilateral), 44 patients had parenchymal disease which was predominantly pyelonephritic scarring (18 unilateral, 20 bilateral but asymmetrical, 6 bilateral and symmetrical), 9 patients had essential or other non renal hypertension including 2 catecholamine producing tumours and 8 patients had been transplanted.

The technique involved the introduction of catheters via the femoral vein under basal sedation or general anaesthetic. Subjects were supine for at least 1 hour before sampling and remained horizontal throughout. No means of pharmacological stimulation of renin release was employed. 0.5 - 1.0 ml blood samples were drawn from the main renal veins and the caudal vena cava below the entry of the renal veins. In the pathological studies, when possible, segmental samples were obtained from the upper, middle and lower zones of each kidney. The transplanted patients underwent sampling from the renal veins, the vena cava, the graft vein and the iliac or femoral vein below the graft. Plasma renin activity (PRA) was measured by radio immuno assay of generated angiotensin I.[18] Precision within assays as represented by the coefficient of variation of duplicates ranging throughout the standard curve was 5%.

Logarithmic transformation was carried out to normalize PRA data and measurements were compared by the student to test. Confidence intervals for R/Rc were calculated by X^2 analysis and details of this are reported elsewhere.[14]

3. NORMOTENSIVE CHILDREN

3.1 Results

There was no significant difference between PRA levels in the renal veins of these children ($P < 0.2$). Regardless of absolute renin values the mean plasma renin ratio of left:right renal vein was 1.03 (95% confidence limits 0.72 - 1.38).

The renal vein PRA was found to be significantly higher than the PRA in the inferior vena cava (IVC) caudal to the entry of the renal veins ($P < 0.001$). The mean PRA ratio of the renal vein over IVC was 1.21 (95% confidence limits 0.81 - 1.82). Ratios calculated at low, intermediate and high PRA levels did not differ significantly.

Ratios were calculated in analogy with the pathological situation i.e. by dividing the higher renal venous PRA (R) by the value obtained from the contralateral kidney (Rc) and the latter by the value in the caudal IVC (P). A mean R/Rc ratio of 1.16 was found and statistical analysis showed the 95% confidence limit to be 1.41. Three patients had R/Rc ratios >1.40 with the highest value in the series of 1.55. There was a wide variation of Rc/P ratios with a mean of 1.15 (95% confidence limits of 0.78 - 1.62). Ten subjects had Rc/P ratios of >1.3 and thirteen had ratios of <1.0.

3.2 Comment

From this data it was concluded that 1.5 was a reasonable upper limit of normality for R/Rc if this is defined by 95% confidence limits. Although 20% of the subjects had an Rc/P ratio of >1.3 it was not felt that this necessarily afforded evidence against Stockigt et al's [2] suggestion of contralateral feed back inhibition of renin release since in the children studied there was no pathological stimulus from either kidney to suppress contralateral renin production. For more detailed discussion the reader is referred to Gerdts et al, 1979.[14]

4.   HYPERTENSIVE CHILDREN

4.1   Results (R/Rc)

Excluding the studies on transplanted patients there were 50 studies
in which the R/Rc ratio was > 1.5 and 43 in which values of < 1.5 were
obtained.

4.1.1.   Renovascular disease.   There were 37 studies on 34 patients.
Ratios of > 1.5 were seen in 15 of those with unilateral disease and in 9
with bilateral disease.   Surgical treatment was undertaken in 11 with unilateral disease (9 with ratios > 1.5) and of those 7 were cured in terms of
blood pressure control, 3 were significantly improved and one died in the
immediate perioperative period at another hospital without it being clear
that the operation had been successful as far as the blood pressure was
concerned.   8 patients had nephrectomies, 3 were revascularized and the
remaining 7 were treated medically.   Of the patients with bilateral disease
5 underwent surgery (4 with ratios > 1.5) and 2 were cured and 3 improved.
Revascularization was undertaken in 4 cases, in one a nephrectomy was
undertaken on one side and the other kidney was revascularized and the
remaining 11 children were treated medically.

4.1.2.   Parenchymal disease.   There were 46 studies on 44 patients.
In 26 patients, R/Rc ratios were > 1.5 but it is noteworthy that none of
these children had symmetrical disease.   10 patients with unilateral and
6 with bilateral asymmetrical disease underwent surgery.   11 were cured and
in 5 a significant improvement in blood pressure occurred.   There were 15
nephrectomies, one nephrectomy coupled with a partial nephrectomy on the
other side and the remainder were treated medically.

4.1.3.   Essential and non renal hypertension.   There were 10 studies
          on 9 patients within this category.   All had R/Rc ratios of
< 1.5.   Medical treatment was undertaken in 8 and 1 patient was cured by
removal of a phaeochromocytoma.

4.2   Comment

Surgery was undertaken in 32 patients of which 20 were cured, 11 improved
and there were no failures in terms of blood pressure control although the
one perioperative death is difficult to classify.   Of these 28 had R/Rc ratios
> 1.5 and 4 < 1.5.   Amongst the latter 3 were improved by surgery and the
remaining patient was the child who died at the time of surgery.   This
gave a 100% surgical success rate if success is considered to be a cure
or significant improvement in blood pressure.   There was 0% false positive

ratios but a 9.6% incidence of false negative values. For further
discussion the reader is referred to Dillon, Shah and Barratt, 1978.[5]

4.3 Results (Rc/P)

In only 14 studies Rc/P ratios of > 1.3 were found. In 10 of these
the disease was bilateral but in 4 apparently unilateral pathology was present.
7 of these patients underwent surgery and of these 5 were cured and 2
improved.

4.4 Segmental vein sampling

Segmental renal vein sampling was undertaken in the course of
47 studies. In 11 of these it provided useful information about local
sources of renin release that main vein sampling alone could have missed.
In 3 children partial nephrectomies have been undertaken on the strength
of these findings with satisfactory outcomes in terms of blood pressure
control.

4.5 Transplanted patients

9 studies on 8 hypertensive transplanted patients were undertaken.
In 2 patients the graft was implicated as the cause of the hypertension,
in 2 the original kidneys and in the remainder the values were equivocal.

4.6 Complications

One child died of a vertebral artery embolus which was considered to
be a complication of an angiocardiographic study that was undertaken at
the same time as the renal vein sampling. Two children became hypovolaemic
at a time when duplicate samples were being removed for comparison with
another method and hence blood loss was considerable.

5. CONCLUSION

(a) A renal vein renin ratio of 1.5 is an acceptable upper limit of
normality when investigating children with suspected renal hypertension.

(b) Surgical treatment of renal hypertension, if feasible, undertaken
on the basis of a renal vein renin ratio of 1.5 or above is likely to
prove successful in terms of blood pressure control.

(c) The Rc/P ratio although possibly alerting clinicians to the possibility
of contralateral pathology in patients with renal hypertension is probably
of dubious value in accurately identifying lack of contralateral renin
suppression.

(d) Segmental renal vein renin measurements are feasible in children and can identify local sources of renin release that main vein sampling may miss.

(e) There may be some value in renal vein renin measurements in the investigation of transplanted patients with hypertension.

ACKNOWLEDGEMENTS

The studies described in this paper were supported in part by the following:- The Kidney Research Aid Fund, The National Kidney Research Fund, The Buttle Trust, The Medical Research Council, The German National Scholarship Foundation and the Joint Research Board of The Hospital for Sick Children at the Institute of Child Health, London. A special word of thanks goes to Mrs Vanita Shah,F.I.L.M.S. who undertook the majority of the plasma renin measurements, Drs K.G. Gerdts and J.M. Savage my co-workers, the staff of the Department of Cardiology who undertook the renal vein catheterization and the paediatricians who referred patients and specimens to me.

REFERENCES

1. Judson WE, Helmer OM. 1965. Diagnostic and prognostic values of renin activity in renal venous plasma in renovascular hypertension. Hypertension 13:79
2. Stockigt JR, Noakes CA, Collins RD, Schambelan M, Biglieri EG, 1972. Renal vein renin in various forms of renal hypertension. Lancet 1:1194
3. Godard C. 1977. Predictive value of renal vein renin measurements of children with various forms of renal hypertension: an international study. Helvetica Paediatrica Acta 32:49
4. Robson AM. 1978. Special diagnostic studies for the detection of renal and renovascular forms of hypertension. Pediats. Clin. North. Am. 25:83
5. Dillon MJ, Shah V, Barratt TM. 1978. Renal vein renin measurements in children with hypertension. Br. Med. J. 2:168
6. Bourgoignie J, Kurtz S, Catanzaro FJ, Serirat P, Perry MH. 1970. Renal venous renin in hypertension. Am J Med 48:332
7. Figueroa JE, Bennett DJ, DeCamp PT, Batson HM. 1975. Experience with renal vein renin ratios in the identification of a pressor kidney. South Med J 68:1200
8. Ernst CB, Bookstein JJ, Montie J, Baumgartel E, Hoobler SW, Fry WJ. 1972. Renal vein renin ratios and collateral vessels in renovascular hypertension Arch Surg 104:496
9. Gunnells JC, McGuffin Wl, Johnsrude I, Robinson RR. 1969. Peripheral and renal venous plasma renin activity in hypertension. Ann Intern Med 71:555
10. Amsterdam EA, Couch NP, Christlieb AR, Harrison JH, Crane C, Dobrzinsky SJ, Hickler RB. 1969. Renal vein renin activity in prognosis of surgery for renovascular hypertension. Am J Med 47:870

11. Marks LS, Maxwell MH. 1975. Renal vein renin: value and limitations in the prediction of operative results. Urol Clin North Am 2:311
12. Sealey JE, Buhler FR, Laragh JH, and Vaughan ED. 1973. The physiology of renin secretion in essential hypertension. Estimation of renin secretion rate and renal plasma flow from peripheral and renal vein renin levels. Am J Med 55:391
13. Maxwell MH, Marks LS, Varady PD, Lupu AN, Kaufman JJ. 1975. Renal vein renin in essential hypertension. J Lab Clin Med 86:901
14. Gerdts KG, Shah V, Savage JM, Dillon MJ. 1979. Renal vein renin measurements in normotensive children. J Pediat 95:953
15. Leumann EP, Bauer RP, Slaton PE, Biglieri EG, Holliday MA. 1970. Renovascular hypertension in Children. Pediatrics 46:362
16. Kaufman JJ, Goodwin WE, Waisman J, Gyepes MT. 1972. Renovascular hypertension in children. Report of seven cases treated surgically including two cases of renal autotransplantation. Am J Surg 124:149
17. Loggie JMH, McEnery PT. 1975. Hypertension in childhood and adolescence. in paediatric nephrology, ed MI Rubin, TM Barratt p417. Baltimore, Williams, and Wilkins.
18. Dillon MJ, 1975. Measurement of plasma renin activity by semimicro radioimmunoassay of generated angiotensin I .J Clin Pathol 28:625

VESICOURETERAL REFLUX AND URINARY TRACT INFECTION: INTRODUCTION TO
SEMINAR

JOHN W. DUCKETT, M.D.--CHAIRPERSON

Further light has been shed on the riddle of the small scarred contracted kidney with the fashionable term "reflux nephropathy". At the
last IPNS meeting in Finland, a great amount of interest was aroused
about the subject, resulting in a work shop conference which convened
in June, 1978 in Bermuda. A monograph of these proceedings was published, edited by Hodson and Kincaid-Smith entitled Reflux Nephropathy
This volume presents a variety of controversial subjects that involve
urologists, nephrologists, radiologists, pathologists, pediatricians,
and other specialists. Unfortunately, emotional and anecdotal
arguments are often injected into these debates. In this seminar we
hope to offer an update on these subjects and focus on the issues of
greatest disagreement. May I first introduce our distinguished panel:

Prof. George A. Richard, University of Florida, Gainesville, FL

Prof. Jan Winberg, Karolinska Hospital, Stockholm, Sweden

Dr. Jean Smellie, University College Hospital, London, UK

Prof. Hermann Olbing, Universitatskinderklinik, Essen, W. Germany

Prof. Robert Jeffs, Johns Hopkins University, Baltimore, MD

Mr. Phillip Ransley, Institute of Child Health, London, UK

This brief introduction and update of the subject may indeed be
confusing and is intentionally so.

Is VUR normal? We used to think that it was distinctly abnormal;
however, a study done by Kollermann and Ludwig in 1967 showed that 30%
of children under three years of age have mild reflux. Animal experiments, by Lenaghan and Cussen in 1968 showed that 80% of pups under
six months of age reflux and Roberts in 1974 showed a high incidence
of reflux in monkeys under three years of age. The concept of "marginal

competence" of the antireflux mechanism in normal children may be valid.

What is the pathogenesis of VUR? Most of us feel it is a congenital anomaly of the UV junction with a laterally displaced abnormal ureteric orifice and a short intramural ureter. If the marginal competence concept is valid, uninhibited contractions seen in young children at the time of bladder training with increased bladder pressures may stress the UV junction and contribute to the development of VUR. Chronic cystitis has been felt to cause reflux, however, there is little evidence that cystograms done with the bladder infected have any higher incidence of VUR then those carried out in uninfected bladders (Leibowitz).

Is reflux nephropathy a useful term? RN is defined as calyceal clubbing, adjacent cortical scarring, and arrest of renal growth. This term, coined by Baily in 1973, as an alternative to chronic pyelonephritis was intended to stress that VUR is essential to the pathogenesis of this lesion. Habib has called this lesion "congential segmental hypoplasia"; the Ask-Upmark kidney may be the same renal lesion.

How does intrarenal reflux fit into the picture? Ransley's "big bang" theory postulates that areas of renal scarring are drained by flat or concave renal papillae which allow IRR. This permits pyelo-tubular backflow with pyelo-interstitial extravasation. While IRR may occur in 5-15% of newborns and infants with reflux, it is rare after four years of age (Rolleston). As the distribution of non-convex papillae is the same in all age groups, the relatively larger size of collecting ducts in infants is thought to be responsible for their higher incidence of IRR (Tamminen). Hodson and Rolleston feel that scarring may be caused by sterile reflux, whereas Ransley finds that infected urine and IRR must additionally be present to cause scarring.

Where does Stephen's "bud theory" for renal scarring fit in the picture? Stephens feels that the site of origin of the ureteral bud on the mesonephric duct is responsible for the renal anomaly; that the renal morphology of the shrunken kidney is congenital and not a result of reflux. A normally sited bud will reach the center of the renal blastema, induce a normal kidney, and be incorporated into the bladder in the A location. An abnormally sited bud reaches more peripheral blastema of poorer quality, induces an abnormal kidney from this, and is incorporated into the bladder in a lateral, C position. Thus, the reflux and scarring are there at birth and infection is superimposed on the congenital abnormality.

We, therefore, have four major mechanisms that may produce reflux nephropathy: 1) sterile reflux, 2) a congenital anomaly associated with reflux, but not caused by it (Stephen's bud theory), 3) the "big bang" theory of VUR plus IRR and infected urine, and 4) the blood-borne infection alone, such as neonatal pyelonephritis.

Are VUR and RN truly a health hazard? Stamey feels that they probably are not; concluding this from only 300 transplants done per year for RN. Theoretical calculations showing that if 1.5% of girls under 12 have bacteriuria and 17.5% of this group have renal scarring and 10% of this group have serious scarring, calculates to 1/4,000 girls under 12 who will have serious scarring or renal failure. In another way, he shows that if 1% of bacteriuria is present in children under four and 30% of these have VUR and 6% of these have IRR than 1/5,555 of children under four will have IRR. Since there are about 20 million little girls under 12, that means 5,000 of them progress to renal failure,

of children under four, 2,500 of them have IRR. Heale in New Zealand
in a report of the 25 year natural history of VUR, showed that of 1,000
children with urinary tract infection, 13% would develop severe scarring, 7% uremia, 4% hypertension, and 2% chronic renal failure. That
calculates to 6000/yr. in the USA of girls under 12 years. There are
2000 leukemias a year in children in the USA.

Smellie, Normand, and Edwards at University College Hospital in
London have clearly shown that 85% of normal ureters and 41% of dilated
ureters will cease to reflux with time alone. The rate of cessation
was 10-15% per year.   Puberty was not associated with spontaneous cessation. They also showed that thorough medical follow-up and suppressive antibacterial control avoids renal scarring. On the other hand,
intermittent antibacterial therapy does result in scarring (Lenaghan
and Filly).

There is a good bit of confusion with regard to renal growth and
VUR. Subnormal growth rates have been noted with sterile reflux (Lyon,
Redman). Resumption of renal growth when infection was eliminated has
been reported (Kelalis). Depressed renal growth in the presence of VUR
has been shown to return to normal after antireflux surgery (Scott and
Stansfeld, Bauer and Retik). Yet another study found renal growth was
not influenced by the correction of VUR (Tamminen and Parkkulainin).
One study even showed that physical growth was retarded with VUR fol-
lowed by a growth spurt after surgical correction of VUR (Merrell and
Mowad).

Winberg, Claesson et al in 1979 reported an interesting follow-up of
22 patients who had experienced one episode of neonatal pyelonephritis
treated early and appropriately. Although 40% of these had reflux,

only 5% had a high grade. All kidneys showed significant growth
retardation (-.56 SD thickness) but no focal scars were seen and the
grade of reflux did not seem to make any difference. They also showed
in another group of 38 kidneys with focal scars that the damaged kidney
had growth retardation, while the healthy kidney showed compensatory
hypertrophy. These changes were not related to the grade of VUR and
interestingly enough the GFR was greater than 100 in all but five of
these cases.

VUR is related to hypertension. Smellie demonstrated that 20% of
patients with established scarring will develop hypertension. Williams
found in a group with surgically corrected VUR that hypertension
eventually developed in 18.5% of those with bilateral and 11.3% with
unilateral RN. Most of these children have normal renal function while
some have a high plasma renin, Savage has shown that 9% of normotensive
patients also have an elevated renin. Although elimination of reflux
does not seem to protect against hypertension (Stecker and Williams),
Woodward has shown improvement in hypertension control after surgical
correction.

Williams reported in 1968 on 100 patients who had untreated urinary
tract infections during pregnancy who were followed up four to six
months after delivery. Thirty-two percent were found to be still
infected. Twenty-one percent had VUR, and of those with reflux 62%
were infected. Thus, reflux which is permitted to persist into the
child bearing years is assoicated with a high rate of urinary tract
infection during pregnancy. This is of particular concern because
maternal UTI's have been shown to produce increased infant morbidity.

Finally, as VUR is a condition which is very <u>readily correctable by surgery</u>, the pediatric urologist is able to give a persuasive argument for correcting the more severe forms of VUR. In 98% of cases reflux is corrected. One to four percent develop obstruction, but this may be successfully corrected without damage to the kidney if careful postoperative monitoring is carried out. Although UTI's may continue to recur after antireflux surgery, the infection will be confined to the bladder and the kidney spared.

In conclusion, VUR seems to be a significant health hazard. Neither the lesions of RN the mechanism of VUR are yet established or fully understood. They can be controlled in many cases with conscientious medical surveillance. Surgical correction in good hands is also very successful. Therefore, the decision for surgery over medical therapy remains a difficult one. We have much to learn—let us see what new light we may shed on the subject today.

REPORT ON THE INTERNATIONAL VESICOURETERAL REFLUX
STUDY IN CHILDREN (IRSC)

H. OLBING

INTRODUCTION

The previous presentations and discussions of this symposium
and recent unbiased review articles (8) document that there
is no convincing evidence whether surgical or nonsurgical
management of children with nonobstructive moderate vesico-
ureterorenal reflux (VUR) is superior (1,3,4,5,6,7,8,9). The
only published randomised trial, which showed no convincing
differences, does not meet present standards of nonsurgical
management and present possibilities of evaluation of renal
parenchyma (10). Therefore, groups of pediatric nephrologists,
urologists, and radiologists cooperating in great hospitals
as well in the United States as in Europe decided independently
from each other to perform a randomised collaborative therapeutic trial. After some time of independent preparations, both
groups joined and assimilated their protocols to such a degree
that parallel studies with the possibility of data pooling
could be started.

QUESTION OF THE STUDY

Among the many important problems, we decided to confine ourselves to one question which can be expressed in the following
two ways:

Is there any difference in
    renal growth and scarring,
    renal function,
    risk of hypertension

between surgically and nonsurgically treated children with
moderate VUR ?

Does sterile moderate VUR
    prevent normal renal growth,
    cause renal damage,
    cause hypertension ?

ELIGIBLE AND EXCLUDED PATIENTS

First of all, we had to define moderate VUR. We worked out a
reflux grading system, adopting those published by Heikel and
Parkkulainen and by Dwoskin and Perlmutter to the present knowledge on the pathogenesis of reflux-correlated renal damage.
Grade I and II are not dilatating; grade I goes only into the
ureter, grade II into the renal pelvis. Clubbing of all calices
to such an extent that no papillary impressions remain demonstrable is defined as gross VUR (grade V). In the United States,
only children with grade IV which means with calyceal blunting
but with remaining of at least some papillary outlines have
been defined as eligible for the study. In Europe, beyond the
first year of life also children with grade III, that is dilatation of renal pelvis and calices with clearly visible papillary
outlines without calyceal blunting are eligible.

Regardless of their reflux grade, children with conditions listed in the following table are excluded from the study:

    Previous operations on the urinary tract, except
        meatotomies, urethral dilatation or internal
        urethrotomies.
    Obstruction of urine flow other than
        in males: meatal stenosis;
        in females: "bladder neck", meatal or urethral stenosis.
    Malformations of kidney or urinary tract.
    Solitary kidney.
    Neurogenic bladder disease.
    Clinical evidence of severe bladder dysfunction.

Anorectal anomalies.

Calculi.

Renal insufficiency.

Age more than 10 years.

The patients will be stratified for age, sex, condition of their renal parenchyma, and in Europe for reflux grades III and IV as well as history of previous UTI.

STUDY GROUPS

With these very restrictive criteria for patient selection, patient numbers big enough for statistical analysis can only be collected in a collaborative study. The USA study group consists of the following 17 major teaching institutions:

Albert Einstein College Hospital, Bronx, New York
Babies Hospital, Columbia University, New York, N.Y.
Childrens Hospital Medical Center, Boston, Mass.
Childrens Hospital, Chicago, Illinois
Childrens Hospital, Detroit, Michigan
Childrens Hospital, Philadelphia, Pennsylvania
Childrens Hospital, St. Louis, Missouri
Childrens Hospital, National Med. Center, Washington, D.C.
Downstate Medical Center, Brooklyn, N.Y.
Emory University, Atlanta, Georgia
Georgetown University, Washington, D.C.
John Hopkins School of Medicine, Baltimore, Maryland
Mayo Clinic, Rochester, Minn.
Texas Childrens Hospital
University of California School of Med.,Los Angeles,Calif.
University of California, San Diego, California
Childrens Hospital and Health Center, LaJolla, California
University of Florida, Gainesville, Florida,

PATIENT COLLECTION

144

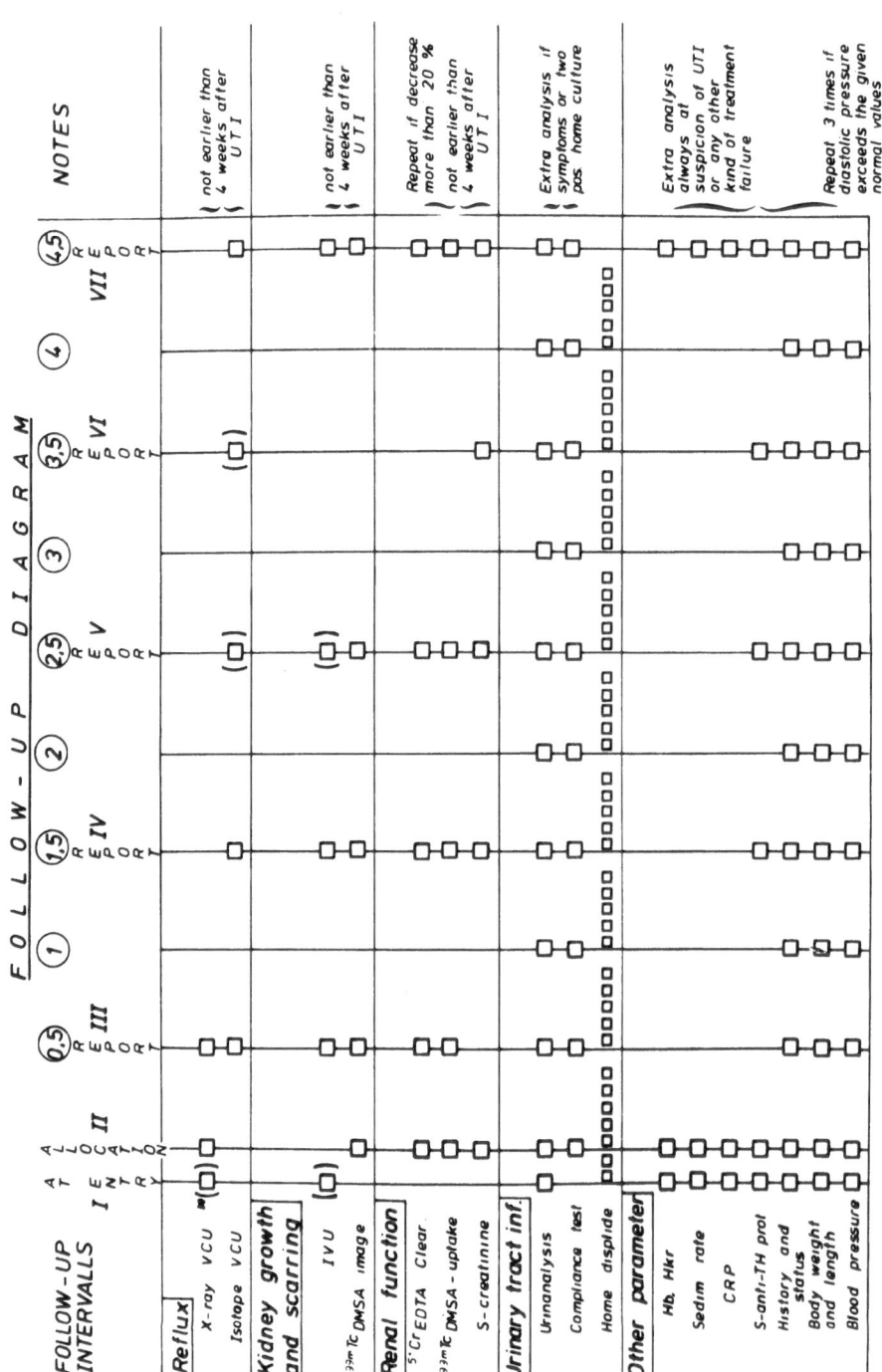

the European study group of the following 8 university hospitals:

Universitätsklinikum Essen, W.Germany

Östra Sjukhuset, Göteborg, Sweden

Universitätskliniken Graz, Austria

Universitätskliniken Hamburg, W.Germany

Medizinische Hochschule Hannover, W.Germany

University Childrens Hospital, Helsinki, Finland

Karolinska hospital, Dept. Ped. Surgery)
St. Göran's Childrens Hospital   )
Huddinge Sjukhuset, Stockholm   ) Stockholm,Sweden
Sach'ska Barnsjukhuset   )

Cliniques Universitaires de Bruxelles,Hopital Erasme,Belgium.

We expect that this structure of the two parallel study groups
will enable us to collect representative data instead of predominantly severe cases accumulating in so highly specialised
referring institutions as Stanford or, on the other side, more
favourable courses as obtainable only in places with ideal conditions of primary patient care as in Goeteborg.

STANDARDISATION OF METHODS AND RESULTS

Of course, we standardised the techniques and the expected results of the methods essential for the characterisation of the
primary state of our patients as well as their further course
under randomised management; this was rather easy for the techniques of X-ray- and isotope voiding cystourethrograms, i.v.-
urograms, urinalysis, urine culture and blood pressure measurements. Urograms and X-ray voiding cystograms will be centrally
evaluated; as an example I mention the method selected for
renal parenchymal measurement, published by Claesson,Jacobsson,
Olsson and Ringertz (2); by evaluating the ratio between the
height of L1 to L3, renal length, renal area and the thickness
of renal parenchyma in the upper and lower pole and at the
lateral margin, it seems to be possible to record very early
and to follow reliably renal parenchymal damage; particularly,
significant differences between both kidneys can be early
documented.

Cystoscopy, although not mandatory for nonsurgically treated
patients, is also standardised.

Global kidney function will be followed by measurements of
serum creatinine, in Europe additionally by single-injection
^{51}Cr-EDTA-clearances. The standardisation of the evaluation of
single kidney function was more problematic. In Europe we decided to use the ^{99m}Tc-DMSA-uptake test which, although newer,
is regarded as acceptable by our group.

PATIENT FOLLOW-UP

Regardless of surgical or nonsurgical management, identical
standardised examinations will be performed at the entry as
well as at prefixed dates during the follow-up of each patient.
Urinary tract infection will be treated adequately with antibiotics. At entry into the study, continuous antibiotic prophylaxis will be started and continued until six months after
the reflux has disappeared in the surgical as well as in the
nonsurgical group, drug compliance will be evaluated.

ETHICAL IMPLICATIONS

A randomised trial dealing with such dangerous conditions as
ours has to meet the highest ethical standard. Informed consent of parents and, if old enough, of children, is required
before randomisation. The following definitions of treatment
failure have been worked out, allowing free decision about
further treatment regardless of the previous randomisation.

1. Alarming Renal Failure

    The ^{51}Cr-EDTA-clearance of a single kidney
    is less than 50 % of its former value
    (estimated with ^{99m}Tc-DMSA uptake %).

2. Medical Failure

    2 pyelonephritic or }
    6 non-pyelonephritic) } bacteriuric episodes

    during follow-up

3. Surgical Failure

    Postoperative obstruction requiring
    reoperation

    Non-changed or worse reflux after
    operation.

The study protocol has been approved by the ethical committees
of participating hospitals, if already existing, and by the
reviewers of our sponsors. An external monitoring committee
follows our work and the literature so that the study can be
either changed or stopped, if necessary.

SAMPLE SIZE

The end points on which judgement of success or failure of
the two therapeutic regimens will rest are

    the development of new scars,
    the inhibition of renal growth,
    the development of hypertension,
    the development of renal failure.

Also, the changes of preexisting scars and recurrence rates
of urinary tract infection will be documented and analysed,
although the significance of these parameters may remain
less conclusive.

For an alpha error of 0.05 and a beta error of 0.80, and
assuming a difference of 10 % in the efficacy of the two
therapeutic regimens, 125 patients in each group will be
required. Estimates based on the patient numbers observed
during the last years in the participating hospitals indicate
that two years will be necessary to accumulate this number of
patients. The patients will be followed at least 5 years and,

148

if possible and necessary, 10 years. The data from the United
States are collected and analysed in the Albert Einstein College of Medicine, New York, those from Europe in the University Hospital Essen; the identity of most parts of our protocol allows pooling of most of the data.

Patient collection has been started in most participating
European hospitals during January 1980, by the others in
Europe and in the US during May 1980.
At the 20th September, 1980, the number of reported patients
was 54 in Europe and 7 in the US.
Probably, I can present first meaningful results during the
IPN-symposium after the next.

I hope that all of you and also I myself will be lucky enough
to see that day.

REFERENCES

1. Aladjem,M, Boichis H, Hertz M, Herzfeld S, Raviv U:
   The conservative management of vesicoureteric reflux:
   A review of 121 children. Pediatrics 65,78-80(1980)
2. Claesson,Jacobsson,Olsson,Ringertz: A computerized system
   for handling renal size measurements. Acta Radiol. 1981
   (accepted for publication).
3. Coleman JW, McGovern JH: Ureterovesical reimplantation
   in children.Surgical results in 491 children.
   Urol.XII,514(1978).
4. Friedland GW: Post-reimplantation in renal scarring.
   In: Hodson J,Kincaid-Smith P(Eds.): Reflux Nephropathy.
   Masson Publishing USA,Inc.1979,299-305.
5. Kincaid-Smith P, Becker,G: Reflux nephropathy and chronic
   atrophic pyelonephritis: A review. J.Infect.Dis.138,774(1978)
6. Marberger M,Altwein JE,Straub E,Wulff HD, Hohenfellner
   R: The Lich-Gregoir antireflux plasty:experiences with
   371 children. J.Urol. 120, 216 (1978).
7. Normand C,Smellie J.: Vesicoureteric reflux: The case for
   conservative management. In: Hodson J, Kincaid-Smith P
   (Eds.): Reflux Nephropathy.Masson Publ.USA Inc.1979,281-286.
8. Ransley PG: Vesicoureteric reflux: Continuing surgical
   dilemna. Urology 12, 246-255 (1978).
9. Strohmenger P, Mellin P, Olbing H: Die Bedeutung der Harn-
   stauung für das Ergebnis von Antirefluxoperationen.
   Urologe A, 10, 195 (1971).
10. Scott JES, Stansfeld JM: Treatment of vesico-ureteric re-
    flux inchildren. Arch.Dis.Child. 43, 323-328 (1968).

THE NATURAL HISTORY OF VESICO-URETERIC REFLUX

J.M. SMELLIE AND I.C.S. NORMAND

DEPARTMENTS OF PAEDIATRICS, UNIVERSITY COLLEGE HOSPITAL, LONDON
AND UNIVERSITY OF SOUTHAMPTON

The potential consequences of an incompetent vesico-ureteric valve are the transmission to the renal pelvis of organisms colonising the bladder and the intra-vesical voiding pressure. In addition residual urine will accumulate when refluxed urine returns to the bladder and is likely to facilitate recurring infection.

If vesico-ureteric (VUR) and urinary tract infection (UTI) are both present, the papillary morphology allows intrarenal reflux (IRR) and the renal pelvic pressure is sufficient to reverse the urine flow at the calyco-tubular junction, infection of the papilla can result. If treatment of the infection is delayed or inadequate, scarring may follow. Contraction of such a scar may deform adjacent papillae, thus leaving these areas susceptible to further damage (1).

In the obstructed urinary tract, the transmission of uninfected urine under high pressure may in itself cause the uniform thinning of renal tissue and blunting or clubbing of the calyces characteristic of obstructive atrophy. Although an important cause of impaired renal function, this aspect will not be considered further here.

All of these effects appear to be of greater significance in infancy and early childhood when the kidney is growing rapidly, a higher proportion of children are likely to have incompetent VU valves and because of mechanical factors the bladder voiding pressures may be higher.

In order to examine some of these hypotheses we have made prospective clinical and radiological observations over periods of 2-22 years on more than 200 children without overt obstruction who presented with symptomatic urinary infection and were found to have VUR. The management routine designed to keep the refluxing urinary tract free from infection has been continued so long as VUR has persisted and has been unchanged apart from

the introduction of newer antibacterial drugs. It consists of regular
complete bladder emptying,attention to bowel habits and fluid intake and
continuous low dosage prophylaxis while reflux is present and for a further
year. Urine cultures are performed three-monthly and limited radiological
studies every two years. Renal growth is assessed by relating serial renal
length measurements to the child's height (2).

PROSPECTIVE STUDY OF UNINFECTED VUR

In the first 75 children managed in this way, renal growth was within
normal limits in over 90% of kidneys and fresh scarring was minimal.
However there was a significant association of impaired renal growth in
kidneys drained by refluxing ureters and recurrence of infection during
follow-up (3).

We then examined renal growth in a larger group of 201 children
including 70 of these first 75 and excluding those with duplex kidneys.
302 kidneys with reflux were observed over a total of 1712 kidney years.
In 214 kidneys, 24 of which were scarred initially and 33 with severe
reflux with ureteric dilatation, there was no recurrence of urinary
infection. The increase in renal length fell short of expectation by more
than one centimetre over the whole period in only one kidney, and by 0.5
to 1 cm in 6 kidneys. Growth overall proceeded normally in 207 kidneys
including 21 with scarring and 30 with severe reflux. No fresh or extension
of scarring was seen in any of these kidneys.

Infection was not completely prevented by the medical regime outlined
and during the same period of observation 88 kidneys, 24 of these also
being scarred, were exposed to a recurrence of infection, 80 of them single
episodes. In 16 kidneys, 10 scarred, overall growth was slowed by one
centimetre or more and in a further 7 growth was slightly unsatisfactory.
This difference in renal growth from that seen when the urine remained
sterile is highly significant. Renal growth was normal in 65 of these
kidneys. Two fresh scars developed in this group in which infection recurred.

During these observations reflux has tended to improve progressively
and disappear (3). Cessation of reflux was most closely related to its
severity on presentation, VUR stopping in 85% of undilated and 40% of
dilated ureters. No significant relationship was found between infection
and the tendency for VUR to disappear. However this was least likely to
happen in kidneys which were small, scarred, drained by dilated ureters

and in which URI had a greater tendency to recur.

UNILATERAL REFLUX

Renal growth was also studied in 96 children with unilateral reflux.

When both kidneys were structurally normal, no significant difference in growth was found between the kidney with reflux and that without. The mean renal growth of 77 pairs of kidneys was +1.2mm and +1.0mm respectively in relation to the expected growth over the period of observation. When the unilateral reflux drained a scarred kidney, there was a significant difference in the growth of the two kidneys, the mean difference from that expected in 19 scarred kidneys with reflux being -1.2mm and in the unscarred kidneys without reflux being +8.8mm. This difference was highly significant as was the hypertrophy of the normal kidney in relation to expected growth (p < 0.001). A fresh scar appeared in two of these scarred kidneys, both associated with infection.

VUR disappeared on follow-up in 79 of the 96 refluxing ureters. In children with normal kidneys, reflux stopped in 90% of the ureters and in all of those followed for more than 5 years. It stopped in over half of those draining scarred kidneys.

VUR AND RECURRENT INFECTION

Divergent views have been held regarding the role of VUR in the aetiology of recurrent UTI and so we looked at the rate of recurrence of urinary infection in three groups of children who had close clinical and bacteriological follow-up for at least one year after stopping antibacterial therapy. In 22 children with radiologically normal urinary tracts, no further antibacterial treatment was given after a 7-10 day initial course, when the mean age of the group was 6.5 years. 46% were recurrence-free at the end of one year. Another group of 25 children with normal urinary tracts received 12 months' low-dosage antibacterial prophylaxis after their initial treatment. 68% of these children were recurrence-free 12 months after stopping prophylaxis at the mean age of 7.4 years (4). 105 children in whom VUR ceased received prophylaxis while the reflux was present and for one further year, that is for 3-12 years. The mean age of stopping prophylaxis was 11.7 years and one year later, 101 (96%) were recurrence-free.

The low recurrence rate in the group with VUR might be due to the longer period of prophylaxis, or to the children being slightly older when antibacterial treatment stopped. It might also suggest that a major cause of the earlier recurrent infections in these children has been removed with the disappearance of reflux, whereas other causes such as constipation and faulty bladder emptying had persisted or recurred in the children with radiologically normal urinary tracts.

RENAL SCARRING

Renal scarring is usually already established by the time the child presents and more severe scarring is usually seen in the younger children with more severe reflux. The "obstructive atrophy" type of scarring is most often seen in infant boys with gross reflux, though irregular focal scarring can be identified at any age and with any severity of VUR (5).

Fresh scarring both in our experience and in most published reports has followed infection in the refluxing urinary tract. No new scars developed in 214 children with sterile reflux, though 2 scars developed in 88 kidneys with reflux which were exposed to further infection. Three other children were observed to develop a scar as a result of them presenting symptomatic infection. In the Cardiff-Oxford study no scarring developed in bacteriuric schoolgirls with VUR and normal kidneys, although new scars developed in a number of schoolgirls with reflux and covert bacteriuria who already had scarred kidneys (6).

VUR tends to be transient but the potential effects of its association with infection in the young child are permanent and may lead to later hypertension.

Ransley and Risdon (7) have shown experimentally in the piglet that the development of scars may be modified by antibacterial treatment. Thus it is essential to recognise early and treat adequately all UTI in infants and young children. Prevention of recurrent infection can readily be accomplished in the unobstructed urinary tract by detailed attention to voiding, drinking and bowel habits together with continuous low-dosage antibacterial prophylaxis.

CONCLUSION

We have not obtained evidence from these studies that VUR is damaging either to the child's health or to his renal growth or structure unless it is accompanied by either raised bladder pressure or infection.

If an unobstructed urinary tract in which reflux occurs can be kept free from infection (and this is possible with modern prophylaxis and good compliance in about 90% of children) then normal renal growth can be expected in almost every kidney and scars will not develop or extend.

Infection had no significant effect upon the likelihood of VUR stopping which will happen in time in over 80% of undilated and 40% of dilated ureters and in almost every child with unilateral reflux into a normal kidney. Infection did have a significant association with impaired renal growth if VUR was present. This association was mainly seen in kidneys which were scarred at the outset. The only new scars which developed followed infections in a refluxing urinary tract.

Nevertheless in a study of 302 kidneys with reflux in children managed conservatively, renal growth overall was within one centimetre of that expected in 94%.

An optimal programme for the care of children with VUR must take into account many factors such as age, severity of VUR, complexities of temperament and compliance of both the child and his family. Raised bladder pressure due to obstruction is largely a surgical problem and infection is mainly a problem for the paediatrician. The most satisfactory result for the individual child and his kidneys will emerge from the informed understanding collaboration between the paediatrician and the surgeon such as is becoming well established within the International Vesico-ureteral Reflux Study.

REFERENCES

1. Ransley PC, Risdon RA. 1978. Reflux and renal scarring. British Journal of Radiology: Supplement No. 14.
2. Hodson CJ. 1979. Reflux nephropathy: scoring the damage. In Reflux Nephropathy ed. Hodson J. and Kincaid Smith P. Masson Publishing U.S.A. Inc. 29-47.
3. Edwards D, Normand ICS, Prescod N. Smellie JM. 1977. Disappearance of vesico-ureteric reflux during longterm prophylaxis of urinary tract infection in children. Brit.Med.J. 2:285-288.
4. Smellie JM, Katz G, Grüneberg RN. 1978. Controlled trial of prophylactic treatment in childhood urinary tract infection. Lancet 2:175.
5. Smellie JM, Edwards D, Hunter N, Normand ICS, Prescod N. 1975. Vesico-ureteric reflux and renal scarring. Kidney International 8:S65.
6. Cardiff-Oxford Bacteriuria Study Group. 1978. Sequelae of covert bacteriuria in schoolgirls - A four year follow-up study. Lancet 1:889.
7. Ransley PG, Risdon RA. 1980. Proceedings at the Fifth International Symposium of Pediatric Nephrology.

CONTROLLED CLINICAL TRIALS - INTRODUCTION

HENRY L. BARNETT

The goal of this symposium on controlled clinical trials in pediatric nephrology and urology is two-fold. First, to present the design and, when possible, some results of several surveys and trials in progress. Second, to seize the opportunity to stress the importance of medical surveys and controlled clinical trials and, perhaps, most importantly, to examine some of the principles and practices of their design and methods. We are very fortunate in having Dr. Curtis Meinert as a participant in the symposium. Dr. Meinert is Editor-in-Chief of the new Journal, Controlled Clinical Trials, the official Journal of the newly-found Society for Clinical Trials. We have asked Dr. Meinert to discuss design and methods for controlled clinical trials, drawing examples, wherever possible, from the studies presented by the other participants.

One comment before we begin. Sir Thomas Lewis, in 1933[1], suggested that clinical research should be extended to include the statistical study of large groups of patients for the purpose of determining prognosis and treatment as an essential part of what he termed clinical science. He, as well as Bradford Hill, in 1937[2], included in their concept of this aspect of clinical science medical surveys as well as controlled clinical trials. The sudden and continuing flow of new and powerful remedies since 1940 has required that the focus be on controlled clinical trials, perhaps to some neglect of medical surveys. If so, it is unfortunate, since properly designed and conducted surveys can serve to refine the questions asked in clinical trials. For example, medical surveys may identify more homogeneous subgroups within a heterogeneous diagnostic category. A controlled clinical trial of treatment of patients in such a subgroup may very well detect differences that would not have been revealed in a trial on all patients in the more heterogeneous diagnostic category. In addition, medical surveys may disclose associations that provide clues concerning pathogenesis and etiology that raise new questions for investigators in other areas of biomedical research.

In the program to follow, the design of two controlled clinical trials and one medical survey will be presented together with a discussion of some selected problems encountered in the studies of the International Study of Kidney Disease in Children (ISKDC). These presentations will be followed by Dr. Meinert's discussion and a period for questions and comments from the audience.

REFERENCES

1. Lewis T. 1933. Clinical Science. Brit. Med. J., ii, 717.

2. Hill AB. 1937. Principles of Medical Statistics

3. CLINICAL SURVEY OF HEPATITIS B ANTIGENEMIA ASSOCIATED NEPHRO-
PATHY IN CHILDREN

A Report of the Asian Study of Renal Disease in Children

INTRODUCTION

Since a case report of HB antigenemia associated nephropathy
(abbr.:HB NP) in an adult,occuring after a blood transfusion(Combes
,B.et al.,1971)(1),information on this nephropathy has been increa
sing. The first pediatric patients were reported by Brozosko,W.J.
et al.(1974) in 18 children(2). Although the high incidence of renal diseases in HB positive Japanese children was emphasized by
Shingo,S.(1973)(3),the first description of HB NP in Japanese child
-ren was reported by Uraoka,Y. et al.(1977)(4). Since then the
number of reports of HB NP in pediatric patients is increasing.

Hattori,S. and Matsuda,I.et al. presented the first nationwide
survey of HB NP(5)(1978) which motivated us to initiate this cooperative medical survey.

Contact with the International Study of Kidney Disease in Child-
dren (ISKDC) was made through its director,Barnett,H.L.,when he
was invited to The 14th Annual Meeting,Japanese Society of Pediatric Nephrology,Kurume,Japan,1979 as a guest speaker on "Controlled
Clinical Trial".

The purpose of the survey was to study the epidemiology,natu-
ral history,clinical feature and the pathogenesis of this nephropathy. We did not start a clinical trial at this time for three
reasons:(1) The natural history was not clear;(2)Membranous nephropathy,the most frequent form of the associated glomerular diseases
has high spontaneous remission rate*in children;(3)The effects of
steroids on the host with HB antigenemia and possibly on some form
of immunodeficient state were not elucidated.(*Habib,R.et al.)(6)

PATIENTS AND METHODS

The distribution of 40 HB NP patients in 10 centers in Japan and in Korea is shown in Table 1.

Table 1. Distribution of patients in participating centers

Centers		Directors	Number of cases
#1	National Nishi-Sapporo H.(Sapporo)	Kadowaki,J.	0
2	Tokyo Metropolitan Children's H.(Tokyo)	Ito,H.	6
3	Nihon Univ.Surugadai H.(Tokyo)	Kitagawa,T.	0
4	Kitasato Univ.Hospital(Kanagawa)	Sakai,T.	2
5	Nihon Medical College H.(Tokyo)	Murakami,M.	2
6	National Medical Center H.(Tokyo)	Yamaguchi,M.	2
7	Niigata Univ.Hospital(Niigata)	Sakai,K.	1
8	Kurume Univ.H.(Kurume)	Yamashita,F.	11
9	Kumamoto U.H.(Kumamoto)	Matsuda,I.	9
10	Seoul Univ.H.(Seoul)	Ko,K.W.	7

The criteria for selection of patients were (1)The presense of the evidences of renal abnormalities in a patients with positive HB_s antigenemia with or without abnormal liver function judged by elevated serum GOT and GPT more than 41 Karmen units;(2)Exclusion of other causes for the renal abnormalities.

METHODS

Light (HE,PAS and PAM) and electronmicroscopic examinations were performed.in renal biopsy specimens.Immunofluorescent staining(IF) was processed in local laboratories,except the staining of e-antigen which was done by Mayumi,T.,Tokyo Metropolitan Insttitute for Clinical Medicine and Jichi Medical College.

Serum HB antigens and antibodies were also analyzed by Maymi, T. and in local laboratories. Serum C3 was analyzed by Partigen,(Behringer).For the determination of circulating immune complex, Raji Cell and/or C1q binding assay were used.

RESULTS

1. THE DISTRIBUTION OF PATIENTS AMONG HISTOLOGICAL CATEGORIES, AGE AND SEX (Table 2)

Of the 40 patients with HB NP,24 (60%) had Membranous Glomerulonephritis(MGN) and 8 (20%) had Minimal Change(MC).There were 4 patients with Membranoproliferative Glomerulonephritis(MPGN), 2 with Proliferative Glomerulonephritis (PGN) and one each

with Focal Global Sclerosis(FGS),and Advanced Glomerulonephritis
(Adv.). The ratio of male to female was 35 to 5 for the entire
series;it was 23:1 for patients with MGN and 5:3 for those with
MC. The difference in the male and female ratio in patients with
MGN and MC was statisticaly significant(p= $\geq$ 0.05).

Table 2. HB NP by histology,age and sex

Histology	N(%)	Sex	Age:3-5	6-8	9-11	12-14	15-18	Total	(%)
MGN	24	(60)	M	5	4	5	2	7	23	(95.8)
			F					1	1	(4.2)
							Total		24	(100)
MPGN	4	(10)	M		1	1	1	1	4(no female)
PGN	2	(5)	M		1				1	
			F			1			1	
MC	8	(20)	M	1		1	1	2	5	(62.5)
			F		1	1	1		3	(37.5)
							Total		8	(100)
FGS	1	(2.5)	M		1				1(no female)
Adv.	1	(2.5)	M					1	1(no female)
			M	6	7	7	4	11	35	(87.5)
			F		1	2	1	1	5	(12.5)
			Total	6	8	9	5	12	40	(100)

2.MODE OF DETECTION (Table 3)

The presenting findings at the detection among 40 patients
were urinary abnormalities during screening of school children or
by the chance in 47.6%,edema in 35.7%,macrohematuria in 12 %,and
urinary abnormalities found in patients with hepatitis in 4.8%.

Table 3. Mode of detection of HB NP patients

Mode of detection	Histology:MGN	MPGN	PGN	MC	FGS	Adv.	Total	(%)
During hepatitis	1			1			2	(4.8)
As a career							0	
Macroscopic hematuria	2*	1		1		1*	5	(11.9)
Chance proteinuria	2		1	2			5	(11.9)
Chance hematuria	1			3			4	(9.5)
Chance proteinuria & hematuria	7	3	1				11	(26.2)
Edema	12*			1	1	1*	15	(35.7)
Total Items	25*	4	2	8	1	2*	42*	(100)

In Table 3,total number of item was counted as 42 instead 40 which was the actual number of patients,because one of each with MGN and Adv. were detected by the appearance of both macrohematuria and edema.

3.CLINICAL FEATURES

Urinalysis at the time of detection(Table 4)showed hematuria combined with proteinuria in 25 of toal 40 patients and in 20 of 24 MGN(83.3%).Isolated hematuria or proteinuria was observed only in the patients with MC.The amounts of proteinuira were variable.

Table 4.Urinary findings at the time of detection

Urinary findings / Histology:	MGN	MPGN	PGN	MC	FGS	Adv.	Total(%)
isolated proteinuria	2	1	2	1	1		7 (17.5)
isolated hematuria	2			6			8 (20.0)
combined(hematuria & protein- uria)	20	3	0	1	0	1	25 (62.5)
Total number	24	4	2	8	1	1	40 (100)

The nephrotic syndrome sometime occured during the course of the disease in 22 of 40 patients. In 20 of those it was persistent. In the remaining 2 it was transient. Kidney function judged by BUN and serum creatinine concentration was within normal limits in all patients. Serum GOT and GPT were abnormaly high in about half of the patients(Table 5,6).

Table 5.Nephrotic syndrome by histology

Nephrotic syndrome	Histology:MGN	PGN	PGN	MC	FGS	Adv.	Total(%)
persistent	14	1	1	2	1	1	20 (55)
transient	2						2 (5)
non-nephrotic	8	3	1	6			18 (62.5)

Table 6. Liver function

GOT or GPT:	30-40	41-60	61-100	101-200	200-1000	Total
GOT	15	8	6	6	1	36
(%)	(41.6)	(22.2)	(16.7)	(16.7)	(2.8)	(100)
GPT	21	3	6	5	2	37
(%)	(56.8)	(*.1)	(16.2)	(13.5)	(5.4)	(100)

4.IMMUNOLOGICAL FINDINGS

e-Antigenemia was present in 11 of 18 patients with MGN;3 of 4 with MPGN;2 Of 7 with MC. The differences between MC and MGN and between MC and MPGN were both statisticaly significant.Anti-eAntigen was present in 6 of 30 patients(Table 7).

Table 7.HB antigen,antibody in serum by histology(positive/N)

Antigen/antibody Histology	MGN	MPGN	PGN	MC	FGS	Adv.	Total(%)
HBs	24/24	4/4	2/2	8/8	1/1	1/1	40/40(100
Anti-HBs	0/21	0/3	0/1	1/8	0/1	0/1	1/35(2.9
e Antigen	11/18	3/4	1/2	2/7	-	-	17/31(54.8
(%)	(61.8)	(75)		(28.6)			
Anti-e	3/17	1/4	0/2	2/7	-	-	6/30(20.C
Anti-HBc	9/9	1/1	-	4/5	-	-	14/15(99.3

HBs antigenemia and e-antigenemia disappeared in 8 of 40(20%) and in 3 of 7(17.6%) respectively. Anti HBs appeared in 2 of 40 (5%),antiHBc in 2 of 35(6.7%) and anti-e was 3 of 24(12.5%). Subtype of HBs antigenemia was divided in adr(N=9),adw(N=3) in 12 patients examined without the deviation in histological categories

Low levels of serum C3 were found(Table 8) in 6 of 40(15%). There was no significant difference among the histological catego-ries.

Table 8.Serum complement(C3) by histology

Level of serum C3/Histology:	MGN(%)	MPGN	PGN	MC	FGS	Adv.	Total(%)
low(M-2SD) (≦50)	3(12.5)	2	1				6 (15)
Borderline(M-1SD)(≦70)	4(16.7)	1		2			7 (17.5)
normal (≧ 71)	17(70.8)	1		1	6	1	1 27 (67.5)
Total (%)	24(100)	4		2	8	1	1 40 (100)

Circulating immune complexes were detected in 12 of 15 or 80 % of patients in whom it was measured.They found in 7 of 9 or 77.8 % of patients with MGN.

Immunostaining of renal biopsy specimens was positive for IgG in 16 of 24 patients,for IgA in 3 of 24,for IgM in 11 of 22,for C3 in 16 of 24,for HBs antigen in 2 of 20 and for e-antigen in 8 of 13(Table 9).

e-antigen,C3,IgG,A,and IgM were stained at glomerular basement membrane mainly in diffuse,granular pattern with few exception. HBs antigen was positive only in 2 patients,one each with MC and MGN.

Table 9 Immunostaining of renal biopsy specimen

Stainings	−	±	+	++	+++	N(examined)	+/N (% positive)
IgG	8		7		9	24	16/24(66.7)
IgA	21		2		1	24	3/24(12.5)
IgM	11		11			22	11/22(50)
C3	7	1	9	1	6	24	16/24(66.7)
HBs Ag	17	1	2			10	2/10(20)
e−Ag	5		8			13	8/13(61.5)

5. STAGE OF MGN AND THE TYPE OF MPGN

Sixteen patients with MGN showed the stage II in 4; II-III in 2; III in 7 and III-IV in 3. Three patients with MPGN were classified in type III and it was unknown in remaining one patient with MPGN.

6. CLINICAL EVOLUTION

Among 7 patients with hematuria alone, 3 impoved and 4 were stationary in urinary findings. Among those presenting with both hematuria and proteinuria, 3 of 9 improved and 6 were stationary (Table 10).

Table 10. Clinical evolution: improvement in urinary findings

Urinary findings /Histology:		MGN	MPGN	PGN	MC	FGS	Adv.	Total (%)
Hematuria	improved	1			2			3 (42.9)
	stationary					4		4 (57.1)
Proteinuria	improved			1				1
	stationary		1					1
Combined	improved	2	1					3 (33.3)
	stationary	4	2					6 (66.7)

Nineteen of 22 nephrotic patients were treated with steroid. Complete remission occured in 12 of 19, 9 of whom had MGN. Four patients had partial remission, 2 with MGN, and one each with MPGN and Adv. (Table 11). One patient with FGS responded but had frequent relapses. One patient with MGN was stationary and one other died of hepatic failure.

Table 11.Steroid response in nephrotic patients with HB NP

Responses or course/Histology:	MGN (%)	MFGN	PGN	MC	FGS	Adv.	N (%)
complete remission	9(69.2)		1	2			12(63.2)
"proteinuria only"	1(7.7)	1				1	3(15.8)
imcomplete remission	1(7.7)						1(5.3)
stationary	1(7.7)						1(5.3)
frequent relapser					1		1(5.3)
death	1(7.7)						1(5.3)
total	13(100)	1	1	2	1	1	19(100)

DISCUSSION AND SUMMARY

We would like to emphasize the following features observed in this series of 40 patients with HB NP. (1)Half of the patients were detected by chance mainly by urinary screening in school.(2) The male -female sex ratio of 7to 1 is higher than that reported in any other type of renal diseases in children. (3)High proportion of patients had MGN which accounted for 24 or 6o% of 40. (4) Nineteen of 20 patients who had nephrotic syndrome at some time during the course were treated with steroid and of these 19,12 had complete remission.(5)There was high incidence of e-antigenemia,of positive circulating immune complexes and of positive e-antigen stainings in renal tissues.(6)These results suggests that e-antigenemia might have important role in the pathogenesis of HB NP, especially in those with MGN and MFGN in whom the frequency of e-antigenemia was higher than in patients with MC.

Tekekoshi,Y.et al (1978)(7) speculated that MGN in Japanese children is mainly caused by HB virus because they found the high incidence of positive HBs antigenemia in MGN(11/11:100%) compared with other types(4.6%) in 163 biopsied specimens.These results were confirmed by Yamashita,F.et al.(1979)(8),Hattori,S.,Matsuda,I. and Ito,H.et al.(1979)(9),Same results were reported from France (Kleinknecht,et al.,1979)(10). Tekoshi,Y,and Mayumi,M.et al.,proposed that e-antigen and antibody immune complex might play important role in the pathogenesis of MGN in children,because e-Ag IC was positive in glomerular capillary wall in 2 renal specimens (1979) (11). Ito,H.,Matsuda,I.,Hattori,Mayumi,M.et al*confirmed the high incidence of positive e-Ag by IF in glomeruli in MGN in more larger series(1980)(12,13)*.(Those patients were included in this survey)

HB Nephropathy will be a good model to elucidate the pathogenesis of the MGN and other glomerulonephropathy in children.Further detailed investigation including the observation of the correlation of the behaviour of HB virus associated antigen or antibody and the clinical sign and symptoms will be necessarily.
(Asian Study of Renal Disease in Children:ASRDC

Members:Kadowaki,J., Ito,H.,Kitagawa,T.,Sakai,T.,Murakami,M.,

Yamaguchi,M.,Sakai,K.,Yamashita,F.,Matsuda,I.,Ko,W.K.,

Consultants:Barnett,H.L.,(New York),Bernstein,J,(Pathology,

Detroit),Okada,M.(Pathology,Tokyo),Sakaguchi,H.(pathology,Tokyo),

Kim,Y.I.(Pathology,Seoul),Mayumi,M.(Virology,Tokyo)

Coordinator:Yamashita,F.Dep.of Ped.,School of Medicine,Kurume Univ..

67,Asahi-machi,Kurume City,Japan 830)

REFERENCES

1.Combes,B.et al.,Glomerulonephritis with deposition of Austrarian antigen-antibody complexes in glomerular basement membrane, Lancet,2:234-237,1971.
2.Brozosko,W.J.,et al.Glomerulonephritis associated with hepatitis B surface antigen immune complex in children,Lancet,2:477-481,1974.
3.Shingu,T.,Austraria antigen and nephritis,in Gendai-Shonikagaku Taikei,Supp.(1972 a)pp 366-387,1973(in Japanese),Nakayama Shoten, Tokto.
4.Uraoka,Y.et al.,A infant with MGN in the family with positive HB antigen,Shonika,18:1063-1068,1977(in Japanese)

5.Hattori,S.,Matsuda,I.,et al.Nationwide survey on HBs nephropathy,The 14th Annual Meeting of Japanese Society of Pediatric Nephrology,Kurume,1978
6.Habib,R.et al.,Membranous glomerulonephritis in children,Edelman,C.M.,Jr. ed. Pediatric Kidney Disease,Little Brown,Boston,1978
7.Takekoshi,Y.et al.,Strong association between membranous nephropathy and hepatitis-B surface antigenemia in Japanese children, Lancet,2:1065-1068,1978
8.Yamashita,F.Matsuo,H.et al.,HB antigen associated nephropathy in children,The 1st Asian Pacific Congress of Nephrology,Tokyo, 1979
9.Hattori,S.,Matsuda,I.,Ito,H. et al.,Clinicopathological study in children with positive HB antigen(Abstract,in Japanese),The 22nd Annual Meeting of The Japanese Society of Nephrology,Tokyo, 1979.
10.Kleinknecht,C.et al.,Membranous nephritis and hepatitis surface antigen in children,J.Ped.,95:946-952,1979.
11.Takekoshi,Y,Mayumi,M.et al.,Free "small" andIgG-associated "large hepatitis B e antigen in the serum and glomerular capillary walls of two patients with membranous glomerulonephritis,New Eng. J.Med.,300:814-819,1979

12.Ito,H.et al.,The role of HB e antigenemia in the pathogenesis of HB associated membranous nephritis',The 5th International Symposium on Pediatric Nephrology,Philadelphia,1980
13.Hattori,S.Furuse,A.et al.,Membranous Glomerulonephritis and HB e antigen,ibid.,1980

CYCLOPHOSPHAMIDE VERSUS CHLORAMBUCIL IN THE TREATMENT OF
FREQUENTLY RELAPSING AND STEROID-DEPENDENT NEPHROTIC
SYNDROME.
A co-operative study of the "Arbeitsgemeinschaft für
pädiatrische Nephrologie".

H.P. KROHN, Hanover, West Germany.

Several patients with steroid responsive minimal change
nephrotic syndrome (MLNS) must be treated with cytotoxic
drugs because of side-effects of previous steroid therapy.
The aim of the study reported here is to compare the
effectiveness and the side-effects of the two most widely
used cytotoxic drugs, Cyclophosphamide (CP) and
Chlorambucil (CHL), in these patients. (1)

The definitions of nephrotic syndrome, relapse,
remission and the therapeutic regimen in this study are
determined according to the International Study of Kidney
Disease in Children (2). As a result of our previous
Steroid Study I (3), however, in the present study the
group of "frequently relapsing nephrotic syndrome" is
sub-divided into patients with frequently relapsing
nephrotic syndrome without steroid dependency, and in
those with steroid dependency. The first group will be
referred to as "frequent relapsers" (FRNS), the second
group as "steroid dependent" (SDNS).

By definition, a patient is steroid dependent when 2
consecutive relapses occur during standard relapse therapy
or within 14 days after cessation of steroid therapy
(fast relapse), or when 2 out of 4 relapses within a
period of 6 months are fast relapses. Patients, qualified
for the study, were recorded in the central office
(Hanover) and each of the two groups, FRNS and SDNS, were
randomised separately. The allocation of the patients
was selected by chance.

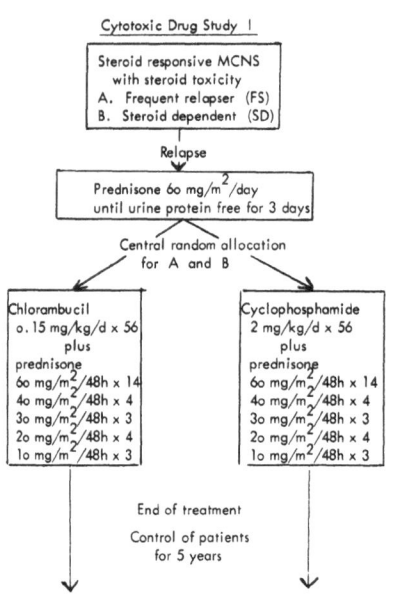

Figure 1.
Protocol of the study.

Remission of nephrotic syndrome was induced in the single patient with standard relapse Predni-sone therapy (Figure 1). After urine was protein-free for 3 days, cytotoxic therapy consisting of Cyclophosphamide 2.0 mg/kg body weight or Chlorambucil 0.15 mg/kg body weight was started and steroid therapy was tapered down consecutively. All therapy was discontinued after 8 weeks, and the patients were to be followed for proteinuria and side-effects over a period of 5 years.

The duration of remission of nephrotic syndrome following cytotoxic therapy is used as the only criterion of the effectiveness of cytotoxic therapy. Acute side-effects of the therapy are recorded as blood smear alteration, hemorrhagic cystitis, alopecia and infections. Long-time side-effects, such as gonadal toxicity, should be monitored over a period of 5 years.

53 patients entered the study. 16 of them had suffered from frequent relapses, 37 were steroid dependent. In the group of FRNS 8 patients were treated with Chlorambucil, 8 with Cyclophosphamide. In the group of SDNS 17 children were treated with Chlorambucil, 20 with Cyclophosphamide. Of the latter group 3 patients had to be withdrawn because their treatment did not follow protocol. The groups were comparable in sex, age and duration of

nephrotic syndrome before entry into the study.

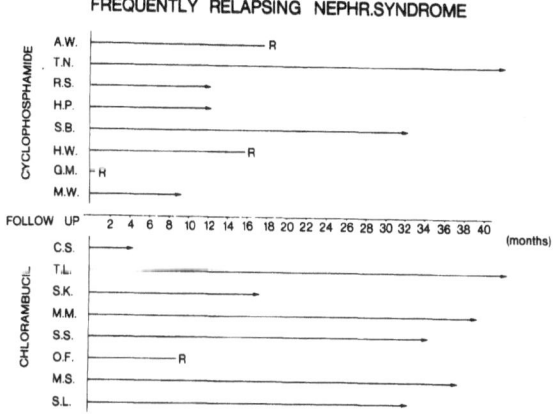

Figure 2.
Course of 16
patients with
FRNS following
cytotoxic
therapy.
R = relapse
→ in remission

The clinical course of all patients with FRNS following
cytotoxic therapy is documented in Figure 2. In the group
of CP-treated patients 3 patients had a relapse 1, 16 and
18 months after cessation of cytotoxic therapy. 5 patients
are in remission after 9, 12, 32 and 42 months without
therapy. In the CHL-treated group only 1 out of 8 patients
relapsed 9 months after the end of therapy. 7 patients
remained in remission up to 42 months. Life table
analysis shows that there is no significant difference
in the outcome between CP and CHL treatment in FRNS.

The course of nephrotic syndrome in patients with
SDNS is depicted in Figure 3. Following CP therapy 13 out
of 18 patients suffered a relapse of nephrotic syndrome,
most of them within 6 months after cessation of therapy.
A remission of nephrotic syndrome lasting longer than 12
months is documented in only 2 patients. After cessation
of CHL therapy 11 out of 16 patients suffered a relapse
of nephrotic syndrome within 6 months. Only 1 patient
has remained in remission of NS for a period of more than
12 months. There is no difference in the duration of
remission of nephrotic syndrome following Cyclophosphamide
or Chlorambucil therapy in patients with SDNS. Only 20 %

168

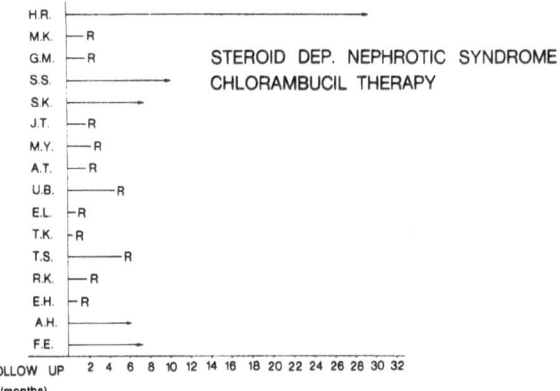

STEROID DEP. NEPHROTIC SYNDROME
CHLORAMBUCIL THERAPY

Figure 3.
Course of 34
patients with
SDNS following
cytotoxic
therapy.
R = relapse
→ in remission

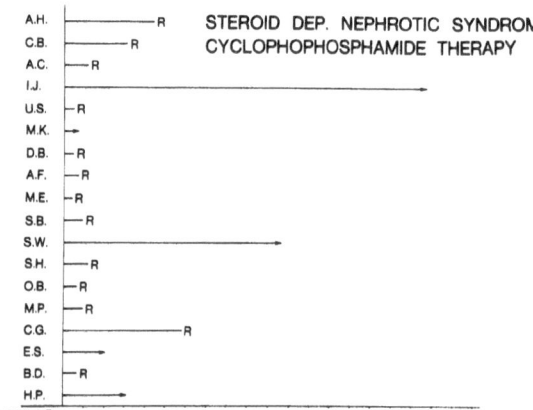

STEROID DEP. NEPHROTIC SYNDROME
CYCLOPHOPHOSPHAMIDE THERAPY

of patients
remain in re-
mission 2 years
after therapy.

Figure 4.
Remission
of Neph-
rotic
Syndrome
following
cytotoxic
therapy
in FRNS
and SDNS
documen-
ted as
life sur-
vival rate

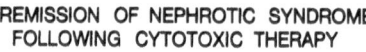

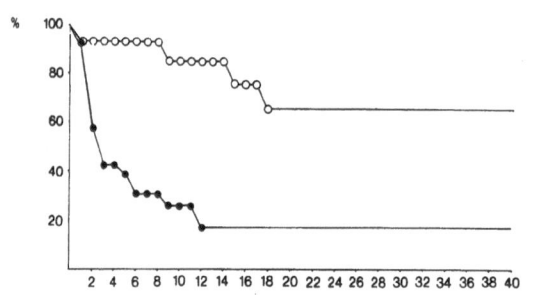

REMISSION OF NEPHROTIC SYNDROME
FOLLOWING CYTOTOXIC THERAPY

• STEROID DEPENDENT NEPHROTIC SYNDROME
○ FREQUENTLY RELAPSING NEPHROTIC SYNDROME

If one compares the effectiveness of the same cytotoxic therapy (CP and CHL) in patients with FRNS and in
those with SDNS (Figure 4), there is a significant difference in the response. There is a long-lasting effect
in patients with FRNS, i.e., 66 % of patients were still
in remission 2 years after treatment. Some patients suffered relapses after a period of remission lasting 10 to
12 months and only 1 patient had a relapse 1 month after
cessation of therapy. On the contrary, patients with SDNS
continued to suffer from frequent relapses within 3 to 6
months after cessation of cytotoxic therapy and only 3 had
remissions after more than 20 months.

Acute side-effects of Cyclophosphamide and Chlorambucil therapy were recorded rarely in both groups.
Alterations in blood smear such as leucocytopenia (less
than 3,000 per mm^3) (n = 6), thrombocytopenia (less than
100,000 per mm^3) (n = 8) or lymphocytopenia (less than
1,000 per mm^3) (n = 21) were reversible within some weeks.
Hemorrhagic cystitis was never seen. Mild alopecia and
infections were documented in a few patients treated with
both drugs. Differences in acute side-effects of Cyclophosphamide and Chlorambucil therapy were not significant.
In 3 patients cytotoxic therapy had to be interrupted for
up to 14 days, but in no case were side-effects severe
enough to require cessation of therapy.

The results of the cytotoxic drug study of APN
document that Cyclophosphamide and Chlorambucil, when given
for 8 weeks in a dosage of 2 mg/kg or 0.15 mg/kg per day
respectively, are effective in producing long-lasting
remissions in patients with FRNS without steroid dependency
but are ineffective in patients with SDNS. No difference
could be found in the effectiveness of the two drugs
studied in respect of the prevention of relapses, and
there were no differences in the acute complication rate.

LITERATUR:

1. BRODEHL, J.:
   Steroide oder Zytostatika beim kindlichen nephrotischen
   Syndrom.
   Klin. Pädiat. <u>184</u>, 241 (1972).

2. ABRAMOWICZ, C.M., ARNEIL, G.C., BARNETT, H.L., BARRON,
   B.A., EDELMANN, C.M., GORDILLO-P G., GREIFER, I.,
   HALLMANN, N., KOBAYASHI, O., TIDDENS, H.A.:
   Controlled trial of azathioprine in children with
   nephrotic syndrome.
   Lancet I : 959 - 961 (1970).

3. Arbeitsgemeinschaft für Pädiatrische Nephrologie (1979):
   Alternate-day versus intermittent prednisone in
   frequently relapsing nephrotic syndrome.
   Lancet I : 401 - 403 (1979).

ANTICOAGULANT VERSUS NO SPECIFIC TREATMENT IN CHILDHOOD HEMOLYTIC
UREMIC SYNDROME. A RANDOMIZED PROSPECTIVE STUDY.

W. PROESMANS, P. BINDA KI MUAKA, B. VAN DAMME, J. VERMYLEN,
R. VLIETINCK and R. EECKELS. University of Leuven, Leuven, Belgium

1. INTRODUCTION

The appropriate management of fluid and electrolyte disturbances has led to a dramatic decrease of acute mortality in childhood
hemolytic uremic syndrome (H U S). The value of additional anticoagulant therapy therefore has been seriously question. ed but
whether or not anticoagulants are useful especially with regard to
the long-term evolution of kidney function in the surviving patients
has not been established. We have approached this problem by a
prospective at random study which started in June 1976 and is still
in progress now. Thirty-nine patients have entered the study so far.

2. PATIENTS, MATERIALS, METHODS

All patients, up to the age of 15, entering the University
Childrens'Hospital during the acute phase of the H U S, are allo-
cated at random (sealed envelopes system) to one of two different
therapeutical schedules : the one consists of supportive therapy
only (to be referred to as the CONTR group) the other comprises in
addition the administration of heparin and dipyridamole (further
to be referred to as the +ANT group). All other therapeutic measures are standardized as much as possible as described in the protocol. Dipyridamole is given intravenously, twice daily at a dose
of 1 mg per kg body weight per day. Heparin is given four-hourly as
an intravenous shot, starting with a dose of 2 mg per kg body
weight. The dose is adjusted according to the clotting time which
is maintained between 10 and 15 minutes. This allows, after
72 hours to estimate the daily heparin requirement which is given
in four intravenous injections, the clotting time being assessed
from now on only once a day, four hours after the first morning

injection.

Anticoagulants are started as soon as the diagnosis is established. They are withdrawn when the number of platelets exceeds 150,000 per mm^3 together with a normalization of the fibrin/fibrinogen degradation products in blood and urine.

Before dismissal, a percutaneous renal biopsy is performed which is examined by conventional light microscopy and immunofluorescence. The pathologist analizes the biopsies without knowledge of the clinical history or the therapy.

3. RESULTS

The CONTR group is made of 20 infants and children, the + ANT group of 19 patients. Both groups are almost identical with regard to the following features : prodromes, age distribution, hematological data, serum creatinine level on admission, number of transfusions, number of cases treated with peritoneal dialysis and hemodialysis and the duration of the hospital stay. They were, however, striking differences in 1) the severity of the disease (more severe cases being found in the + ANT group) and 2) in blood pressure (severe hypertension was present in 7 patients of the CONTR group but in none of the + ANT group)(Table 1). The duration of the anticoagulant therapy varied from 4 to 22 days with a median of 11 days. Complication of the anticoagulant therapy have been few and in one patient severe enough to necessitate temporary interruption of the drugs.

3.1. Immediate outcome

Despite vigourous symptomatic therapy, there has been one death in the CONTR groups and 2 in the + ANT group, the former after four weeks of ongoing hemolysis and progressive renal insufficiency, the latter two 6 hours and 3 days after admission respectively. Death in these two patients was not related to the anticoagulant therapy.

Three patients in the CONTR group had an unusually prolonged course of their illness with life-threatening hypertension. The first died, the second still has arterial hypertension after 18 months, the third is in chronic hemodialysis. Such evolution was never seen in the + ANT group.

3.2. Kidney biopsies

Thirty-five percutaneous kidney biospies have been performed between 10 and 32 days after admission. It should be emphasized that only one of the three children from the CONTR group with a prolonged course, could be biopsied.

The following histological lesions have been scored on a scale of 0 to 3 : glomerular changes (sclerosis, necrosis, congestion, segmental solidification, crescents and basal membrane thickening); arteriolar lesions (thrombi, necrosis, intimal proliferation);

interstitial lesions (edema, fibrosis, infiltration); tubular changes (casts, necrosis, atrophy). The mean scores for fifteen out of
the seventeen types of lesions studied are higher in the CONTR
group, suggesting a beneficial effect of the anticoagulants.
When the differences are analysed using the Kruskal-Wallis test
for non parametric data, they were found not to be statistically significant.

3.3. Long-term outcome

Seventeen patients of both groups have made a reasonably quick
recovery from their illness. One child had a second episode of
H U S 10 months after the first and recovery was each time complete.
Long-term follow-up - to a maximum of three years in only a small
number of them - shows that kidney function, as judged from the
serum creatinine levels and the creatinine clearance values   completely normalised within one year after the acute phase of H U S
and this applies to both series of patients (Table 2).Hematuria
and proteinuria are exceptionel and hypertension absent (with one
exception) after one year.

4. CONCLUSIONS

1. The administration of anticoagulants does not   influence
the acute mortality of infants and children with H U S, as expected.

2. When one analizes the different aspects of the disease in the
control patients as compared to the patients who received anticoagulants, two striking features emerge which are clearly in favour
of the anticoagulant therapy especially if the higher incidence of
severe cases in the ANT group is taken into account. First of all,
7 out of the 20 control patients had to be treated for severe hypertension which never occurred in the + ANT patients. Secondly, from
the 20 control patients, three had a very severe course with malignant hypertension leading to hypertensive encephalopathy in all
three and necessitating the use of very active hypotensive drugs
such as diazoxide, minoxidil and captopril for weeks or months.
One of these patients died presumably from cerebral hemorrhage
after four weeks of progressive renal failure. The second patient
stayed in the hospital for almost four months and after 18 months
his blood pressure is still difficult to control. The last child
went into terminal renal failure and is presently in regular hemodialysis. Such unusual mode of evolution was not observed in the
+ ANT group.

3. The biopsies of the patients from the control group have an
higher average score for most of the lesions observed as compared
to the + ANT group. The differences, however, are not statistically significant. It must be stressed, however, that two of the
three patients from the CONTR group with prolonged courses could
not be biopsied in the weeks following the onset of the disease
and on the other hand it should be recalled that this group also
comprises quite a lot of mild cases. The conclusions therefore
must be considered as tentative the more so as the data of the
immunofluorescence study are not yet included in the analysis.

4. On the long run, kidney function normalises indifferently
in both groups in as far as it concerns patients who recovered
from the acute illness within the three weeks after the onset.

Table 1. Prospective H U S study. Data on admission.

		CONTR	+ ANT
Patients			
number		20	19
age	mean	1 9/12	1 7/12
	range	1/12-9 11/12	3/12-12 7/12
prodromes			
	intestinal	20	19
Hematological data (mean values)			
platelets/ µl	$\overline{m}$	50,400	53,600
hemoglobin g/dl	$\overline{m}$	7.4	7.5
fragmentocytes %°	$\overline{m}$	39	46
haptoglobin mg/dl	$\overline{m}$	12	9
Renal manifestations			
hypertension	absent	11	16
	moderate	2	3
	severe	7	0
diuresis	normal	15	8
	oliguria	1	2
	anuria	4	9
serum creatinine mg/dl $\overline{m}$		3.7	4.3
Severity of disease			
	mild	7	3
	moderate	6	5
	severe	7	11

Table 2. Long-term outcome

		CONTR	+ ANT
Serum creatinine mg/dl	6 mo	0.62	0.61
mean values	12 mo	0.63	0.66
	24 mo	0.57	0.61
	36 mo	0.67	0.66
Creat. clearance	6 mo	83 ± 21	84 ± 29
ml/min per 1.73 sq.m.	12 mo	94 ± 23	103 ± 24
mean values ± SD	24 mo	105 ± 23	115 ± 20
	36 mo	112 ± 23	115 ± 30

Principles and Practices of Controlled Clinical Trials

Curtis L. Meinert, Ph.D.

I am pleased to have an opportunity to participate in this Symposium. I am especially delighted to see that a section of the program is devoted to clinical trials. As one who has spent his entire professional career in the design and conduct of such trials, I am impressed with the importance of the trial as an evaluation tool. Often they provide the only reliable answer to vexing treatment questions. It is no wonder Dr. Frederickson, now Director of the NIH, referred to the trial as the indispensible ordeal.(1) The question is not whether we should have trials, but rather how we should carry them out. It is this latter point I wish to discuss in the time allotted to me.

A universal problem has to do with the number of patients available for study. The fact of the matter is that most trials are too small to answer the question they were designed to deal with. About half the trials funded by the NIH have less than 50 patients per treatment group.(2) To be sure, some of these are mounted as feasibility studies and were not designed to provide definitive results, but the lions share do not fall into this category. Incidentially, we should delete the term definitive from our vocabularly when speaking of trials in the planning stage. Nearly every investigator I know sets out to perform a definitive trial but few turn out to achieve this goal.

The recent article by Friedman et al (3) in the New England Journal of Medicine provides graphic evidence of the sample size problem present in trials. Among 71 articles which were negative and in effect concluded in favor of the null hypothesis of no difference, over 80% had less than a 50-50 chance of detecting a 25% beneficial treatment effect!

No trial should be undertaken without a sample size calculation to indicate the number of patients required to detect a specified difference at a given type I and II error level or the level of error protection which can be expected for a given sample size. A type I error, as you will recall, occurs when the null hypothesis is rejected when in fact it is true. Whereas a type II error is made when the null hyposthesis is accepted when in fact it is false. One minus the probability of a type II error is the power of a test, and is the probability of correctly rejecting the null hypothesis. Virtually all of the papers reviewed by Friedman and colleagues failed to recognize the importance of power and the danger of making a type II error.

So what can we do to solve the sample size problem? First, we should not start a trial if it is clear the numbers available for study will be too small to answer the question. I, like many others, am of opinion that it is unethical to perform a trial which exposes humans to risks, however small, if the trial has no chance of detecting an important difference, if one exists.

In many cases it is just not possible for any one clinic to recruit the desired number of patients, at least not within a lifetime of work. In such cases it is necessary to turn to the multicenter trial with several clinics, all following the same study protocol. The study described by Dr. Goldsmith involves this kind of design. The multicenter trial, while logistically more difficult to mount and carry out than is a trial confined to a single center, provides advantages which simply are not possible with the small scale single center trial. Some of these will be addressed in a paper scheduled to appear in the next issue of Controlled Clinical Trials.(4)

Unfortunately, we still tend to shy away from the multicenter trial because of real and imagined obstacles. There is no question that they are difficult for investigators to initiate, in part because funding mechanisms, especially those available through NIH, were not designed for collaborative activities of this kind. The demise of the planning grant some years ago has made it difficult for investigators to convene to plan the study and develop a viable funding proposal. In addition, the reward system, as reflected by the promotion criteria of most academic insititutions, places more emphasis on smaller more individualized projects than on collaborative endeavors. All other things being equal, I expect an individual who develops his curriculum vitae by carrying out a series of small scale studies, even if they are useless, is likely to move up the academic ladder faster than an individual with an equal number of publications from collaborative projects, but where that individual's contribution is obscured because of the way in which the papers are authored, e.g., under the study name without anyone listed as senior author.

In addition, we should be realistic about the numbers of patients that can be recruited into a trial. It does no good at all to have an elaborate sample size calculation if the recruitment goal derived from the calculation can not be achieved. Investigators are unbelievably bad at predicting recruitment performance. Estimates made during the design phase of a trial are almost always much higher than the number of patients who can actually be enrolled in the study. Unless the estimates are based on actual record reviews, where the exclusion criteria of the study have been taken into account, the projections must be seriously downgraded, sometimes by a factor of four or more, to get a realistic idea of how long it will actually take to do the study.

We need to recognize that there are strengths in the collaborative multidisciplinary approach to a problem which are usually impossible to achieve in the small scale trial. I continue to be impressed by the chemistry of collaborating groups, where indeed the whole is greater than the individual parts. In addition, there is evidence that the multicenter trial is better designed and executed than the smaller scale single center counterpart.(5) The level of statistical expertise is often higher and there is usually more attention to quality control of the data collection process in such trials than is possible in the small scale trial.

Every trial, small and large alike, must be concerned with data integrity. The collection of data without ongoing

ongoing quality checks is an invitation to disaster. Trials
in which it is possible to identify costs associated with data
intake, editing, and analysis suggest that this component may
represent anywhere from 10 to 20% of the total budget of the
study.(6) I am skeptical of any trial which overlooks the
need for such basic support.

Quality control is only one aspect of data intergity.
The structure of the trial itself can have an impact on the
way the trial is viewed by the public. Structural defects
can lead to conflicts of interest which may compromise the
study results. For example, it is important to make certain
that those responsible for carrying out and analyzing the
trial are independent of the sponsor, especially if the sponsor
has a prioriety interest in the treatment being tested. The
Anturane Reinfarction Trial has been critized because of
its failure to provide this separation in the area of data
analysis.(7) The data center for that study was part of
the corporate structure of the firm which produced Anturane.
Investigators should be very wary of any arrangement, whether
it involves a single center or multiple centers, in which a
drug firm assumes a major responsibility for data analysis.
Arrangements which restrict or deny the rights of investigators
to perform data analyses, as they see fit, should be rejected.
At the same time investigators should forego any financial
relationship which can be perceived as influencing their
objectivity. It is important to make certain that those
carrying out a study involving a prioriety product do not have
any financial interest in the product under test. For example,

the National Cooperative Gallstone Study,(8) an NIH funded tiral, requires all its investigators, including the oversight committee, to disclose financial arrangements which could constitute a conflict of interest.

The recent series of articles in the Boston Globe (9,10) involving falsification of data in a multicenter cancer trial should raise concerns for all of us, even if such events occur only rarely; certainly such reports can not help but raise doubts in the public sector regarding the value of research in general and clinical trials in particular. There are built-in mechanisms to detect fraudulant data in most areas of science, because of the tendency to withhold judgement regarding a procedure until it has been replicated several times. This option does not always exist in clinical trials, particularly when they require years to carry out and costs millions of dollars to perform. It is unlikely that there will be any replications of some of the nations more expensive trials.

I would like now to touch upon a couple of analysis problems common to most trials. One of these was noted by Dr. Goldsmith in the question "who do we count?" The basic analysis in any trial should include everyone entered into the study and the group in which an individual is counted should be determined by that individual's original treatment allocation. This is the only analysis justified by the randomization process. The selective removal of patients after treatment, whether or not the trial is masked, has the potential of making the study groups non-comparable in various and subtle ways which can not be corrected by any analysis technique. A forthcoming paper from the Coronary Drug Project provides evidence to suggest that patients who comply to a treatment are different from those who do not.(11)

The approach proposed has the advantage of being conservative in that it may obscure a treatment difference when one actually exists. The notion that problems arising from noncompliant patients and those who dropped out of the study can be eliminated by simply recruiting new patients to make up for such deficiencies is a serious misconception. The only reliable way to avoid difficulties is to minimize compliance and dropout problems by careful patient selection and through use of follow-up procedures which help to insure high patient compliance to the study treatments.

The approach to analysis proposed does not, of course, preclude additional analyses focusing on selected subgroups of patients. There is certainly nothing wrong with a report that includes other analyses involving selected subgroups of patients. For example, added analyses in the University Group Diabetes Program (UGDP) were carried out in which mortality in the tolbutamide treated group was compared with that in the placebo treated group in the subgroup of patients who had high levels of adherence to the assigned study treatment.(12) This analysis, while subject to intrepretational problems, was helpful in understanding the results of the study.

The last issue I want to touch on deals with the way in which results are presented. Even a cursory review of published reports reveals a great attention to the question of whether or not a particular finding is significant. If a difference yields a p value of 0.05 or less it is regarded as statistically significant, otherwise it is not and the difference is ignored. There is certainly nothing magical about the 5% level of significance. The needs of the scientific community would be better served if more attention was paid to intrepretation of the data and less to the question of whether a given result is statistically significant. It may surpise some to learn that the mortality findings of the UGDP, which led to termination of the use of tolbutamide in that study, did not achieve statistical significance even at the 10% level. Use of the drug was stopped, as it should have been, when it became clear it was not beneficial. In fact, it is ethically untenable to consider continuing a trial until a significant difference is observed in the negative direction. Trials are designed to test the question of efficacy, not to establish toxicity.

The slavish adherence to the 5% level of significance in the literature is a result of undue emphasis on hypothesis testing. Such overemphasis can, and sometimes does, lead to rediculous conclusions in which a great deal is made of a clinical by irrelevant finding because it is statistically significant. The larger the sample size the smaller the difference required to reject the null hypothesis.

The information supplied in most manuscripts on methods used for data collection and analysis is usually inadequate for an informed evaluation of the study design. Part of the reason for the sketchy nature of this information is due to space limitations imposed by journals. Authors faced with such limitations usually prefer to use available space for their

their results and discussion rather than for a description of methods. Nevertheless, the conscientious investigator will find ways around the space restrictions through supplemental publications, or by making a detailed description of the study design and methods available through some depository, such as the National Technical Information Service. The paper I referred to earlier, scheduled to appear in the forthcoming issue of <u>Controlled Clinical Trials</u> (4), provides a listing of key items of information which should be included in reports from clinical trials.

A key item of information has to do with the method of randomization. Some authors will use the term random, but mean haphazard, The validity of the results can be adversely effected if patients were assigned by some psuedo random allocation scheme, such as hospital number, particularly if the investigator knows the treatment to which a patient will be assigned prior to completion of the necessary eligibility examinations. Such schemes are almost certainly subject to selection biases which may render the study group non-comparable from the outset. Sufficient details regarding methods should be provided so readers are not in the dark on the allocation procedure.

The problems involved in designing and carrying out a trial are many and complex. It is certainly true that clinical trials, as noted by Frederickson:

> "...are indispensable. They will continue to be
> an ordeal. They lack glamor, they strain our resources
> and patience, and they protract the moment of truth to

excruciating limits. Still, they are among the most

challenging tests of our skills. I have no doubt

that when the problem is well chosen, the study is

appropriately designed, and that when all the populations

concerned are made more aware of the route and the goal,

the reward can be commensurated with the effort. If, in

major medical dilemmas, the alternative is to pay the

cost of perpetual uncertainty, have we really any choice?"

I think not and so we must all strive to make the trial a

better more effective evaluation tool for present and future

use.

REFERENCES

1. Fredrickson DS: The field trial: Some thoughts on the indispensable ordeal. Bull N. Y. Acad Med, 44: 985-993, 1968.
2. National Institutes of Health Clinical Trails Committee: NIH Inventory of Clinical Trials, Fiscal Year 1978. NIH Research and Evaluation Branch, Division of Research Grants, Bethesda, Md., (in press).
3. Freiman JA, Chalmers TC, Smith H Jr, Kuebler RR: The importance of Beta, the type II error and sample size in the design and interpretation of the randomized clinical trial: Survey of 71 "negative" trials. N. Engl J Med 299:690-694, 1978.
4. Meinert CL: Toward more defenitive clinical trials. Controlled Clinical Trials (in press).
5. Personal Communication with T. Chalmers and based on analysis of design features of a large array of trials.
6. Meinert CL: Cost Profiles of Data Coordinating Centers. Presented at the Fifth Annual Symposium on Coordinating Clinical Trials, Arlington, Virginia, May 25-26, 1978.
7. Doubts about Anturane. Lancet, Vol. II:206-307, 1980.
8. National Cooperative Gallstone Coordinating Center, Cedar-Sinai, Los Angeles, California.
9. Boston Sunday Globe, June 29, 1980.
10. The Boston Globe, June 30, July 1-3, 1980.
11. Coronary Drug Project Research Group: Influence of adherence to treatment and response of cholesterol on mortality in the Coronary Drug Project. NEJM, Vol.303, #13, October 30, 1980.
12. Meinert CL, Knatterud GL, Prout, Klimt CR: The University Group Diabetes Program: A study of hypoglycemic agents on vascular complications in diabetes with adult-onset diabetes: II. Mortality results. Diabetes 19(suppl 2): 787-830, 1970.

PROBLEMS OF LONG TERM DIALYSIS IN CHILDREN.

Michel BROYER, Marie-France GAGNADOUX, Jean-Louis BACRI,
Kathleen LABORDE.
Hôpital des Enfants Malades. Paris, FRANCE.

If iterative hemodialysis has become now a routine treatment for children in terminal uremia, this approach is usually considered for a short period of time as kidney transplantation is the first choice treatment in this age group. Unfortunately for different reasons some children have to be treated by hemodialysis during long periods of time. Many problems could occur in these patients and the purpose of this paper is to report on the complications and difficulties registered in the specialised pediatric dialysis centre of the Enfants Malades Hospital in a ten year period (1969-1979).

Patients and methods.
More than 200 children and adolescents had been referred to the dialysis unit of the Enfants Malades Hospital in the period 1969-1979. Among this pool of patients 138 aged 1 year 4/12 - 15 years 5/12 had been treated by hemodialysis longer than 3 months, these patients have been used for building actuarial survival curve. Out of them 107 patients had been treated by hemodialysis longer than 1 year and the long term complications reported here apply to this population for which the mean follow up is 2.9 years. The growth study recently published (1) applies to 76 patients from this pool observed between 1969 and 1978. Details of dialysis treatment and medications given were reported in this last study (1).

Survival.
Actuarial survival of children on LTD was respectively 93, 88, 85 and 80 % at 1, 2, 3 and 4 years and after. These figures are calculated taking in account all patients and all deaths

during hemodialysis treatment including nephroblastoma and patients coming back dialysis after transplantation failure.

This survival is similar to that given in the EDTA registry
for specialised pediatric centres and clearly above the survival
of children treated in non specialised centres (2).

Causes of death were the following : cerebral hemorrage 1,
pulmonary edema 1, myocardial ischemia or infarction 2, pulmonary
embolism 1, iatrogenic hypernatremia 1, cardiac arrest on dialysis 2, in 3 cases death was related to the causal disease : oxalosis in 1 and nephroblastoma in 2, finally in 2 cases the cause of
death remained unknown. Analysis of death rate in function of
initial renal disease shows that nephrotic syndrom with focal hyalinosis represents a high risk group of patients (4/11 versus
9/127). These deaths are illustrative of some of the problems
encuntered during hemodialysis treatment but also of the progresses performed with time, 9 of these 13 deaths occured before
1975 and most of them could have been avoided.

Vascular access and related problem.

Since 1971 internal fistula replaced systematically external
shunt for the vascular access in all patients accepted for a dialysis programme in our institution whatever the age. In this
chapter we report data on fistula concerning the 138 patients
treated at least 3 months. Three patterns of blood access were
used, a) end to end distal fistula between the radial artery and
the cephalic vein ; b) end to side proximal fistula between bra-
chial artery and the cephalic or the basilic vein ; c) vascular
graft with saphenous vein, bovine carotid or PTFE interposition.

The survival rate of these fistulae appeared similar to that
observed in adults : 84 % for distal fistula and 77 % for proximal fistula after 1 year for smallest children and 84 % and 79 %
respectively in largest ones versus 86 % for all distal fistula in
a series of adults (3). Psychological stress of repeated veini
puncture was not as great a problem as one would fear. Only in
2 children was this stress so important that it seemed intolerable
to the staff. The acceptance of the puncture pain was not worse
in younger than in older children.

Thrombosis was almost the only complication of internal fistula : 42 % of fistula were thrombosed at 2 years in the smallest patients (< 20 kg BW) versus 27 % in the others but incidence of thrombosis differed according to the pattern of the fistula : low in distal fistula (10 % at 1 & 2 years) it was high in vascular graft (87 % at 1 year for the smallest and 56 % for the others. Thrombosis did not always result in loss of blood access : 6 out of 8 thrombosed distal fistulae in small children could be used again after resection of the thrombosed part. Other complications were rare and never life threatening : 3 local infections (in 2 of these cases hemorrages occured and lead to closure of fistula), 4 false aneurysms leading to 2 resections and 1 ligature.

Two episods of cardiac failure requiring closure or banding of fistula occured during a 330 patient year of follow up. In 2 other cases banding of fistula was performed preventively as the flow was too high. Out of the 107 children dialysed longer than 1 year, 16 remained at least once without any vascular access during a period of time long enough to need peritoneal dialysis, usually performed with a permanent catheter. Some children switched alternately from hemodialysis to peritoneal dialysis and inversely 1 or 2 times. Thanks to this approach no one child died from vascular access shortage.

Problems occuring during the dialysis sessions.

In spite of a careful procedure and monitoring children are more prone to adverse symptoms than adults during dialysis sessions. Out of 3.230 sessions recorded in 1979 we have noted hypotension in 25.2 %, headaches in 11.6 % and vomitings in 13.7 % of the sessions, but cramps were only observed in 1.8 %.

Special mention has to be made of marked hypotension occuring in some patients not only during the dialysis sessions but also between them. We have observed 5 such patients all but one were bi-nephrectomized and all had been dialysed for longer than 4 years when this syndrome began. Hypotension persisted in spite of weight excess and increase of Extracellular water and continues at the present time to raise problems.

Bone disease.

The frequency of renal osteodystrophy is different from one series of patients to another one probably in relation with the treatment prescribed. Out of the 107 patients followed longer than 1 year, 18 developped bone disease on LTD, but we must consider separately 4 of them who had oxalosis. That is to say a frequency of bone disease in dialysed children of 14 %. Medical treatment including adapted doses of 25 OH D3, 1 α OH D3 or 1-25 $(OH)_2$ D3 calcium and aluminium gels allowed a good control of osteodystrophy in 9 cases, but 5 patients had to be parathyroidectomised. Note that bone disease was much more frequent in very young children (5/10 patients under 4 years) and in non compliant patients not taking vit D derivatives and/or aluminium gel.

The risk of Aluminium intoxication adds a new problem to the dialysis patient and we decided to stop aluminium gel in children who had plasma aluminium above 100 ng/l, with the consequence to increase their plasma phosphorus and then to favour hyperparathyroidism.

Hypertension.

HT could be a vital problem in some patients on dialysis either from salt and water overload in non compliant patients or from hyperreninism. The differential diagnosis between this 2 types of HT is not always obvious and needs eventually water compartments measurement. In the past we were quite large about the indication of bilateral nephrectomy in the second type HT (24/138). At the present time, it would be possible to avoid this operation, thanks to hypotensive drugs like Captopril[R] and bilateral nephrectomy is now replaced in our centre by unilateral left nephrectomy in preparation to transplantation.

Growth.

Growth failure remains one of the major problem of children on long term dialysis. Growth data from this series of patients are available for 76 cases. Statural growth expressed as standard deviation score (SDS) was very variable. Sixteen children showed a normal length increment for chronological age but 18 had a severely decreased growth rate (SDS > -0.5/year). The mean annual loss of height for age was 0.39 SD/year and was comparable in boys and girls. Growth rate was much less severely impaired in the more growth-retarded children at onset of dialysis, and height increment was inversely related to initial length expressed as SD. Bone maturation rate was also markedly decreased in almost all patients, and the mean loss in bone maturation score for age was 0.54 SDS/year. In most of the children studied before they reached a bone maturation score corresponding to a bone age of 13 for boys and 12 for girls, skeletal maturity and statural growth were equally retarded, resulting in an unchanged growth potential.

The mean values of biochemical, clinical and nutritional data regularly checked during therapy have been compared in the group of children growing normally versus the group of growth retarded children. The substances considered as indicative of uremic toxicity were slightly higher in the second group but the difference reached significance for creatinine only. Calorie intake was slightly lower in the second group but was associated with an increased skinfold thickness, suggesting that patients with growth failure utilise the calories ingested more to increase adipose tissue than for statural growth. The available data afforded no evidence for a relation of either calorie intake or number and duration of dialysis to growth. Osteodystrophy even severe was consistent with a normal growth increment provided that no bone distorsion developped but it resulted in a loss of growth potential. Parathyroidectomy and administration of 1 α or 1.25 OH cholecalciferol were often associated with a gain in growth potential.

During pubertal age, a complete growth arrest was rare, but a normal growth spurt was never observed. A relative increase in growth rate occured when bone age reached 13-14 years for boys and 12 years for girls. Growth remained slow, but was often prolonged beyond the normal age resulting in a limited though not negligible catch-up. During this period however, which corresponded to sexual development, a marked loss of potential growth was almost constantly observed and finally the ultimate height as far as it was known remained generally small.

P   Problems related to the etiology of renal disease.

If we except general processes as LED or PAN, two diseases could had symptoms or complications of their own on long term dialysis : cystinosis and oxalosis.

Cystinosis : only 6 patients of the present series are cystinotic but we have informations about 10 other patients. Two complications should be pointed out : recurrent epistaxis and severe hypertension. Six of 16 cystinotic dialysed patients (4) have had frequent epistaxis sometimes severe. Epistaxis occured both during dialysis sessions and interdialytic period, often favoured by minor trauma. Careful naso pharyngeal examination revealed no vascular abnormalities and iterative cauterisation of mucosa did not provide improvement, this symptom disappeared after transplantation.

Severe hypertension remained or appeared after the first months of dialysis in 3 out the 16 cystinotic patients which responded poorly to UF, but subsided after bilateral nephrectomy. One can add that ocular involvement worsened in 3/16 cases with severe sight defect.

Thyroxin supplementation was needed in all but 2 cases. Finally hepato and splenomegaly was found in respectively 7 and 5 patients and 2 patients had bleeding from oesophageal varices. Live biopsy did not show symptom of cirrhosis but a heavy load of Kupfer cells.

Oxalosis : 4 patients had oxalosis and was dialysed 2.5 to 6 years. All developped severe disabling bone disease in spite of parathyroidectomy. Bone X Rays were peculiar with densification of all metaphyseal areas. Fractures of femoral neck were noted in all patients. This complication was also noted in 14 out of 15 oxalotic patients treated more than 2 years in the last report of EDTA (5).

Psychological incidence.

Psychological incidence of LTD in children has been extensively worked out in many groups. It cannot be summarized easily as the problems are quite different from a patient to another one. Nature and importance of psychologic disturbences depend essential ly on two factors : the quality of familial support and the quality of life allowed by the treatment. In absence of medical complications with a good hemoglobin level, an acceptable height for age and easy dialysis sessions, the child on LTD could have few problems specially if he is treated at home and if the family supports him strongly on the way of getting his autonomy. But this situation is rather rare and usually in spite of an apparently acceptable tolerance, obvious perturbations at the subconscious level are objectived by appropriate tests.

School attendance is a good index of psychologic adaptation. Some children are able to attend full time schooling and progress regularly year after year but the majority has difficulties to follow the standards of education. At the present time out of 19 children of school age treated by LTD in our unit, 13 are attending school regularly, 4 less regularly and 2 have no school attendance. Progression of the level remains in the standards for 6 children but a delay of 2 to 4 years is noted in the 13 others. Schooling is obviously better with home dialysis and all the 7 children treated at home attend full time school.

Neurological complications.

There were few neurological complications. Repeated measurements of nerve conduction velocity never shown a significant decrease except in the only case of polyneuritis in a child with oxalosis. For that reason we have at the present time given up this investigation.

More than 1 convulsion occured in 12 out of 107 patients that is to say a frequency of 11 %. Phenobarbital in appropriate dosage always succeeded to avoid recurrence of seizures.

Aluminium encephalopathy was not really observed in our series but one child who took a large amount of aluminium gel before dialysis was referred to us with the first symptom of dialysis dementia after 2 or 3 dialysis in a centre with a non free aluminium water. The symptoms disappeared in few weeks. Aluminium intoxication is a real hazard and must be regularly looked for in children on LTD.

Myocardiopathy.

Some children on long term dialysis developped cardiomegaly and symptoms of cardiac failure. It is difficult to determine in these symptoms the respective role of extra cellular overload, of hypertension, of chronic anemia, of arterio venous fistula or of uremia itself. In order to assess the frequency of cardiomyopathy a systematic study of echocardiography was undertook in 30 dialysed patients. Fourteen of them were in the limits of the normal but 16 had an obvious cardiomyopathy. Three patterns have been found : a) hypertrophy and hyperkinesy of myocardium : 12 cases ; b) hypertrophy but hypokinesy of the myocardium : 2 cases ; c) dilatation of ventricules and hypokinesy : 2 cases. The abnormal patterns were seen either in severely uremic patients at the onset of dialysis or and more frequently after a long time on dialysis.

Patients treated by hemodialysis longer than 5 years.

We reviewed the files of the 17 patients younger than 15 years at the beginning of the treatment (1 year 8/12 - 14 year 6/12) and who received long term dialysis for a period longer than 5 years and up to 11 years. Two died at the 60th month of treatment one at age 17 6/12 from an accidental cardiovascular overload and the other at age 11 9/12 from an early complication of transplantation.

Five are presently living with a functionnal transplant and 10 remain on dialysis. The total follow up on dialysis of this group of patients reaches 110,5 year. Five out these 17 patients got difficult problems of vascular access at least once and needed several operation for maintening a usable fistula, but no one died or was transplanted in emergency for that reason.

Among complications of uremia, a marked osteodystrophy was observed in 5 patients with a good evolution in 3 of them (1 parathyroidectomy, 2 treatment with $1 \alpha 25 (OH)_2$ vit D). Three (anephric) needed to be frequently transfused. Only one had clinical cardiac failure which improved after the banding of a high flow humeral fistula. Three developped seizures and were maintened on phenobarbital. Interestingly 4 of the 10 dialysed patient at the present time have permanent hypotension in spite of fluid overload and severe hypotension during dialysis.

Note that 2 developped large cytotoxic antibodies which prevent them to be transplanted.

If we except two patients with a low IQ, out of the 15 surviving subjects 4 are working full time after obtaining a diploma or professionnal qualification, 5 are continuing schooling or professionnal training but 3 did not attend school regularly and are poorly rehabilitated, one of these patients has oxalosis and a severe disabling bone disease.

In conclusion, in spite of a low mortality rate and of technical progresses, many problems may occur or persist in children on long term dialysis. There is no doubt at the present time that kidney transplantation remains a better alternative for this age group.

REFERENCES.

1. KLEINKNECHT C. BROYER M. GAGNADOUX MF et al.
   Growth in children treated with long term dialysis. A study of
   76 patients.
   in advances in Nephrology vol 9, year book med. publ. Chicago,
   1980, p 133-163.

2. CHANTLER C. DONCKERWOLCKE R. BRUNNER F.P. et al.
   Combined report on regular dialysis and transplantation of
   children in Europe 1978.
   in proceeding of the Europ. Dial and transpl. Ass. vol 16,
   Pitman Medical Tunbridge Wells. 1979, p 74-104.

3. GAGNADOUX M.F. PASCAL B. BRONSTEIN M et al.
   Arterioveinous fistulae in small children.
   Dialysis and transplantation 1980, 9, 318-320.

4. BROYER M. GUILLOT M. GUBLER M.C. et al.
   La cystinose infantile, réévaluation des symptomes précoces et
   tardifs.
   in Actualités de l'hôpital Necker 1980 Flammarion Médecine
   Sciences, Paris, p 127-157.

5. CHANTLER C. DONCKERWOLCKE R. BRUNNER F.P. et al.
   Combined report on regular dialysis and transplantation of
   children in Europe 1979.
   in proceed. of the Europ. Dial. and transpl. assoc. vol 17
   in press. Pitman Medical Tunbridge Wells.

DEVELOPMENTAL ASPECTS OF PERITONEAL DIALYSIS

A.Y. ELZOUKI, A.B. GRUSKIN, H.J. BALUARTE, J.W. PREBIS AND M.S. POLINSKY

The use of the peritoneal membrane for removing uremic solutes was first reported in 1923 (1). Since then many investigators have contributed to bringing peritoneal dialysis (P.D.) from an experimental technique conducted in animals to its present state of clinical prominence. Although the technique of peritoneal dialysis is being used with increased frequency in children, relatively few studies dealing with dialysis kinetics have been performed in children and/or the developing animal.

The purpose of this presentation is two fold. Firstly, a few general principles and theoretical considerations related to peritoneal dialysis kinetics will be reviewed. Secondly, we will report our experience in evaluating those factors which might explain age related differences in dialysi kinetics.

GENERAL PRINCIPLES OF PERITONEAL DIALYSIS

The peritoneal membrane functions as a passive semi-permeable membrane (1). Consequently, the movement of solutes across the peritoneal membrane is a resul of diffusion along concentration gradients and solvent drag. Since the permeability of most physiological solutes is inversely related to its molecula radius, larger molecular weight solutes move by diffusion more slowly than smal ones, and as such will show lower membrane permeability. Because the exact area of the peritoneal membrane that participates in solute exchange is not precisely known, it is not possible to determine actual mass transfer coefficients for solutes moving across peritoneal membranes. Solute movement is evaluated by measuring either clearance and/or dialysance. Both are a function of membrane area as well as permeability.

Although the determination of peritoneal clearance is a clinically useful technique, its measurement is not ideally suited for comparative studies of differences in dialysis mechanics, membrane area, or membrane permeability. Comparative studies of the peritoneal membrane require that determinations of peritoneal dialysance be made with dialysis mechanics, i.e. dwell times and dialysate volumes held constant. The formula for peritoneal dialysance follows(2):

$$D= -\ln \left[\frac{1 - SD \frac{(V_D + V_B)}{S_B V_B}}{T} \right] \cdot \frac{V_B \cdot V_D}{V_B + V_D} \quad \text{where}$$

D= dialysance in ml/min; S_D= solute concentration in dialysate; S_B= solute concentration in blood; V_B=assumed volume of distribution within the body of urea or inulin, 60% and 20% of BW respectively); V_D= volume of dialysate in ml returned at the completion of an exchange; and T= time in minutes from initiation of inflow until the completion of drainage.

The peritoneal dialysance of a solute may be defined as the rate of solute removal per unit driving concentration between plasma and dialysate, or the instantaneous clearance at time zero of a dialysis exchange. The peritoneal dialysance of solutes have been shown to be a combined function of peritoneal permeability and peritoneal surface area. Thus, when changes in dialysance occur in comparatively performed studies it may be concluded that an alteration in one or both of these factors have occurred (3).

Changes in the dialysance of urea, a small molecular weight solute has been shown to reflect alterations in peritoneal surface area. Changes in the dialysance of inulin a large molecular weight solute reflects an alteration in either surface area and/or peritoneal permeability.

The formula for determining the dialysance ratio follows (1,4):

$$D_R = \frac{D_I}{D_U} + \frac{\text{permeability inulin}}{\text{permeability urea}} \times \frac{\text{membrane area}}{\text{membrane area}}$$

The dialysance ratio or permeability index provides a dimensionless index of permeability as the term for surface area cancels out in mechanically identically performed comparative studies. Change in the dialysance ratio of two solutes of widely differing molecular weights, such as urea and inulin, indicate that an alteration in peritoneal permeability has occurred.

We have calculated the theoretical effect on urea dialysance of varying each of the factors known to influence dialysance. These calculations demonstrated that 1) when dwell times are altered; 2) when the volume of dialysate is altered, i.e. the dialysate flow rate is altered, and 3) when permeability changes occur as reflected by an altered dialysate to blood ratio, major changes in dialysance of urea occurs, if dialysance is expressed in ml/min/kg.

Changes in the volume of distribution of solute within the body have only a minimal effect on dialysance. Consequently differences in the extracellular space and total body water associated with growth and development will have only a minor effect on dialysance. How does dialysance change with weight assuming a fixed exchange times and fixed volume of dialysate in relation to the volume of distribution of solute within the body? Our calculations showed the dialysance per kg/bw will be constant at all weights for any given solute given a similar degree of peritoneal permeability and functional size of the peritoneal membrane, as reflected by a constant dialysate to blood ratio of solute (5).

Thus, if dialysis mechanics i.e. exchange time and dialysate volume per kg/bw are maintained constant, any differences occurring in the dialysance of urea, inulin or dialysance ratio with increasing age must reflect intrinsic developmental differences in either the relative peritoneal surface and/or intrinsic peritoneal permeability.

The published data dealing with the developmental aspects of peritoneal dialysis suggest that this technique may be more efficient in children than in adults (6,7). Efficiency may be defined in many ways--removal of solute, rate of decrease of blood levels, or the rate of movement of solute across the peritoneal membrane. When evaluating the kinetics of peritoneal dialysis in the young, four factors need to be considered: 1) peritoneal surface area; 2) permeability of the peritoneal membrane; 3) the dialysate flow rate, i.e. dwell times and dialysate volume; and 4) peritoneal capillary blood flow.

Two studies in which the anatomical surface area (SA) of the peritoneal membrane was actually anatomically measured in infants and adults demonstrated that the peritoneal S.A. relative to body size in newborn is approximately twice that of adults (7,8). Such observations do not necessarily imply that the functional size of the peritoneal membrane which participates in exchange is greater in the young (4).

EXPERIMENTAL STUDIES

In order to critically evaluate other factors known to influence peritoneal dialysis kinetics in the young and to determine whether solute transfer during P.D. is age related, we performed dialysance studies of urea as urea C_{14} and inulin as inulin H_3 in a group of puppies less than one month of age and in a group of adult dogs (5,9,10). The mechanics of each study was identical i.e. dialysate volume instilled into the peritoneal cavity in ml/kg and dwell times. The dialysance of both urea and inulin solutes was significantly higher in the puppies. Urea and inulin dialysance was increased 65% and 125% respectively (p<0.01).

Also, the dialysance ratio or permeability index, i.e. DI/DU was greater in the puppy. This ratio was 70% higher in the puppies than in the adult (p<0.05).

DISCUSSION

Since exchange time and dialysate volume was held constant in each experiment the differences in dialysance between adults and neonates can only be explained as reflecting changes in the functional peritoneal surface area and/or the permeability of the peritoneal membrane. If the differences were due only to age related differences in surface area then DI and DU would be higher in the neonate as found, but the DI/DU ratio would be similar in both groups. The finding that the dialysance ratio also changed with age can be explained only by an age realted change in peritoneal permeability.

Another major factor which plays a major role in peritoneal dialysis efficiency in clinical care and influences the transperitoneal movement of solute during P.D., other than peritoneal S.A. and permeability is the Dialysate Flow Rate (Q.D.) (11,12). Several studies have demonstrated that when Q.D. is increased, the clearance of small solutes e.g. urea will also increase. When Q.D. was increased to 200 ml/min (12 l/h), the urea clearance increased to 40 ml/min in comparison to a urea clearance of 20 ml/min when the Q.D. dialysis exchange was 30 ml/min (2100 ml/70 min). We have also performed dialysance studies in puppies and adult dogs using two different volumes of dialysate. As expected, the dialysance of urea varied with changes in dialysate flow rate. Dialysance of inulin, a large molecular compound, did not change significantly with changes in dialysate volume.

A number of studies reported by other investigators in infant and young animals suggest that the peritoneal membrane in the young permits a greater rate of transfer of solute than does the peritoneal membrane of adults (6,7). Although this conclusion is correct the conclusions may have been derived accidentally. The available studies permit alternative explanations because the dwell time as well as the quantity of the dialysis fluid utilized was not necessarily kept constant.

If one assumes, for example, that 70 cc/kg of dialysate fluid per exchange were used in a 3.0 kg newborn with a total exchange time of 70 minutes, then the Q.D. would be 210/70=3 cc/min and Q.D.kg would equal 3/3=1 cc/min/kg in the newborn. If a similar exchange were performed in a 70 kg adult using 2100 cc of dialysate volume per 70 min then Q.D.=2100/70=30 cc/min and Q.D./kg=30÷70 or 0.42 cc/min/kg.

Assuming that the transperitoneal movement was such that a similar dialysate to blood ratios of solute occurred in both infants and adults approximately 2.5 times as much solute would be removed per kg/bw in the neonate. Such a finding would not demonstrate that the peritoneum functions differently in the young than in the adult, but would merely show that the solute in the extra cellular compartment was exposed to a larger sink into which it could diffuse. In short, the differences would be due to the influences of dialysis mechanics and not reflect intrinsic differences in the peritoneal membrane per se.

In summary, our various studies have addressed three of the four variables involved in the kinetics of peritoneal dialysis: permeability, functional surface area, and dialysate volume. They demonstrate that the peritoneal permeability as well as the functional surface areas of the peritoneum is greater in infants than in adults, and that changes in dialysate volume influence peritoneal dialysance. The practical implications of these studies on peritoneal dialysis kinetics in the young are that the rate of removal of solutes is quicker in the young than in the adult for a given set of dialysis mechanics. Any differences in dialysis mechanics in the young as compared to the adult would further serve to augment any differences reflecting the intrinsic characteristics of the peritoneal membrane. Finally, the removal of larger molecular weight compounds, i.e. middle molecules, may occur more rapidly in the young because the peritoneal membrane in the young is more permeabile to larger molecules.

REFERENCES

1. Henderson, L.W.: Peritoneal Dialysis. in Massry, S.G. and Sellers, A.L. Clinical Aspects of Uremia and Dialysis, Charles C. Thomas, Springfield, Ill., Chapter 19, pp. 555-582.
2. Henderson, L.W. and Nolph, K.D.: Altered permeability of the peritoneal membrane after using hypertonic peritoneal dialysis fluid. J.Clin.Invest. 48:922-1001, 1969.
3. Henderson, L.W.: The problem of peritoneal membrane area and permeability. Kidney Int. 3:409-410, 1973.
4. Henderson, L.W. and Kintzel, J.E.: Influence of antidiuretic hormone on peritoneal membrane area and permeability. J.Clin.Invest. 50:2437-2443, 1971.
5. Elzouki, A.Y., Gruskin, A.B., Baluarte, H.J., Polinsky, M.S. and Prebis, J.W.: Developmental Aspects of Peritoneal Dialysis Kinetics in Dogs. In Press. Pediatric Research.
6. Feldman, W., Baliah, T. and Drummond, K.N.: Intermittent peritoneal dialysis in the management of chronic renal failure in children.
7. Esperance, M.J. and Collins, D.L.: Peritoneal dialysis efficiency in relation to body weight. J.Pediatr.Surg. 1:162-169, 1966.
8. Putiloff, P.V.: Materials for the study of the laws of growth of the human body in relation to the surface areas of different systems; the trial on Russian subjects of planigraphic anatomy as a means for exact anthropometry one of the problems of anthropology. Report of Dr. P.V. Putiloff at the Meeting of the Siberian Branch of the Russian Geographic Society. October 29, 1884, QMSK, 1886.
9. Elzouki, A., Gruskin, A., Prebis, J.W., Baluarte, H.J. and Polinsky,M.S.: Age Related Changes in Peritoneal Dialysance, Abstract National Kidney Foundation, 9th Annual Clinical Dialysis and Transplant Forum, November, 1979.
10. Elzouki, A.Y., Gruskin, A.B., Baluarte, H.J., Polinsky, M.S. and Prebis, J.W.: Age related changes in peritoneal dialysis kinetics. Pediatr. Res. 14:618, 1980.
11. Tenckhoff, H., Ward, G. and Boen, S.T.: The influence of dialysate volume and flow rate on peritoneal clearance. Prox.Europ.Dial.Transpl. Assoc. 2:113-117, 1965.
12. Nolph, K.D., Popovich, R.P., Ghods, A,J, and Twardowski, A.: Determinants of low clearances of small solutes during peritoneal dialysis. Kidney Int. 13:117-123, 1978.
13. This research was supported in part by NIH Grant IRO1 HL 23511-01, General Clinical Research Center Grant RR-75 and in part by the Ministry of Education, Libya.

PROTEIN-ENERGY REQUIREMENTS OF CHILDREN AND ADOLESCENTS ON CAPD.PRELIMI-
NARY RESULTS OF NITROGEN BALANCE STUDIES

N.G.De Santo,G.Capodicasa,M.Pluvio,D.Giugliano,R.Torella and C.Giordano
Chair of Nephrology and Institute of Medical Pathology,1st Medical Faculty
University of Naples,Naples,Italy

INTRODUCTION

Recent data from this laboratory have demonstrated that adult uremic
patients under CAPD keep a positive nitrogen balance when receiving a
diet providing 1.2 g/kg of protein(1).

In managing children with intermittent peritoneal dialysis it has been
stressed the fact that they should eat as much they wish(2).However it
it has to be mentioned that only 2 patients of the pediatric-adolescent
age have been studied carefully.Lindner and Tenckhoff(3) treated 2
girls aged respectively 13 and 16 years eating 1.5 g/kg of protein.Both
were on positive nitrogen balance.These data of course do not apply to
CAPD.

Here we report our preliminary experience with children on CAPD.The
data collected indicate that also for this age a positive nitrogen balance may be obtained.

METHODS

Patients

The study was performed in 3 patients of our CAPD program,hospitali-
zed one at time,in our metabolic ward for 3 weeks.

Table I includes all the pertinent data related to these patients:
sex,age,weight,underlying renal disease,daily urinary volume,residual
glomerular filtration rate,BUN,plasma phosphate and potassium,peritoneal
urea clearance,blood pressure,months of CAPD treatment.

Table I: Characterization of patients participating to the study

	Pat.no.1	Pat.no.2	Pat.no.3
Sex	M	F	M
Age(years)	13	15	12
Weight(kg)	29.5	36	12.5
Blood pressure(mmHg)	120/80	90/70	110/70
Renal disease	CG	Unknown	CP
Urine(ml/day)	1,100	900	950
Residual GFR (ml/minx1.73sq.m.)	4.07	3.90	4.7
BUN(mg/dl)	35	32	28
P (mg/dl)	3.91	3.97	3.86
K (mEq/L)	4.10	4.20	4.15
Peritoneal Urea Clear. (ml/min x 1.73 sq.m.)	15.25	16.00	15.00
Months on CAPD	11	7	10

CG= chronic glomerulonephritis, CP = chronic pyelonephritis

Catheters

The patients had been implanted with a permanent peritoneal catheter which was of the Goldberger type(4) for patient no.1,of the TWH type 2 for patient no.2(5) and a TWH for patients under 15 kg in patient no.3 (6).The TWH catheters were kindly provided by Mr.G.Zellerman,Bio-Engineer,Accurate Surgical Instruments,Toronto,Canada.

Dialyzate

The composition of the dialyzate,which was contained in bottles for patient no.1 and in plastic bags for patients nos.2 and 3,was the following:Sodium 132 mEq/L,Potassium 0-4.5 mEq/L,Magnesium 1.5 mEq/L, Calcium   3 mEq/L,Acetate 35 mEq/L,Chloride 101.5 mEq/L.The dextrose concentrations was of 1.5 g/dl(4 liters) and 4.25 g/dl(4 liters for patients nos. 1 and 2,while for patients no.3 only a dextrose concentration of 1.5 g/dl was used.

Table II:Various sources of energy for patients participating in the study

Patient No.	Glucose utilization from dialyzate g/day	Energy from diet kj/kg	Energy from dialyzate kj/kg	Total daily energy input kj/kg
1	113.4	188	54.7	242.7
2	140.0	188	55.3	243.3
3	30.0	419	33.5	452.5

Diets

Two weeks before hospitalization the patients who were on free diets were asked to take note of food intake.On these records,at the time of hospitalization,a diet was devised containing variable amounts of energy (Table II) and of proteins(Table III).

The energy derived in part from the diet and in part from the dialy-zate(7).Dextrose utilization from the dialyzate was of 113 g in patient no.1,of 140 g in patient no.2 and of 30 g in patient no.3.Total daily energy input was of 242.7 kj for patient no.1,of 243.3 kj/kg in patient no.2 and of 452.5 kj/kg in patient no.3.The protein intake was of 1.2 g/kg in patient no.1 and of 1.5 and 2.0 g/kg respectively for patients nos.2 and 3.

Nitrogen balance

It was measured by the kjeldhal procedure by usual laboratory methods (8) by analyzing all excreta(dialyzate,urine,feces).Nitrogen balance was calculated by subtracting the output from the intake.Foods were analyzed on 3 occasions namely on day 8,15 and 21.The patients were on stable BUN so that no correction was needed.Nitrogen losses in the skin (9) and in the espirated air(10,11) were not taken into consideration.

RESULTS

Table III reports the outcome of the study in the course of 63 days of nitrogen balance(21 days for each patient).Nitrogen balance was positive in all cases.In patient no.1 it was positive for 0.100 ± 0.050

g/day while retention averaged .340 +.100 g/day in patient no.2 and
2.1 ± 0.2 g/day in patient no.3.

Table III: protein intake and nitrogen balance in the patients participating in this study

Patient No.	Protein intake g/kg	Nitrogen balance g/day
1	1.2	0.100 ± 0.050
2	1.5	0.340 ± 0.100
3	2.0	2.100 ± 0.200

DISCUSSION

Nutrition in peritoneal dialysis has not received adequate investigation so that there are difficulties in devising a diet for patients
on this regimen.The difficulty is increased by the scanty information
of patients described in the literature usually lacking of details such
as urine volume,residual glomerular filtration rate,generation rates for
urea and creatinine,protein losses(1,2).

The data in Table III indicate that adolescents and children on
CAPD may achieve a positive nitrogen balance.This finding is in good
keeping with our previous study(1) in adult patients thus indicating
the anabolic role of this dialytic regimen.The data of course still
preliminary do support the concept that CAPD removing toxics at the
time they are generated is the least catabolic form of dialysis.

ACKNOWLEDGEMENT

Supported in part by NIH,Bethesda,USA,Contract No.1-AM-9-0066,
National Institute of Arthritis,Metabolism and Digestive Diseases and
by Consiglio Nazionale delle Ricerche,Rome,Italy.

REFERENCES

1. Giordano C,De Santo NG,Pluvio M,Di Leo VA,Capodicasa G,Cirillo D,Esposito R,Damiano M.Protein requirement of patients on CAPD: a study on nitrogen balance.Int J Artif Organs 3:11,1980

2. Giordano C,De Santo NG.Dietary management of patients on peritoneal dialysis.Contr to Nephrology 17:77,1979

3. Lindner A and Tenckhoff H.Nitrogen balance in patients on maintenance peritoneal dialysis.Trans Amer Soc Artif Intern Organs 16:255,1970

4. Goldberg EM,Hill W and Kabins S.Peritoneal dialysis.Description of an improved peritoneal catheter and collecting system.Dialysis and Transpl 6:50,1975

5. Oreoplous DG,Karanicolas S,Fenton JSA.Home Pertoneal dialysis.Dialysis and Transpl 6:70,1978

6. De Santo NG,Capodicasa G,Zellerman G,Giordano C.Description of a permanent peritoneal catheter for CAPD in children weighing less than 15 kg.Book of Abstract Congr Soc Ital Nephrology,Rimini,1980 p.251

7. De Santo NG,Capodicasa G,Senatore R,Cicchetti T,Cirillo D,Damiano M, Torella R,Giugliano D,Improta L,Giordano C.Glucose utilization from dialyzate in patients on Continous Ambulatory Peritoneal Dialysis. Int J Artif Organs 2:119,1979

8. Giordano C.Use of exogenous and endogenous urea for protein synthesis in normal and uremic subjects.J Lab Clin Med 62:231,1963

9. Sirbu ER,Margen S and Calloway DH.Effect of reduced protein intake on nitrogen loss from human integument.Am J Clin Nutr 20:1158,1967

10. Costa G,Ullrich L,Kantor F and Holland JF.Production of elemental nitrogen by certain mammals including man.Nature(London) 218:546,1968

11. Giordano C,De Pascale C,De Santo NG,Esposito R,Balestrieri C,Fürst P. L'Utilizzazione dell'azoto atmosferico per la sintesi degli amminoacidi.Bioch Appl 15:551,1968

12. Giordano C,De Pascale C,De Santo NG,Fürst P,Stangherlin P,Esposito R. Use of different sources of nitrogen in uremia.Arch Intern Med 126:781, 1970

CLINICAL ASPECTS OF RENAL OSTEODYSTROPHY

I.B.HOUSTON and   R.J.POSTLETHWAITE

The bone disease associated with chronic renal failure in the past
has often been allowed to progress to the point of producing grotesque
skeletal malformations. It is doubtful whether this attitude was ever
entirely justifiable but with recent developments both in the treatment
of chronic renal failure and in the production of Vitamin D metabolites,
it is certainly indefensible now. It is important therefore, to
identify renal osteodystrophy at an early stage in its development so
that appropriate treatment can be given which will prevent the pain and
disability of the advanced disease.

Therefore, some years ago we decided to improve the early
identification and treatment of this condition and much of the data
contained in this report have been obtained by Dr.R.J.Postlethwaite and
Dr.L.Hill, working jointly from the Department of Child Health and the
Department of Medicine in Manchester.

Identification of early bone disease

Thirty-one children have been studied who exhibited all degrees of
chronic renal failure but were not being dialysed and had not been
transplanted; nor did they have renal tubular diseases as the primary
cause of their chronic renal failure.

Of these 27 children, 17 showed histological evidence of renal
osteodystrophy on bone biopsy. Increased osteoclastic activity was an
almost universal finding but many also had thickened osteoid seams and
evidence of a calcification defect. Twelve of these 17 histologically
proven cases showed radiological evidence of bone disease. Twelve
patients also showed serum parathormone concentrations > 1 ng/ml
(11 exceeded 2 ng/ml), and all of these had evidence of radiological

abnormalities. A parathormone level of < 1 ng/ml was regularly associated with normal radiological appearances even if there was biopsy evidence of bone disease.

Serum parathormone concentrations correlated rather poorly with serum inorganic phosphate levels. Correlation between serum alkaline phosphatase concentrations and severe bone disease was somewhat better but there were several examples of hyperparathyroidism accompanied by levels of alkaline phosphatase which fell within the wide range of normality for children. Thus neither phosphate nor alkaline phosphatase concentration in the serum is a good predictor of bone disease when one looks at cross-sectional data of this type. However, if serum alkaline phosphatase concentrations are measured sequentially on individual patients, increasing levels (even within the normal range) may be better indicators of developing bone disease.

There was a good correlation between serum parathormone levels and serum creatinine concentrations, $(R = 0.82)$ and serum creatinine concentrations of > 1 mg/dl were not associated with high serum parathormone levels (Postlethwaite et al 1976); Chan & DeLuca (1979) obtained rather similar data.

These studies demonstrated that short of doing a bone biopsy, serum parathormone concentrations were one of the earliest indicators of bone disease. However, careful examination of x-rays of the hands and wrists, especially a search for sub-periosteal erosions was almost as sensitive. Moreover, such early radiological changes commonly preceded any clinical evidence such as bone pain or deformity and for clinical as opposed to research purposes, our present procedure is to rely heavily on radiological diagnosis of early but distinct disease and to use this as our indication for starting therapy. Of course this attitude assumes that histological bone disease and hyperparathyroidism without radiological changes are innocuous as well as presymptomatic situations. There have been reports (Chesney et al, 1980) that appropriate treatment of renal osteodystrophy improves growth substantially and if it could be shown that this growth improvement were present even in the pre-symptomatic stage of the disease then much earlier detection and treatment would be needed. It is also conceivable that an increased

serum concentration of parathormone may itself have deleterious effects
on cellular function in many parts of the body (Massry 1980); if this
were accepted then the need for much earlier treatment would need to be
carefully re-evaluated.

1α-hydroxycholecalciferol treatment

A consideration of the pathogenesis of renal osteodystrophy shows
that therapeutic intervention is possible in several places. Successful
renal transplantation of course is highly effective and dialysis may
also be helpful; though the latter may also cause additional problems.
Parathyroidectomy has been reported in a number of patients in the past
and may be essential to control the hypercalcaemia which may otherwise
result from the use of Vitamin D and its metabolites. So far this has
not been necessary in our patients though we are of course reporting
experiences of a relatively short duration and in patients not
receiving dialysis. Certainly parathyroidectomy is a form of treatment
which needs to be kept in mind.

Low concentrations of inorganic phosphate in association with renal
tubular disease or in certain dialysed patients (Pierides et al,1976)
may exacerbate bone disease, but the more common problem in the
non-dialysed, is the excessive retention of phosphate and
hyperphosphataemia. This may be directly responsible for some
parathyroid stimulation and it is certainly associated with increased
risks of metastatic calcification during treatment with Vitamin D
metabolites. Control of serum inorganic phosphate levels with oral
phosphate-binders such as oral aluminium hydroxide therefore is a vital
part of any treatment. It may help to control the hyperparathyroid
element in the bone disease and it certainly adds to the margin of
safety when treatment with Vitamin D metabolites is undertaken.

A Vitamin D metabolite, 1α-hydroxycholecalciferol (1αHCC)˙ became
available to us a few years ago. We have demonstrated (Postlethwaite
and Houston, 1977) as have others (Nielsen et al, 1980), that
administration of 1α-hydroxycholecalciferol in doses likely to lead to
near physiological levels of 1,25-dihydroxycholecalciferol is effective
treatment. Balance studies have shown that it rapidly converts the
negative calcium and phosphate balance of renal osteodystrophy into

positive balances. This improvement in intestinal absorption of calcium and phosphate may not be its only mode of action but it is certainly an important one. In passing, it should be noted that the increased phosphate absorption makes control of the serum phosphate level with phosphate binders even more important.

Treatment with 1αHCC (40 ng/kg/24 hours) increased serum calcium and phosphate concentrations to normal within a few weeks; alkaline phosphatase concentrations fell, but took 6-9 months to attain their minimum values. During this period there was radiological healing of both metaphyseal lesions and sub-periosteal erosions and where measured, parathormone concentrations returned to normal. No examples of tertiary hyperparathyroidism (in which hyperparathyroidism continues despite treatment of the bone disease and normalization of serum calcium) have been encountered as yet.

1αHCC is preferred to ordinary calciferol because of the greater predictability of response to a standard dose and because of its much shorter pharmacological half-life. While hypercalcaemia must be carefully avoided by regular measurement of serum calcium concentration and appropriate adjustment to 1αHCC dosage, we have observed no acceleration in the rate of deterioration of glomerular filtration rate with this treatment. However, even mild and transient hypercalcaemia has a depressant effect upon glomerular filtration rate and must be avoided if at all possible; the short half life of 1αHCC is very helpful in this respect. We have no experience of using 1,25-dihydroxycholecalciferol but on theoretical grounds we would expect that its advantages and disadvantages would be very similar to those of 1αHCC.

Conclusions:

1. Children with advanced chronic renal failure are at risk from the complication of bone disease; they should be carefully and regularly checked for early radiological evidence of it. In the present state of knowledge we recommend starting treatment as soon as the earliest but distinct radiological signs appear; these are usually subperiosteal erosions.

2. Even earlier detection of presymptomatic bone disease by the use of bone biopsy and serum parathormone concentrations may prove desirable if, in the future, it can be demonstrated that growth or another aspect of the patient's well-being is improved by such early treatment. This area urgently needs further work.

3. The use of phosphate binders such as aluminium hydroxide is very important as an adjunct to successful therapy.

4. Calciferol or its metabolites are effective in improving calcium absorption and correcting radiological bone disease; 1αhydroxy- (and probably 1,25-dihydroxy)-cholecalciferol are more predictable and probably safer than ordinary calciferol. However, regular measurements of serum calcium concentration must be made to identify and deal with any episodes of hypercalcaemia which may occur.

REFERENCES

1. Chan,J.C.M., DeLuca,H.F.(1979) "Calcium and Parathyroid Disorders in Children. Chronic Renal Failure and Treatment with Calcitriol". J.Amer.med.Assoc., 241, 1242-1244.

2. Chesney,R.W.,Moorthy,A.V., Eisman,J.A., Jax,D.K., Mazess,R.B., DeLuca,H.F.(1978) "Increased growth after long-term oral $1\alpha,25$-Vitamin D_3 in childhood renal osteodystrophy", New Engl.J.Med., 298, 238-242

3. Massry,S.G. (1980) Proceedings of 5th Intl.Symp. of Paediatric Nephrology.

4. Neilsen,H.E., Rømer,F.K., Melsen,F., Christensen,M.S., Hansen,H.E.(1980) "1αhydroxy vitamin D_3 treatment of non-dialyzed patients with chronic renal failure. Effects on bone, mineral metabolism and kidney function". Clin. Nephrol, 13, 103-108.

5. Pierides,A.M., Ellis,H.A., Simpson,W., Dewar, J.H.: Ward, M.K., Kerr,D.N.S., (1976) "Variable response to long-term 1α-hydroxycholecalciferol in haemodialysis osteodystrophy", Lancet, i. 1092.

6. Postlethwaite,R.J., Hill,L.F., Houston,I.B.(1976) "Detection and management of bone disease in children with chronic renal failure", Melsunger Medizinische Mitteilungen, 50, Suppl. 11, 71-83.

7. Postlethwaite,R.J., Houston,I.B.(1977) "Bone Disease in children with chronic renal failure; therapy with 1αhydroxyvitamin D_3", Clin.Endocrin., 7, Suppl., 1175-1245.

1,25-DIHYDROXYVITAMIN D_3 IN THE TREATMENT OF JUVENILE RENAL OSTEODYSTROPHY

RUSSELL W. CHESNEY, Dept. of Pediatrics, Univ. of Wisconsin, Madison, WI

The discovery of the vitamin D endocrine system and the finding that the kidney is a major site of the synthesis of vitamin D metabolites, provides a theoretical explanation for the vitamin D resistance of uremic osteodystrophy (1). Calcitriol ($1,25(OH)_2D$) and $24,25(OH)_2D$ are predominately synthesized in mitochondria of proximal tubule cells. Because of the reduction in nephron mass in uremia, the synthesis of these metabolites is impaired and circulating levels are low (2). A reduction in calcitriol levels, and possibly in those of $24,25(OH)_2D$, results in diminished gut calcium absorption, secondary hyperparathyroidism and undermineralized osteoid and growing surfaces of bone (3). Ultimately, uremic children develop widened growth plates, bone age retardation and growth failure.

The treatment of juvenile renal osteodystrophy involves dietary phosphate restriction, phosphate sequestering agents, dietary calcium supplementation and the provision of vitamin D. Newer metabolites of vitamin D -- including 25-hydroxy-D (4,5), synthetic 1α-hydroxy-D (6) and calcitriol (7-9) -- have been used in childhood uremia. This paper describes our $5\frac{1}{2}$-year experience using calcitriol. After a discussion of our findings, we will touch on three areas of controversy: 1) the value of calcitriol therapy in increasing growth rate; 2) the possibility that calcitriol therapy impairs renal function, and 3) the role of $24,25(OH)_2D$ therapy.

Twelve patients, aged 3 months to 15 years, were treated with calcitriol because of clinical and radiologic evidence of worsening bone disease despite high-dose vitamin D_2 or dihydrotachysterol (DHT). Only 2 patients were undergoing chronic hemodialysis and 8 patients had experienced renal disease since birth. Most patients had overt augulation of the lower extremities or gait disturbances that prevented normal ambulation. The patients have received calcitriol from 2 to 64 months, and 8 currently receive therapy. These children have received calcitriol for a total of

402 months (mean 33.5 months) or 33 treatment years. Their diagnoses and prior therapy are described elsewhere (10). Renal transplantation was performed in 4 patients, and calcitriol was discontinued but restarted in 2 after rejection. Patient heights were determined using a fixed wall stadiometer, and growth velocity (cm/yr) was calculated only when accurate 12-month growth measurements were available.

The calcitriol used was provided by Hoffman-LaRoche (Nutley, NJ). Each patient received oral phosphate binders, calcium gluconate (1 g/M^2/day) and bicarbonate in the form of sodium and potassium citrate. Bath calcium in hemodialysis patients was 3.5 mEq/L.

Prior to therapy, hypocalcemia was found in 9 patients despite vitamin D and oral calcium. Shown in Figure 1 is the influence of calcitriol on serum chemical values. Hypercalcemia was found in three situations: 1) a single patient with oxalosis and the severe bone disease typical of long-term oxalosis (11); 2) younger patients in whom overdosage with drug is possible, since the smallest capsule is 0.25 µgm, and 3) after radiologic evidence of bone healing had been found and alkaline phosphatase levels fell.

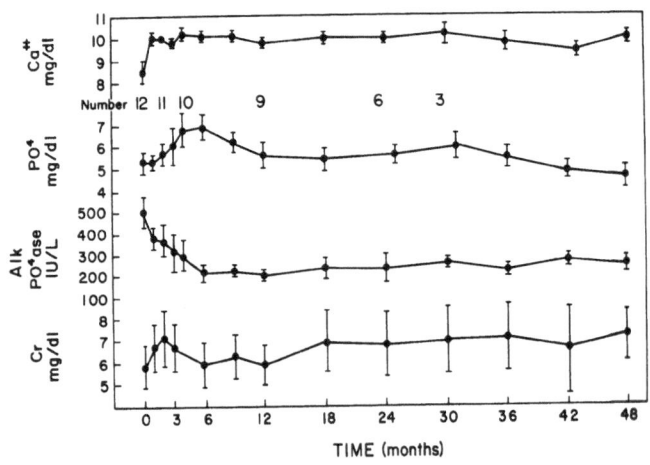

FIGURE 1. Influence of calcitriol on serum calcium, phosphate, alkaline phosphatase and creatinine clearance.

Only in the patient with oxalosis was discontinuation of drug required. Hypercalcemic episodes have been treated with discontinuation of drug for a week, followed by dose reduction. Oral calcium supplements may also be discontinued. Hyperphosphatemia can occur, since calcitriol increases intestinal phosphate absorption. Increased doses of phosphate binding agent are often necessary.

The results of calcitriol on iPTH and serum HCO_3 levels are shown in Figure 2. Although PTH levels fell by 80 percent, supranormal PTH concen-

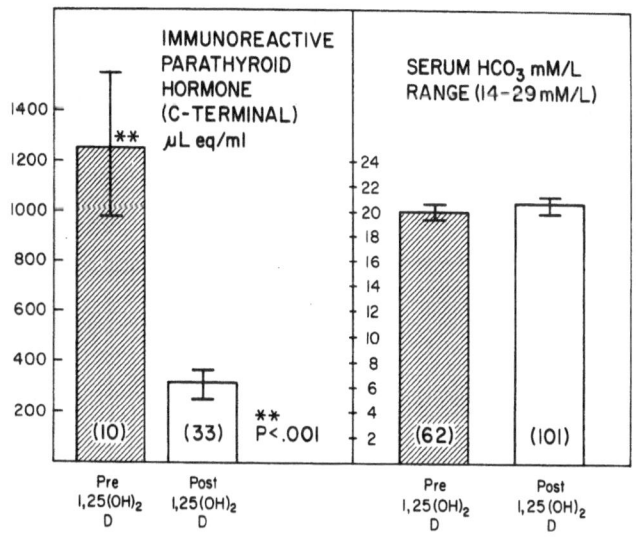

FIGURE 2.
Serum levels
of iPTH and
bicarbonate
(mean $\pm$ SE).

trations remained after calcitriol treatment. The persistently elevated PTH values reflect that the C-terminal fragment of the PTH molecule is being measured, namely that portion which must undergo renal degradation (12). The most dramatic response to therapy was in terms of ambulation and muscle strength. In 5 cases, ambulation was greatly influenced by therapy, and 4 patients unable to walk can now run. Other adult studies have reported a similar influence of calcitriol on gait disturbances and myopathy (13).

Prior to treatment, serum calcitriol levels were measured in these patients and were subnormal in all but one patient, with a mean of 9.0 ± 2 pg/ml (SE). Therapy raised these levels into the normal range. We have examined the relationship of serum calcitriol to creatinine clearance and found a curvilinear relationship. As clearance declines, so does calcitriol concentration. Figure 3 displays the relationship of iPTH to calcitriol concentration, which falls by 87 percent after treatment ($p < .001$). Thus, treatment restores circulating calcitriol and substantially reduces circulating PTH.

We previously reported that growth velocity in 4 patients, evaluated for 12 months pre- and post-calcitriol therapy, increased from 2.6 ± 0.8

212

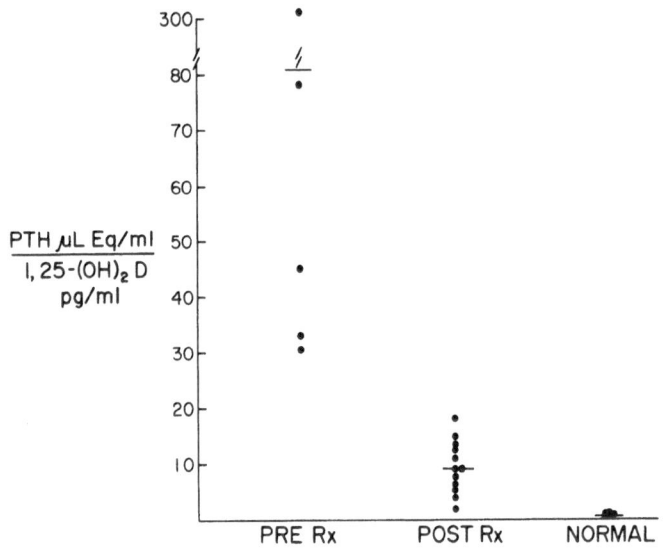

FIGURE 3. The ratio of PTH to calcitriol concentration in serum before and after therapy. The ratio in normal controls is also given.

to 8.0 $\pm$ 3.2 cm/yr (SD) (p < .01). Growth velocity increased from less than the 3rd percentile to the 10th to 97th percentiles post-therapy (9). The long-term growth data available from 10 patients reveals that the mean height velocity increased from 4.2 $\pm$ 1.1 cm/yr (SE) to 7.2 $\pm$ 0.9 after therapy (p < .005) (Figure 4). Growth patterns are shown in Figure 5 and reveal the marked short stature at the start of therapy. After treatment,

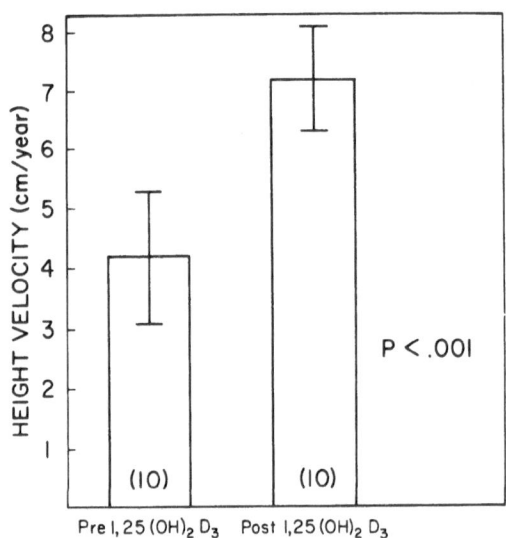

FIGURE 4. Height velocity before and after therapy with calcitriol in 10 patients.

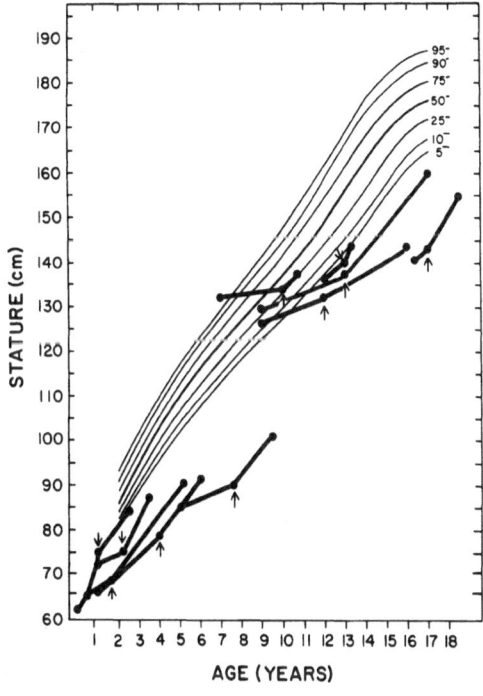

FIGURE 5. Growth patterns before and after calcitriol therapy in 10 patients.

the growth patterns in 9 of the 10 patients parallel the height-vs-age percentile lines. These data indicate that patients start at a height percentile which is 2 to 3.5 SD below the mean for age. After treatment, growth is parallel to that expected for age, but no catch-up growth is evident. It is possible, but as yet unproven, that earlier treatment might prevent this decline in height velocity which occurs early in life.

Various groups have found (6,7,14) or have not found (15-17) height velocity increases after initiation of calcitriol therapy. Although the reasons for these differences are not certain, most patients who have demonstrated increased growth are pre-dialysis. Conversely, children receiving chronic dialysis have not experienced an increased growth rate after therapy. It is tempting to speculate that pre-dialysis patients have more impressive growth after calcitriol therapy, since their cartilage mineralization defect is worse and growth impairment is greater. The child, pre-dialysis, is producing urine containing large amounts of bi-carbonate (reduced Tm_{HCO_3}), uses his bones as a buffer and may have sub-stantial hypercalcuria (3,10). With chronic dialysis, serum calcium, bicarbonate and phosphate are more stable, and, initially, bone disease may be less severe. Accordingly, the increased growth rates found after calcitriol therapy represent improved mineralization of rachitic bones. However, this is an hypothesis until it is proven.

It has been shown that calcitriol is harmful to renal function in non-dialyzed patients (18). This decline in renal function could have occurred because of drug-related hypercalcemia and hyperphosphatemia with intrarenal calcium phosphate deposition, or because PTH-dependent renal blood flow might be depressed (19). When hypercalcemia was avoided, we have found no change in the slope of the reciprocal of serum creatinine ($1/S_{Cr}$) with time and no increase in urine calcium excretion (Figure 6). As shown by

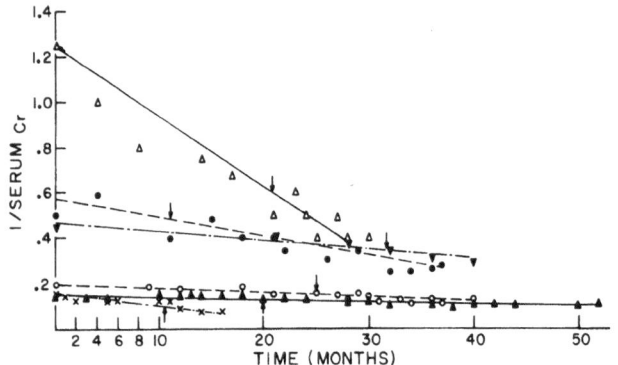

FIGURE 6.
Reciprocal of serum creatinine over time.
Arrow denotes onset of calcitriol therapy.

Nordin (20), a decline in GFR occurs only during hypercalcemic episodes. With correction of hypercalcemia, the GFR reverted to pre-hypercalcemic levels. Since the half-life of calcitriol is so short, the time for reversal of hypercalcemia is actually shorter with this agent than with other vitamin D analogs.

Recent studies in animals have suggested that $24,25(OH)_2D$ may serve as a mineralizing hormone (21). This evidence is summarized in Table I. This experimental evidence to date suggests that $24,25(OH)_2D$ may play a role in the mineralization of bone in animals, although this is not firmly established. It also may be important as an agent given in combination with calcitriol in renal osteodystrophy (35). In our own patients, we find that serum $24,25(OH)_2D$ is subnormal. In patients with a creatinine clearance less than 13 ml/min/1.73 M^2, serum levels are 0.60 ± 0.11 ng/ml

Table I. Role of 24,25(OH)$_2$D in renal osteodystrophy (2,21-34)

---

1. Made predominately in kidney, thus reduced levels in uremia (0.7 vs. 3-4 ng/ml) (Shepard et al)
2. Produced in cartilage and calvaria of <u>rats</u> (Garabedian)
3. Promotes normal ossification of bone when calcium and phosphate are supersaturated in bone ECF in <u>chicks</u> (Edelstein)
4. Reduces iPTH secretion in <u>dogs</u> when given I-V or P-O (Canterbury)
5. Blunts PTH resorption of bone in vitro in <u>rats</u> (Liebenherr)
6. In uremic <u>man</u> (Kanis):
   a) Increases Ca++ absorption
   b) No rise in serum Ca++
   c) Suggests deposition in bone
7. Reversal of "skeletal resistance to PTH" in uremic <u>man</u> by 1,25 and 24,25 (Massry)
8. Combination of 25 and 1,25 or 24,25 and 1,25 best heals osteomalacia in <u>man</u> (Rasmussen)
9. Normal 24,25 and low 1,25 in hypophosphatemic rickets with mineralization defect (Chesney)
10. Subnormal levels in cord blood despite "normal" mineralization

Conclusion: Unique biological role unclear, but may be useful in combination with 1,25. Normal man has 25/24,25/1,25 in 1000/100/1 ratio, and uremia changes this relationship.

(SD) (n=16), in comparison with 1.70 ± 0.11 in children with renal disease and a clearance greater than 50 ml/min ($p < .001$). Accordingly, serum levels of 24,25(OH)$_2$D and calcitriol are reduced in these subjects.

In conclusion, the improvements in medical therapy of childhood uremia, including dialysis and transplantation, have led to the need for comprehensive therapy of renal osteodystrophy and abnormalities of divalent mineral metabolism. Calcitriol is a potent form of vitamin D which can offer considerable benefits, particularly reversing radiologic changes indicative of bone disease, in increasing the height velocity of children before dialysis and in improving muscle weakness.

REFERENCES

1. DeLuca HF. 1979. The vitamin D system in the regulation of calcium and phosphorus metabolism. W.O. Atwater Memorial Lecture. Nutrit Rev 37:161-193.
2. Shephard RM, Horst RL, Hamstra AJ, DeLuca HF. 1979. Determination of vitamin D and its metabolites in plasma from normal and anephric man. Biochem J 182:55-69.
3. Avioli LV, Teitelbaum S. 1978. Renal osteodystrophy. In Edelman CM (ed): Pediatric Kidney Disease. Boston: Little, Brown and Co., p 366.
4. Witmer G, Margolis A, Fontaine O, Fritsch J, Lenoir G, Broyer M, Balsan S. 1976. Effects of 25-hydroxycholecalciferol on bone lesions

of children with terminal renal failure. Kidney International 10:395.

5. Baron R, Norman M, Mazur A. 1979. Dynamic bone histomorphometry in children with chronic renal failure treated with 25(OH)D$_3$. In Norman AW, Schaeffer K, Grigoleit HJ (eds): Proc. of the IVth Workshop on Vitamin D. Berlin: Walter de Gruyter, p 847-852.

6. Chan JCM, Oldham SB, Holick HF, DeLuca HF. 1975. 1α-Hydroxyvitamin D$_3$ in chronic renal failure: A potent analog of the kidney hormone, 1,25-dihydroxycholecalciferol. JAMA 234:47.

7. Henderson RG, Russell RGG, Ledinghan JGG. 1974. Effects of 1,25-dihydroxycholecalciferol on calcium absorption, muscle weakness and bone disease in chronic renal failure. Lancet 1:279.

8. Pierides AM, Ellis HA, Dellagrammatikas H. 1977. 1,25-Dihydroxy-cholecalciferol in renal osteodystrophy: Epiphysiolysis anticonvulsant therapy. Arch Dis Child 52:464.

9. Chesney RW, Moorthy AV, Jax DK, Eisman JA, Mazess RB, DeLuca HF. 1978. Increased linear growth after long-term oral 1,25(OH)$_2$D therapy in childhood renal osteodystrophy. N Engl J Med 298:238-242.

10. Chesney RW, Mazess RB, DeLuca HF. 1980, in press. The long-term influence of calcitriol on growth patterns in childhood renal osteo-dystrophy. Excerpta Medica.

11. Breed A, Chesney RW, Friedman AL, Gilbert E, Langer L, Lattoraca R. 1980, in press. Oxalosis-induced bone disease: A complication of prolonged survival and transplantation in primary hyperoxaluria. J Bone Joint Surgery.

12. Freitag J, Martin KJ, Hruska KA, Klahr S, Slatopolsky E. 1978. Impaired parathyroid hormone metabolism in patients with chronic renal failure. N Engl J Med 298:29.

13. Coburn JW, Massry SG. 1980. Uses and actions of 1,25-dihydroxy-vitamin D$_3$ in uremia. Contrib Nephrol 18:1-217.

14. Chan JCM, DeLuca HF. 1977. Growth velocity in a child on prolonged hemodialysis: Beneficial effect of 1α-hydroxyvitamin D$_3$. JAMA 238:2053.

15. Bulla M, Delling G, Offermann G, Ziegler R. 1980. Renal osteodystrophy in children: Therapy with vitamin D$_3$ or 1,25-dihydroxycholecalciferol. Pediatr Res 14:990.

16. Gilli G, Ritz E, Mehls O, v.d. Linden A. 1980. Effect of vitamin D$_3$ and 1,25(OH)$_2$D$_3$ on growth in experimental uremia. Pediatr Res 14:990.

17. Malekzadeh MH, Ettenger RB, Pennisi AJ. 1977. Treatment of renal osteodystrophy in children on hemodialysis with dihydrotachysterol. In Norman AW, Schaefer K, Coburn JW (eds): Vitamin D: Biochemical, Chemical and Clinical Aspects Related to Calcium Metabolism. Berlin: Walter deGruyter, p 681-683.

18. Christiansen C, Rodbro P, Christensen MS. 1978. Deterioration of renal function during treatment of chronic renal failure with 1,25-dihydroxycholecalciferol. Lancet ii:700-702.

19. Chesney RW. 1980. Does uremic bone disease warrant early treatment with calcitriol? Arch Intern Med 140:1016-1017.

20. Nordin BEC. 1978. Vitamin D analogs and renal function. Lancet ii: 1259.

21. Chesney RW. 1980, in press. Modified vitamin D compounds in the treatment of certain bone diseases. In Spiller GA (ed): Nutritional Pharmacology. New York: AR Liss Co.

22. Garabedian M, Liebenherr M, Corvol MT, Guillozo H, Thil CL, Balsan S. 1979. Cellular location and regulation of the 24,25-dihydroxyvitamin D$_3$ formation in cultured cells from bone and cartilage. In Norman AW, Schaefer K, Herrath D (eds): Vitamin D: Basic Research and Its Clinical

Application. Berlin: Walter de Gruyter, p 391-398.

23. Ornoy A, Goodwin D, Noff D, Edelstein S. 1978. 24,25-Dihydroxy-vitamin D is a metabolite of vitamin D essential for bone formation. Nature 276:517-519.

24. Canterbury JM, Lerman S, Claflin AJ, Henry H, Norman A, Reiss E. 1978. Inhibition of parathyroid hormone secretion by 25-hydroxychole-calciferol and 24,25-dihydroxycholecalciferol in the dog. J Clin Invest 61:1375-1383.

25. Canterbury JM, Bourgoignie JJ, Gavellas G, Reiss E. 1980. Metabolic consequences of oral administration of 24,25(OH)$_2$D$_3$ to uremic dogs. J Clin Invest 65:571-579.

26. Liebenherr M, Garabedian M, Guillozo H, Bailly du Bois M, Balsan S. 1979. Interaction of 24,25-dihydroxyvitamin D$_3$ and parathyroid hormone on bone enzymes in vitro. Calcif Tiss Int 27:47-52.

27. Kanis JA, Cundy T, Bartlett M, Smith R, Heynen G, Warner GT, Russell RGG. 1978. Is 24,25-dihydroxycholecalciferol a calcium-regulating hormone in man? Brit Med J 1:1382-1386.

28. Llach F, Brickman AS, Singer FR, Coburn JW. 1979. 24,25-Dihydroxy-cholecalciferol, a vitamin D sterol with qualitatively unique effects in uremic man. Metab Bone Dis and Rel Res 2:11-15.

29. Massry SG, Turna S, Dua S, Goldstein DA. 1979. Reversal of skeletal resistance to parathyroid hormone in uremia by vitamin D metabolites. Evidence for the requirement of 1,25(OH)$_2$D$_3$ and 24,25(OH)$_2$D$_3$. J Lab Clin Med 94:152-157.

30. Bordier P, Zingraff J, Gueris J, Jungers P, Marie P, Pechet M, Rasmussen H. 1978. The effect of 1α-(OH)D$_3$ and 1,25(OH)$_2$D$_3$ on the bone in patients with renal osteodystrophy. Am J Med 64:101-107.

31. Rasmussen H, Bordier P. 1980. Evidence that different vitamin D sterols have qualitatively different effects in man. Contrib Nephrol 18:184-191.

32. Kanis JA, Cundy T, Smith R, Heynen G, Warner GT, Lorams J, Russell RGG. 1980. Possible function of different renal metabolites of vitamin D in man. Contrib Nephrol 18:192-211.

33. Chesney RW, Mazess RB, Hamstra AJ, DeLuca HF. 1979. Demineralization in hypophosphatemic rickets with normal 24,25-dihydroxyvitamin D and subnormal 1,25-dihydroxyvitamin D levels. Clin Res 27:653A.

34. Hillman LS, Slatopolsky E, Haddad JG. 1978. Perinatal vitamin D metabolism: IV. Maternal and cord serum 24,25-dihydroxyvitamin D concentrations. J Clin Endocrinol Metab 47:1073-1076.

35. Hodsman A, Wong E, Sherrard D, Brickman A, Lee D, Singer F, Norman A, Coburn J. 1980. Use of 24,25-dihydroxyvitamin D$_3$ in dialysis osteo-malacia: Preliminary results. In Cohn D (ed): Endocrinology of Calcium Regulating Hormones. Amsterdam: Excerpta Medica, in press.

THE SPECTRUM OF SKELETAL MANIFESTATIONS IN RENAL OSTEODYSTROPHY

O. MEHLS, E. RITZ, G. GILLI, M. BROYER
Department Pediatrics and Internal Medicine, University of
Heidelberg (Germany; FRG) and Hôpital des Enfants Malades,
Paris (France).

Skeletal complications are a well recognized feature of renal
insufficiency in the child. A number of recent overviews have
covered various aspects of this topic (1-5). The present communication reviews selected topics of clinical interest.

1. Skeletal histology

   On the whole, little information is available on skeletal
histology in uremic children. This may be related to the lo-
gistic and ethical problems with bone biopsies in children.
One common feature of renal osteodystrophy is osteitis fibrosa.
In spongy bone its characteristics are endosteal fibrosis with
replacement of reticular fibers and hematopoetic bone marrow
by dense collagen fibers running parallel to the trabecular
surface (fig. 4). In addition, evidence of ongoing or past re-
modelling activity on the trabecular surface consists in (a)
accumulation of osteoid, covered or not by osteoblasts (active
or inactive osteoid) and (b) resorption lacunae with apparently uni- or multinuclear osteoclasts. In the normal skeleton,
tight coupling between bone apposition and bone resorption is
present and the type of bone deposited consists of regularly
textured lamellar bone. Such tight coupling is lost in advanced
osteitis fibrosa and more primitive bone with inferior texture
and biochemical qualities (woven bone) is deposited. Bone formation may even occur by metaplastic transformation from fibrous
tissue, e.g. in the metaphyseal growth zone (fig. 3). A second
feature, which is not constantly present, is disturbed mineralisation. The problems of evaluating mineralisation in the presence of a high turnover state (i.e. hyperparathyroidism) have
been pointed out elsewhere (6, 7). A defect of primary (7) mine-

Table 1   Morphometric findings in iliac crest spongiosa of uremic children

	Bone volume (mm³/cm³) Vv	Density of osteoid (mm³/cm³) VvO	Surface density (mm³/cm³) of osteoid SvOS	Fraction of surface covered by osteoid (%) HO	Fraction of surface covered with endosteal fibrosis (%) EF
Control (n=21)	187 ± 53	4 ± 2	210 ± 108	0.4 ± 0.8	0
Renal failure, serum creatinine					
2.5 mg/dl (n=7)	229 ± 69	16 ± 15	1139 ± 747	1.6 ± 1.2	14.1 ± 4.4
2-5 mg/dl (n=13)	282 ± 84	30 ± 27	1563 ± 924	7.1 ± 5.8	52.2 ± 34.4
5 mg/dl (n=19)	330 ± 69	64 ± 57	1988 ± 754	8.0 ± 6.1	73.3 ± 31.8
Dialysed children (n=30)	261 ± 84	24 ± 32	1229 ± 735	3.4 ± 2.6	59.9 ± 34.3
Non-dialysed children with epiphyseal slipping (n=8)	337 ± 71	128 ±151	2089 ± 1125	12.3 ± 7.6	88.8 ± 13.3

ralisation can be suspected if an excessive number of non-mineralised osteoid lamellae are present in osteoid seams (fig. 1). The best technique currently available is in vivo labelling of mineralisation fronts with tetracyclin (6). Labelling is invariably absent or defective in osteomalacia.

Skeletal changes may be quantitated with micromorphometric techniques using the principles of stereology. The problem of age corrected normal values has been solved in recent years (8, 9). As indicated in table 1, histological abnormalities are present early and progress in non-treated children with advancing renal failure. Increased volumetric density of bone points to osteoslcerosis of spongy bone particularly in non-dialysed and less in dialysed children. The progressive rise of osteoclastic surface resorption and endosteal fibrosis with renal failure correlates well with increasing iPTH levels (10). It is of note that in dialysed children histological abnormalities are less severe. This may be due to better control of hyperparathyroidism, vitamin D therapy and patient sampling. Particularly noteworthy is the finding that most marked osteosclerosis, endosteal fibrosis and osteoclastic resorption are present in children with slipped epiphyses (10). Although a reasonable correlation between serum chemistry or iPTH and bone histology is found (8), neither the type nor the severity of skeletal lesions can be adequately assessed with serum chemistry. The correlation between skeletal X-ray and bone histology is also less than satisfactory (11). Direct assessment of bone (transiliac bone biopsy; ref. 6) appears indicated whenever therapeutic decisions depend on findings of bone histology (e.g. parathyroidectomy; e.g. detection of severe mineralisation defects, ref. 12).

2.   Histology of the growth zone

The changes in the growth zone of uremic children may be schematically classified as a spectrum from classic rickets to classic osteitis fibrosa (fig. 2). Ricketic changes (13) are not common in advanced renal failure. Classical (13) and more recent (14) studies emphasized the presence of severe osteitis fibrosa in terminal renal failure (fig. 5). Because such histological

features provide a conceptual framework to understand epiphyseal
slipping, a brief discussion appears appropriate. In our studies,
growth cartilage was narrow and provisional calcification of
cartilage ground substance was not defective. However, the normal transition between growth cartilage and metaphyseal bone
was highly abnormal. Vascular invasion was virtually absent and
growth cartilage was often occluded by a bar of dense bone
("Abschlußplatte") and physically separated from metaphyseal
bone. In the metaphysis, trabecules arose de novo by metaplastic
bone formation from primitive fibrous tissue. Such trabecules
were no longer in physical contact with cartilage, were devoid
of a chondroid core and consisted entirely of poorly mineralised
woven bone without the normal trajectorial orientation. The un-
locking between cartilage and bone, therefore, provided a plane
of slipping along which the epiphyses could slip sideways under
the influence of shearing forces. The characteristic subperiosteal resorption zone, as seen in X-rays of metaphyseal cortex,
is due to excessive osteoclastic erosion of cortical bone at
this site of normal "funneling" (7), as shown by histology.

3.   Principles of skeletal X-ray changes

   In cortical bone, resorptive defects may be seen at three
surfaces: periosteal; Haversian (intracortical capillaries)
and endosteal surface. At the periosteal surface, interposition
of fibrous tissue between cortical bone and periosteum may separate a small shell of subperiosteal bone from the mass of
cortical bone proper ("periosteoneostosis"). Resorption along
Haversian capillaries gives rise to cortical striation or cortical speckling. It is our impression that reduction of cortical width from endosteal erosion, which is common in adults
(11), is less common in children. Blurring of the transition
between cortex and spongiosa often results in an apparent
increase of cortical width (fig. 3 and 6).
The amount of cancellous bone may be reduced, normal or even
increased (particularly in the upper metaphysis); but almost
invariably, the numbers and diameters of the trabecules are
increased, their contour and direction are irregular, and their

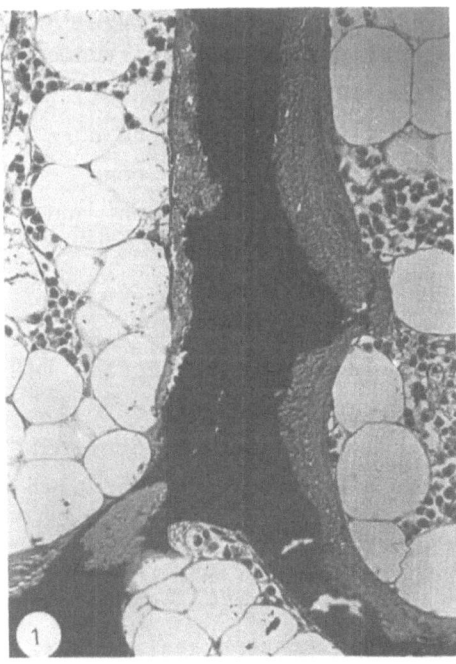

Fig.1: Osteomalacia; iliac crest spongiosa, embedding in methyl-metacrylate, undecalcified section, Van Kossa stain.

Fig.2: Schema of cortical bone changes on X-ray.

Fig.3: Finger of a child with severe osteitis fibrosa. Note periosteoneostosis, subperiostal resorption and cortical speckling. Note also resorptive destruction of ungual tuft.

Fig.4: Osteitis fibrosa; iliac crest spongiosa, undecalcified oection, Masson Goldner stain.

Fig.6: Schema of metaphyseal changes in uremia.

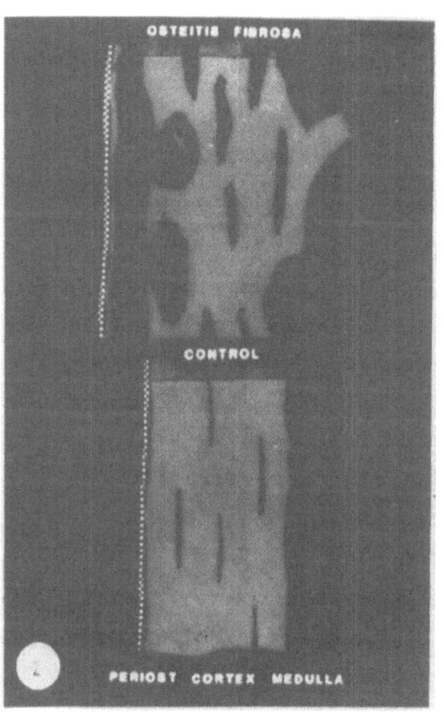

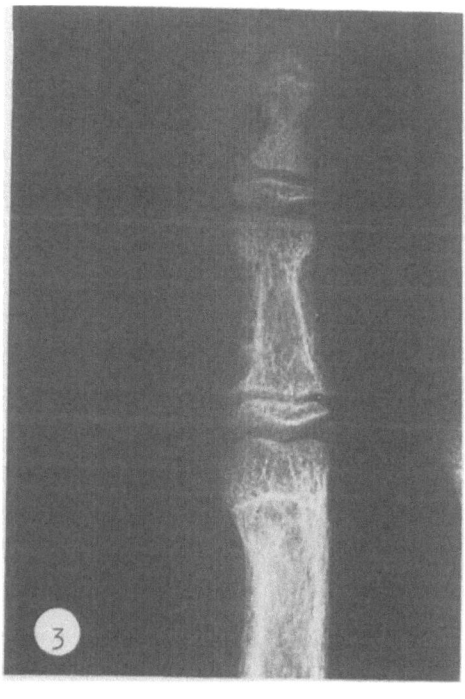

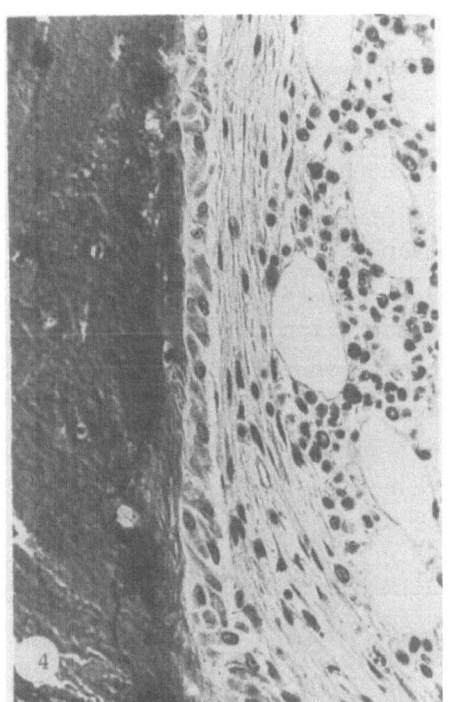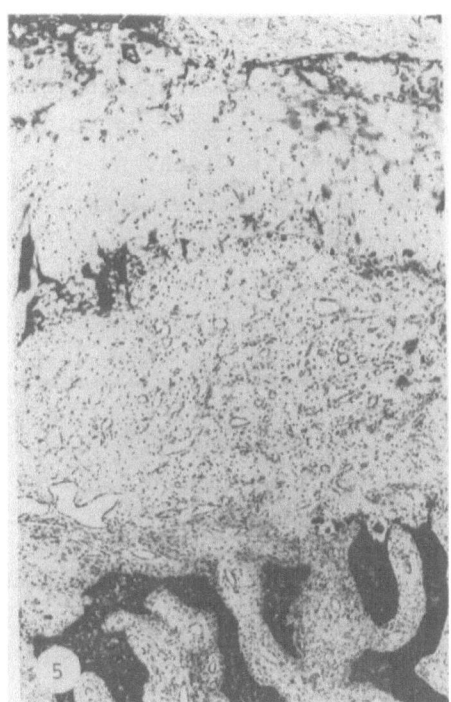

Fig.5: Growth zone of the radius of child with terminal renal failure. Epiphyses and growth cartilage on top, metaphyses on bottom. Note narrow zone of growth cartilage. Underneath growth cartilage dense fibrous tissue. Metaphyseal trabecules, physically separated from growth cartilage and consisting of woven bone.

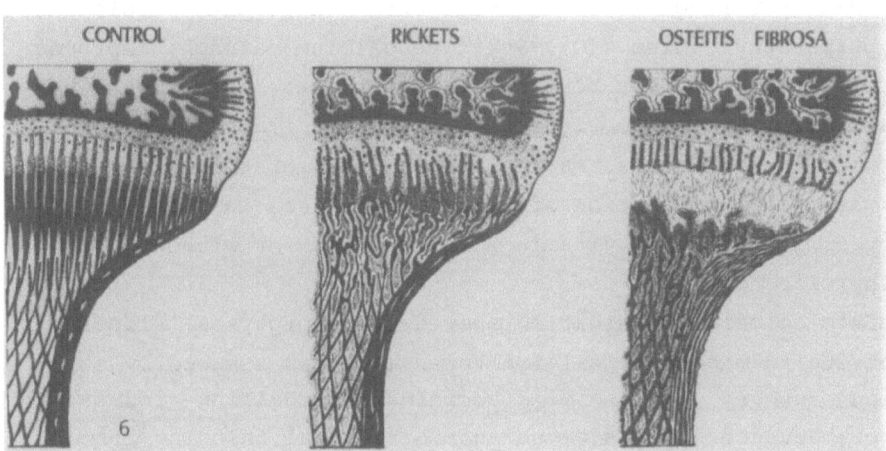

outlines are indistinct and fuzzy.

4. X-ray findings of the growth zone

Accurately aligned X-rays will occasionally show a thin radiolucent zone corresponding to growth cartilage and this is normal
or diminished in width. A broad radiolucent zone underneath is
not due to widening of growth cartilage but due to rarification
in the metaphyseal spongiosa. The metaphysis is the site of intense modelling processes. Depending on the relative prevalence
of mineral resorption (osteoclastic resorption of the metaphyseal trabecules) and mineral apposition transformation of fibrous
tissue into trabecules), cystic defects or a dense "woolly"
pattern may be seen. At the periosteal cortex, a bone resorption
"collar" is seen. These findings have been exhaustively described elsewhere (15, 16).

5. Epiphyseal slipping, epiphyseal necrosis and metaphyseal fracture

The most severe complication of osteitis fibrosa (table 1) in
children is epiphyseal slipping. The sequence and pattern of involvement of epiphyses is age-dependent (17). In prepuberal children, slipping of the forearm epiphyses and particularly slipping
of the femural head are most common and clinically important.
Slipping tends to occur more frequently in congenital renal disease and late in terminal renal failure. Occasionally it super-
venes rapidly within weeks especially in young children. It is
surprisingly infrequent in dialysed children despite persistance
of hyperparathyroidism (10). Positive calcium balance, improved
mineralisation of woven bone in the metaphyses, less severe hyperparathyroidism, more rigorous vitamin D therapy, or a combination of these factors, may be responsible for this clinical
observation. Stabilisation of slipped epiphyses is usually
achieved with adequate vitamin D therapy with or without
parathyroidectomy (5).
Our histological investigation showed that epiphyseal slipping
is not due to macroscopical fractures (14), as assumed by some
previous authors, but due to a coordinated modelling process.
However, advanced bone disease and metaphyseal thinning from

subperiosteal resorption may cause true metaphyseal fractures
(15), presumably from trauma (unpublished own observation).
Of particular interest, and of great clinical importance in
view of its devastating consequences, is the observation of
epiphyseal necrosis, indistinguishable from Perthes disease
(idiopathic femural head necrosis), in children with advanced
renal failure even without antecedant steroid therapy (own unpublished observations). Femural head necrosis in adult patients
on dialysis without steroid therapy is well known (18). The
pathogenesis of the lesion is poorly understood (vascular problems; faulty mechanical loading; traumatic fractures particularly after epileptic fits; hyperparathyroidism?).

6. Extraosseous calcifications

Extraosseous calcifications (vascular, bursal, subcutaneous)
in uremic children are notable by their absence. This contrasts
with findings in adults and is surprising since the Ca x Pi
product in uremic children and adults is comparable (8, 19).
However, visceral (pulmonary, myocardial etc.) calcifications
may be present in uremic children (19).

7. Mineral density of bone

Measurement of whole body calcium, e.g. by neutron activation
analysis, has shown no change or a decrease in adult uremic patients with renal failure and hemodialysis. For obvious reasons,
no such information is available in children. Neutron activation studies showed that redistribution of skeletal mineral
takes place so that mineral density measurements in one reference bone do not unambiguously allow to draw conclusions on
whole body calcium (20). Measurement of mineral density permits
global assessment of mineral content per unit volume within
the periosteal envelope. This global value is dependent on the
relative amount of bone (matrix) mass and on the degree of bone
mineralisation. The measurement does not distinguish between
the two possibilities.
In children specific problems arise with the choice of an adequate base of reference. Results differ markedly when one compares values of uremic children with values normal for age,

226

for height, for body surface or for bone age.

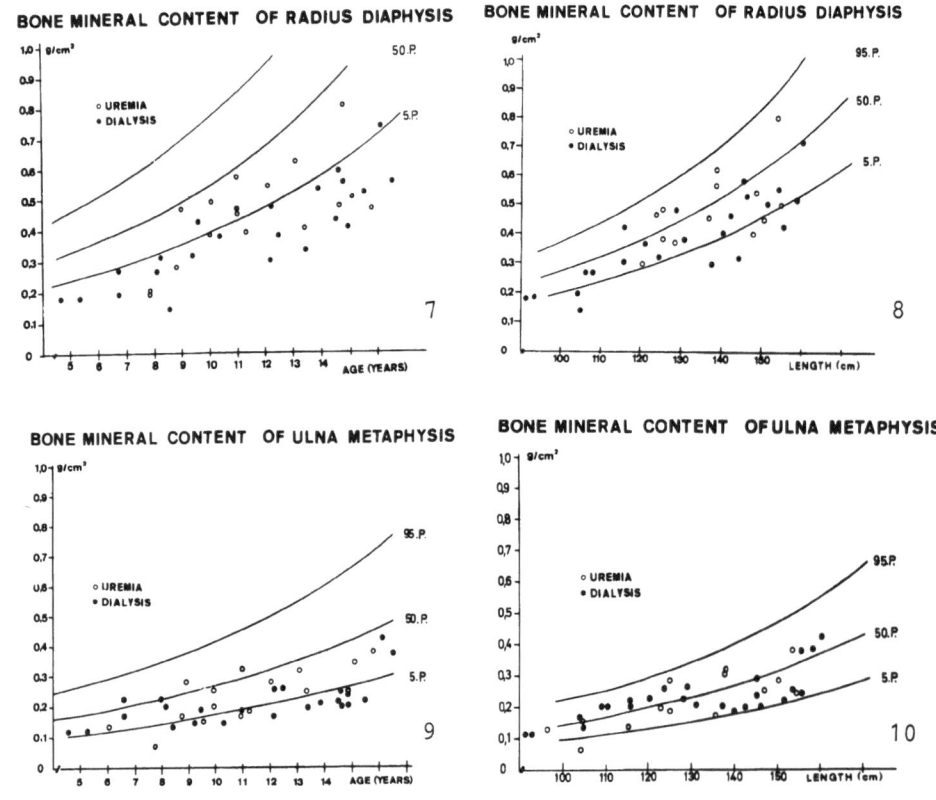

Our own study (fig. 7-11) showed a diminution of mineral density of the radial cortex in non-dialysed, and especially in
dialysed children. The decrease was more marked in the diaphy-
seal than in metaphyseal bone. Diminished radius shaft mineral
density was also reported by Chesney et al. (21).

References:

1. Balsan, S., Royer, P., Mathieu, H.: Les rachitismes et les
   fibroostéolasics destéoclasics des insuffisances rénales
   chroniques de l'enfant. Archives Francaises de Pédiatrique
   23, 769-794, 1966

2. Chan, J.C.M.: Renal osteodystrophy in children. Clinical
   Pediatrics 15, 996-1007, 1976

3. Holliday, U.A.: Metabolism and growth in children with kidney
   insufficiency. Kidney International 14, 299-379, 1978

4. Mehls, O., Ritz, E., Gilli, G., Kreusser, W. Nephron 21, 237-246, 1978 a
5. Mehls, O., Ritz, E., Kreusser, W., Krempien, B. Clin. Endocr. Metab. 9, 151-176, 1980
6. Ritz, E., Malluche, H., Krempien, B., Mehls, O. Calcium Metabolism in Renal Failure and Nephrolithiasis (Ed.) David, D.S., pp. 197-233, New York, John Wiley
7. Ritz,E., Krempien, B., Mehls, O., Malluche, H. Kidney International 4, 116-127, 1973
8. Mehls, O., Krempien, B., Ritz, E., Schärer, K., Schüler, H. Proc. Europ. Dial. Transpl. Ass. 10, 197-201, 1973 b
9. Bulla, M., Stock, G.J., Delling, G., Hofmann, H., Offermann, G. Klin. Wschr. 58, 237-247, 1980
10. Mehls, O., Ritz, E., Krempien, B., Gilli, G., Schärer, K. Vitamin D and Problems related to Uremic Bone Disease (Ed.) Normal, A.W., pp. 551-560, Berlin: de Gruyter, 1975 b
11. Ritz, E., Prager, P., Krempien, B., Bommer, J., Malluche, H.H., Schmidt-Gayk, H. Kidney Int. 13, 316, 1978
12. Prior, J.C., Cameron, E.C., Ballon, H.S., Lirenman, D.S., Moriarty, M.V., Price, J.D.E., Am.J.Med. 67, 583-589, 1979
13. Hamperl, H., Wallis, U. Virchows Arch., Pathol. Anatomie 288, 119-145, 1933
14. Krempien, B., Mehls, O., Ritz, E. Virchows Arch. 362, 129-143, 1974
15. Parfitt, M.A. Calcium Metabolism in Renal Failure and Nephrolithiasis (Ed.) David, D.S., pp. 145-196, New York, John Wiley
16. Mehls, O., Ritz, E., Krempien, B., Willich, E., Bommer, J., Schärer, K. Pediatric Radiology 1, 183-190, 1973 a
17. Mehls, O., Ritz, E., Krempien, B., Gilli, G., Link, K., Willich, E., Schärer, K. Arch. Dis. Childhood 50, 545-554, 1975 a
18. Bailey, G.L., Griffiths, H.J., Mocelin, A.J., Gundy, D.H., Hampers, C.L., Merrill, J.P. Trans.Am.Soc.Artif.Int.Org. 18, 401-403, 1972
19. Ritz, E., Mehls, O., Bommer, J., Schmidt-Gayk, H., Fiegel, P., Reitinger, H. Klin. Wschr. 55, 375-378, 1977
20. Letteri, J.M., Cohn, S.H. Calcium Metabolism in Renal Failure and Nephrolithiasis (Ed.) David, D.S., pp 249-277, New York, John Wiley, 1977
21. Chesney, R.W., Mazess, R.B., Rose, P.G., Jax, D.K., DeLuca, H.F.: Am. J. Roentgenol. 131, 544, 1978

25(OH)D3 IN THE TREATMENT OF JUVENILE RENAL OSTEODYSTROPHY

M. E. NORMAN

GENERAL COMMENTS

The previous speakers in this symposium have clearly and forcefully delineated the major clinical issues confronting pediatric nephrologists when they deal with azotemic renal osteodystrophy in childhood. These are as follows: (1) since chronic renal failure is no longer a fatal condition in children, renal osteodystrophy has emerged as one of its major but treatable complications (Houston, Mehls, Chesney); (2) when evaluated with increasingly sensitive and sophisticated laboratory techniques such as measurement of serum PTH and quantitative bone histology, patterns of subclinical renal osteodystrophy emerge relatively early in the course of chronic renal failure (Houston, Mehls); (3) it remains controversial as to whether or not subclinical renal osteodystrophy should be treated with vitamin D agents, or one should wait for the appearance of clinical abnormalities such as radiologic evidence of hyperparathyroidism (Houston); (4) our information about the spectrum of skeletal manifestations of juvenile renal osteodystrophy, particularly histology, is woefully inadequate and in need of improvement (Mehls); (5) now seems to be the time to test the hypothesis that aggressive therapy with vitamin D agents in very young children (under 5 years) with azotemic renal osteodystrophy may improve long-term growth by a sustained increase in growth velocity (Chesney, Norman); and (6) although each of the major vitamin D metabolites [25(OH)D; $24,25(OH)_2D_3$; $1,25(OH)_2D$] have been shown to improve one or more of the abnormalities in azotemic renal osteodystrophy, we do not yet know how to select the best metabolite or combination of metabolites to treat individual patients. Here the pattern of skeletal histology may play an important role (Houston, Norman).

25(OH)D3 STUDY

As part of our ongoing studies on the evaluation of early diagnosis

and therapy of juvenile renal osteodystrophy in children with varying degrees
of chronic renal insufficiency prior to reaching end-stage renal failure,
we initiated an uncontrolled 4-year therapeutic trial with the vitamin D
metabolite 25(OH)D$_3$ in 1976. I will summarize in this report complete
results after two years of therapy in a portion of the total study population.
In addition to following the usual clinical, radiological and biochemical
parameters, we performed yearly percutaneous transilial bone biopsies.
The trabecular bone was then evaluated by quantitative histomorphometry
(1). This aspect of the evaluation will receive the major emphasis in
this report. Our overall goal was to prevent the progression of clinically
evident renal osteodystrophy (or the emergence of clinical signs of the
disorder if first appreciated while still subclinical in nature), despite
persistence and/or progression of the underlying renal disease. By 1976,
most of the published therapuetic trials with vitamin D metabolites in
azotemic renal osteodystrophy had focused on 1,25(OH)$_2$D$_3$ (2-6). This was
because it was known to be the biologically active form of this sterol and
was believed to be deficient in patients with a reduced functioning renal
mass (see Chesney this Symposium). The reader may then ask, why did we
choose to investigate 25(OH)D$_3$ in 1976? The reasons are listed in Table
I below.

TABLE I.
1. Effects of 1,25(OH)$_2$D$_3$ on bone formation and mineralization were
   unknown (7).
2. Some adults on hemodialysis had undetectable 1,25(OH)$_2$D$_3$ but no
   osteomalacia (8).
3. Some adults on hemodialysis with osteomalacia did not respond to
   physiologic doses of 1,25(OH)$_2$D$_3$ (8).
4. In some adults with CRF, osteomalacia correlated with low serum
   25(OH)D$_3$(9).
5. Osteomalacia in a dog model of CRF responded best to dietary Pi
   restriction and 25(OH)D$_3$ (10).
6. In some adults (11, 12) and children (13) with CRF, osteomalacia
   responded to 25(OH)D$_3$ treatment.

Our study population consisted of 22 children, 19 males and 3 females,
with a mean age of 3 3/12 years. Most were boys with either obstructive
uropathy or congenital nephropathies presenting with chronic renal insufficiency (i.e., GFR $\overset{=}{<}$ 75% of age matched controls) in the first few
years of life. Such children appear to be at greatest risk for developing
severe renal osteodystrophy because of the early onset and slow progression
of their renal diseases (14). Renal osteodystrophy was classified into

230

subclinical and 3 clinical categories on the basis of increasing abnormalities (15). However, in order for a bone biopsy to be performed to confirm the diagnosis, each patient had to first meet at least two laboratory criteria: (1) a glomerular filtration rate $\overset{=}{<}$ 75% of age-matched controls; and (2) an elevated serum iPTH level (C-terminal assay) also compared to age-matched controls (16).

Approximately 1/3 of the children fell into each of 3 categories of renal insufficiency: mild (GFR 50-75% of normal); moderate (GFR 25-50% of normal); and severe (GFR 10-25% of normal). All but 3 of the patients entered the trial with normal serum calcium levels; all had normal serum phosphorus levels, although 16 of 22 were receiving or were begun on phosphate binders. Alkaline phosphate levels varied widely before treatment but the mean level was slightly elevated for age. Seven patients required supplemental calcium to bring their daily elemental calcium intakes to approximately 1.0-1.5 grams/day. Eighteen required supplemental alkali for metabolic acidosis. The mean dose of 25(OH)D3 was 1.7 µg/kg/day with a range of 0.7-2.5 µg/kg/day.

On the figure below are plotted the data for growth velocity expressed in standard deviation units over time. Many but not all patients demonstrated increments in growth velocity although the timing of this improved growth varied between individuals.

Figure 1.

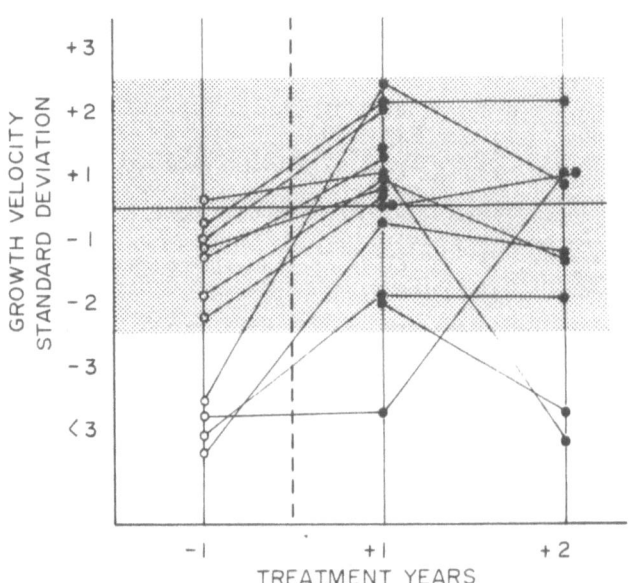

Serum calcium and phosphorus levels fluctuated in the normal range during therapy. Despite the use of pharmacologic doses of 25(OH)D$_3$ in 19 initially normocalcemic patients, only one transient (9 days) and asymptomatic episode of hypercalcemia occurred in over 600 cumulative months! This episode occurred in an 8 year old girl right after a one month winter vacation in Florida during which time 25(OH)D$_3$ therapy was continued. Mean alkaline phosphatase fell during therapy, though levels fluctuated widely between individual patients. Radiologic findings were generally unhelpful either in documenting renal osteodystrophy pre-treatment, or in assessing the response to 25(OH)D$_3$ therapy. Post-treatment PTH levels are presented in Figure 2 (below) as a percent of the pre-treatment control

Fig. 2

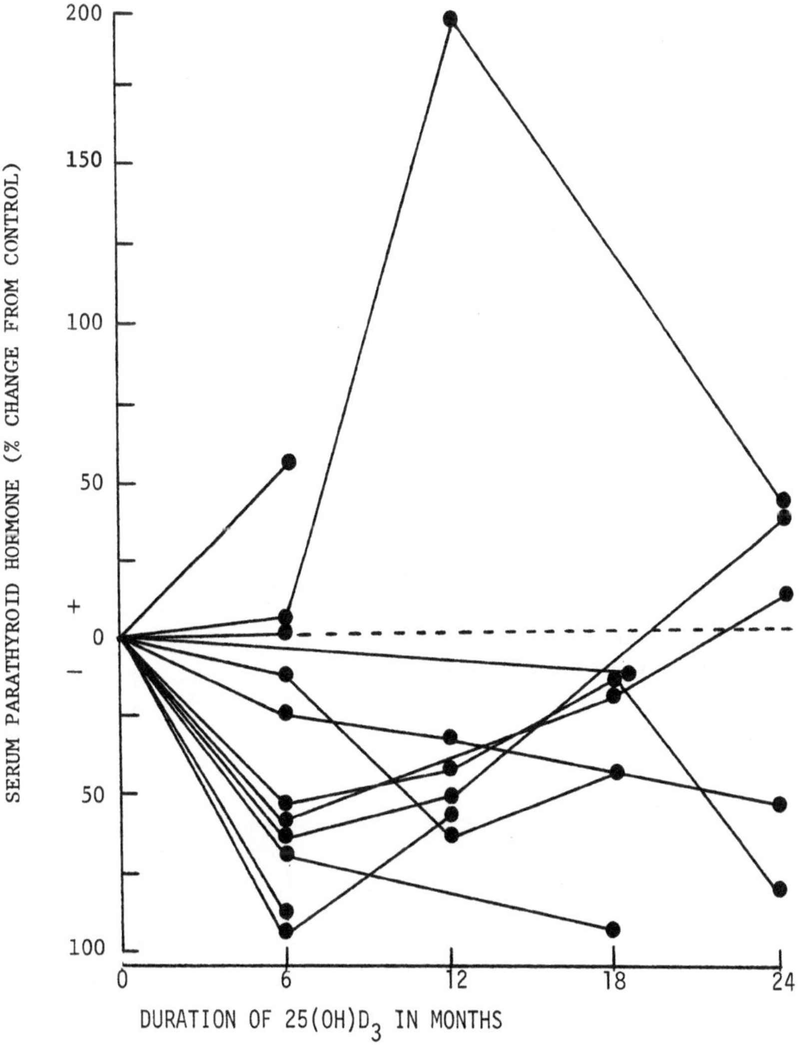

SERUM PARATHYROID HORMONE (% CHANGE FROM CONTROL)

DURATION OF 25(OH)D$_3$ IN MONTHS

232

values for each patient. The general tendency was for PTH levels to fall, though not into the normal range in most patients.

The histologic abnormalities on pre-treatment bone biopsies could be grouped into 3 major categories, a finding similar to that in adults (17). Osteomalacia predominated in approximately 37% of patients, osteitis fibrosa (hyperparathyroidism) in 16%, and a mixed picture in 47%. What follows is a series of representative histologic sections of several biopsies, focusing on trabecular architecture.

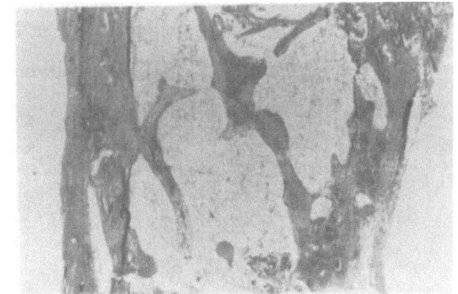

FIGURE 3. Low-power view (25X) of a transilial bone biopsy (normal control). Outer and inner cortical margins are shown at the extreme right and left hand portions of the photograph; islands of trabecular bone and marrow spaces are shown in the center.

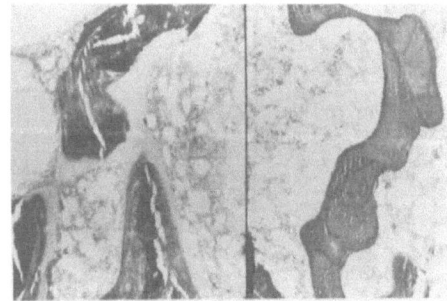

FIGURE 4. Low power view (100X) of a transilial bone biopsy; stain is Toluidine Blue. In this black and white photograph, calcified bone is dark gray or black; unmineralized osteoid light gray. The left hand panel is the pre-treatment biopsy. Note the large mass of unmineralized osteoid (e.g., osteomalacia). The right hand panel is the biopsy after two years of 25(OH)D3 therapy. Most of the trabecular bone surface is calcified and there is little unmineralized osteoid, indicating that osteomalacia has been cured.

FIGURE 5. Low power view (100X) of a transilial bone biopsy; staining is as described in Figure 4. On the left hand (pre-treatment) panel mineralized osteoid is shown in black and unmineralized osteoid in white. There is increased unmineralized osteoid lined by inactive osteoblasts (e.g., osteomalacia) and increased numbers of osteoclasts (e.g., osteitis fibrosa), especially in the upper right hand corner. The right hand panel depicts a normal biopsy 2 years after treatment, with normally calcified osteoid, shown in light gray.

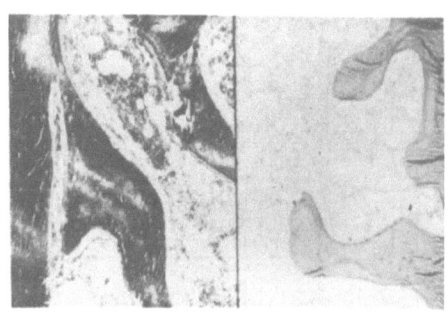

FIGURE 6. High power view (250X) of a transilial bone biopsy; staining is as described in Figures 4 & 5. The left hand panel depicts normal bone. The right hand panel shows a pre-treatment biopsy with only slightly increased unmineralized osteoid but markedly increased numbers of multinucleated osteoclasts which have produced multiple resorption cavities. Thus, the predominant finding here is osteitis fibrosa, a sign of severe secondary hyperparathyroidism.

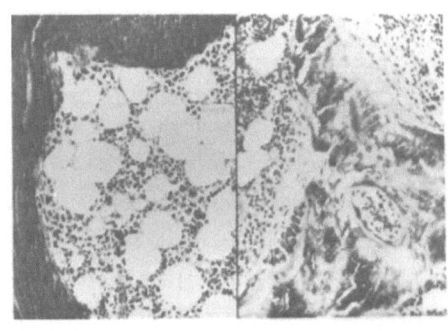

FIGURE 7. High power view (250-300X) of transilial bone biopsy; fluorescent microscopy after double tetracycline labelling. The biopsy was taken after two years of 25(OH)D3 therapy. The extent of the two fluorescent positive (white) bands indicates the calcification front and the width between the bands the calcification rate; both are markedly increased and almost normal (e.g., improved mineralization).

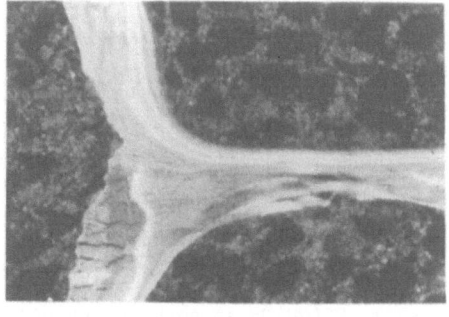

A summary of our findings on biopsies after two years of 25(OH)D3 are presented in Table II.

TABLE II
JUVENILE RENAL OSTEODYSTROPHY

Quantitative Bone Histomorphometry After Two Years of 25(OH)D Therapy

*1. Osteoid Volume:

Elevated in 11 of 12 pre-treatment;
Decreased in 8 of 11 post-treatment

*2. Osteoid Thickness:

Elevated in 7 of 12 pre-treatment;
Decreased in 7 of 7 post-treatment

*3. Osteoblast Surface (as % of total osteoid):

Reduced in 9 of 12 pre-treatment;
Elevated in 8 of 9 post-treatment

**4. Osteoclast Surface:

Elevated in 8 of 12 pre-treatment;
Reduced in 7 of 8 post-treatment

* Measurements for osteomalacia

** Measurement for osteitis fibrosa or hyperparathyroidism

Osteoid volume normalized in 5 of the 8 patients who demonstrated improvement. Osteoid thickness normalized in all 7 patients demonstrating improvement. Osteoblastic surface increased into the normal range in all 8 of the patients who demonstrated improvement. Finally, osteoclast surfaces fell into the normal range in 7 of the 8 patients who demonstrated improvement in this parameter.

In summary, these preliminary data suggest that $25(OH)D_3$, given relatively early in the course of renal osteodystrophy in young children, has a beneficial effect. It appears to heal bone disease, especially osteomalacia, in conjunction with improvements in linear growth velocity and serum alkaline phosphatase levels and PTH levels.

On the basis of available data, the response of the patients described above to $25(OH)D_3$ is perhaps unexpected. $1,25(OH)_2D_3$ is the only identified (and presumably terminal) vitamin D metabolite with known biologic activity at the level of gut, bone and kidney where administered in physiologic doses. Although vitamin D itself and $25(OH)D_3$ can mimic the effects of $1,25(OH)_2D_3$ in vitro and in vivo, the doses required on a weight basis are many-fold higher. Since our patients had mild-moderate chronic renal failure, the responses we observed could be due to conversion of excess $25(OH)D3$ to $1,25(OH)2D3$ by the residual functioning renal tissue. That this is probably not the case is suggested from the preliminary data shown in the last figure.

FIGURE 8.

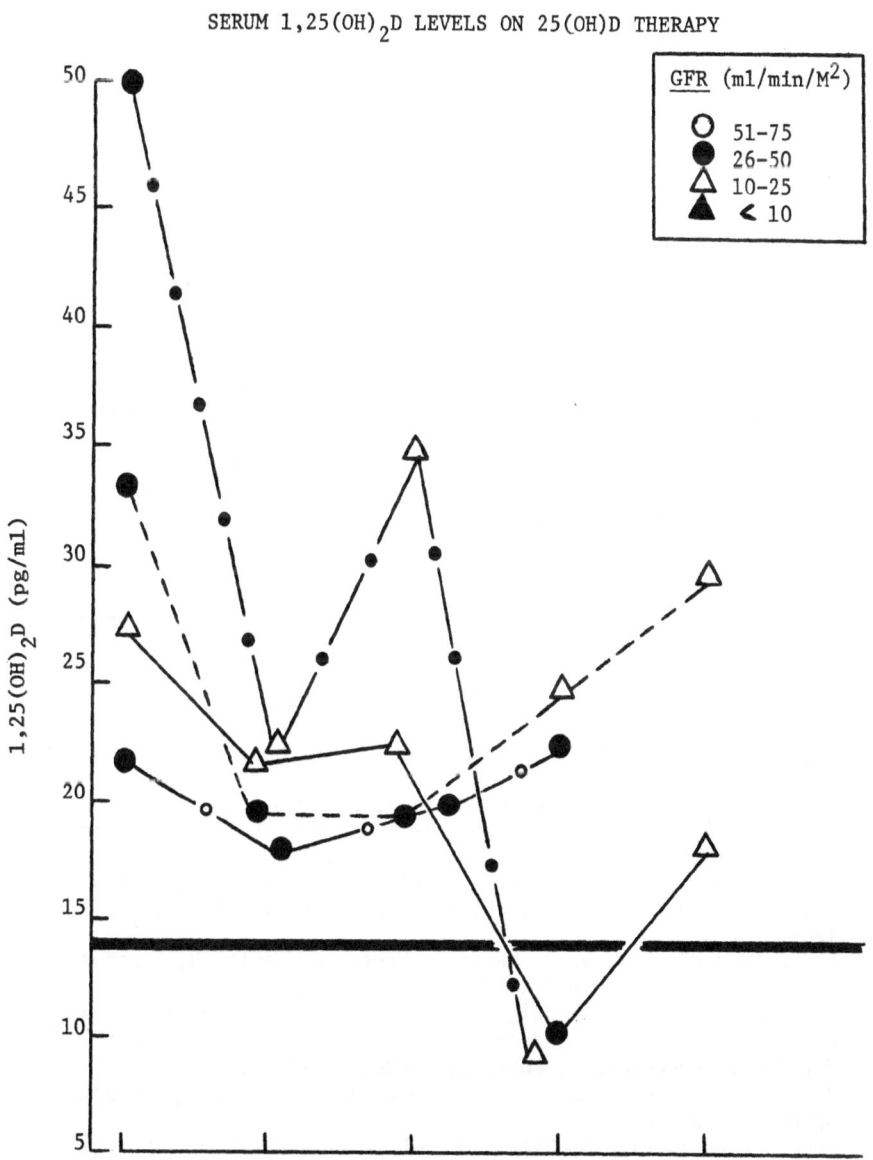

SERUM 1,25(OH)$_2$D LEVELS ON 25(OH)D THERAPY

DURATION OF 25(OH)D THERAPY (YEARS)

236

In this figure, serial $1,25(OH)_2D_3$ levels are presented for four patients with varying levels of GFR both between patients and for the individual patients over time. The corresponding mean serum 25(OH)D3 levels were as follows: pre-treatment, 45 ng/ml; one year, 232 ng/ml; two years, 186 ng/ml; three years, 181 ng/ml. Rather than a rise in 1,25(OH)2D3 levels, there was a general downward trend in the levels. Note also that none of these patients had 1,25(OH)2D3 deficiency at the start of the study as measured in our laboratory (lower limit of normal is given by the heavy horizontal bar). We are presently gathering additional data on the interrelationship of these two metabolites in patients before and after therapy.

REFERENCES

1. Bordier PJ, Chot ST. 1972. Quantitative histology of metabolic bone disease. J Clin Endocrinol Metab 1: 197.
2. Brickman AS, Coburn JW, Norman AW. 1972. Action of 1,25-dihydroxy-cholecalciferol, a potent, kidney-produced metabolite of vitamin D in uremic man. N Eng J Med 287:891.
3. Henderson RG, Russell RGG, Ledingham JGG. 1974. Effects of 1,25-dihydroxycholecalciferol on calcium absorption, muscle weakness and bone disease in chronic renal failure. Lancet 1:279.
4. Brickman AS, Coburn JW, Massry SG. 1974. 1,25-dihydroxycholecalciferol in normal man and patients with renal failure. Ann Intern Med 80:161.
5. Chan JCM, Oldham SB, Holick HF, Deluca HF. 1975 1-alpha-hydroxyvitamin D3 in chronic renal failure: A potent analog of the kidney hormone, 1,25 dihydroxycholecalciferol. JAMA 234:47.
6. Silverberg DS, Bettcher KB, Dossetor JB, Overton TR, Holick MF, DeLuca HF. 1975. Effect of 1,25-dihydroxycholecalciferol in renal osteodystrophy. Canad Med Assoc J 112:190.
7. Rasmussen H, Bordier PJ. 1978. Vitamin D and bone. Metab Bone Dis Rel Res 1:7.
8. Pierides RM, Simpson W, Ward MK, Ellis HA, Dewar JH and Kerr DNS. 1976. Variable response to long term 1,alpha hydroxycholecalciferol in haemodialysis osteodystrophy. Lancet 1:1092.
9. Eastwood JB, Stamp TCB, Harris E, DeWardener HE. 1976. Vitamin D deficiency in the osteomalacia of chronic renal failure. Lancet 2: 1209.
10. Rutherford WE, Bordier P, Marie P, Hruska K, Harter H, Greenwalt A, Blondin J, Haddad J, Bricker N and Slatopolsky E. 1977. Phosphate control and 25-hydroxycholecalciferol administration in preventing experimental renal osteodystrophy in the dog. J Clin Invest 60:332.
11. Recker R, Schoenfeld P, LeteriJ, Slatopolsky E, Goldsmith R, Brickman A. 1978. The efficacy of calcifediol in renal osteodystrophy. Arch Int Med 138:857.
12. Fournier A, Bordier P, Gueris J, Sebert J-L, Marie P, Ferriere C, Bedrossian J and DeLuca HF. 1979. Comparison of 1,alpha-hydroxy-cholecalciferol and 25-hydroxycholecalciferol in the treatment of renal osteodystrophy: greater effects of 25-hydroxycholecalciferol on bone mineralization. Kidney Int 15:196.

REFERENCES (continued)

13. Witmer G, Margolis A, Fontaine O, Fritsch J, Lenoir G, Broyer M, Balsan S. 1976. Effects of 25-hydroxycholecalciferol on bone lesions of children with terminal renal failure. Kidney Int 10:395.
14. Broyer M. 1974. Chronic renal failure in Royer P, Habib R, Mathieu H, Broyer M, Editors, Pediatric Nephrology, Philadelphia, WB Saunders Company, p 358-394.
15. Norman ME, Mazur AT, Borden S, Gruskin A, Anast C, Baron R, Rasmussen H. 1980. Early diagnosis of juvenile renal osteodystrophy. J Pediat 97:226.
16. David L, Anast CS. 1974. Calcium metabolism in newborn infants. The interrelationship of parathyroid function and calcium, magnesium and phosphorus metabolism in normal, "sick" and hypocalcemic newborns. J Clin Invest 54:287.
17. Brickman AS, Sherrard DG, Wong EG, Singer FR, Norman AW and Coburn JW. 1978. Renal osteodystrophy: Separation of types by bone histology and response to $1,25(OH)_2D_3$. VIIth International Congress of Nephrology, Montreal, June 18-23 (Abstr D-29).

TRANSITIONAL NEPHROLOGY

P.A. JOSE

Welcome to the Symposium for Transitional Nephrology. Dr. Eddie Moore will discuss fetal renal physiology followed by a 5 minute discussion, while Drs. Billy Arant, Anita Aperia and myself will present views on the factors influencing postnatal renal function. Overlap in these talks hopefully will bring a clearer view of the subject matter. Questions may be asked after these talks.

Significant strides have been made in the understanding of the physiology of the developing kidney, and I would like to summarize some of the studies that have contributed to this advance.

Last Tuesday, Dr. Jean Robillard (1) presented his data on the relationship among gestational age, glomerulogenesis and glomerular filtration rate (GFR). He demonstrated that the rise in renal blood flow prior to 130 days of fetal life was mainly due to formation of new glomeruli. Thereafter the increase in renal blood flow was mainly due to a fall in renovascular resistance. The site of the increased reno-vascular resistance in newborns has recently been demonstrated by direct micropuncture techniques (2, 3). Ichikawa and Brenner (3) studied rats at 39 days of life and compared them to adult rats. Mean arterial filtration pressure was similar in both groups. Total GFR, superficial single nephron filtration rate, and single nephron blood flow were significantly greater in the older rats. Single nephron filtration fractions, however, were similar. Compared to adult rats, the younger rats (39 days old) had a greater total renovascular resistance which was evenly distributed between the afferent and efferent arterioles. We have suggested previously that the high reno-vascular resistance in the newborn is due to an increased sensitivity of the neonatal renal vasculature to catecholamines (4); the renin angiotensin system was not an important factor (5).

Several authors have emphasized the importance of glomerular plasma flow and the increase in GFR with age (2, 3, 6). We have recently reported that the changes in single nephron filtration distribution in the neonatal dog using the ^{14}C ferrocyanide method paralleled the changes in cortical blood flow distribution. These studies directly demonstrated for the first time a centrifugal pattern of maturation of glomerular filtration in the immediate neonatal period (7) similar to that described for renal blood flow (6, 8, 9, 10, 11, 12).

The intrarenal factors that influence glomerular filtration with age including surface area available for filtration, permeability coefficient and hydrostatic pressure gradients across the glomerular capillary were discussed in the First International Workshop of Developmental Nephrology by Dr. Spitzer (13) and will not be adressed in this talk.

The ontogeny of the endothelial surface, lamina densa and poly-anionic coating was presented by Reeves at the Symposium in Develop-mental Nephrology. I will concentrate on what I consider extrarenal factors that may influence GFR. Several studies have now demonstrated the influence of gestational age and GFR (15, 16, 17). Leake and Trygstad showed that the rise in inulin clearance with gestational age was evident in infants studied less than 24 hours of postnatal age (18) After 2-3 days of extrauterine life, the rise in GFR with gestational age was greatly accelerated. Fawer et al (18) described further the influence of intrauterine and extrauterine environment on GFR. These authors (18) showed that the increase in glomerular filtration rate occurs between the 28th and 35th week of gestation and then levels off up to the end of gestation. Birth is the signal for a marked increase in glomerular filtration rate. The rate of increase in glomerular filtration with age is different in the preterm from the term infant. In the first week of life, the increase in glomerular filtration with age was less in preterm than full term infants (19).

Another extrarenal factor influencing GFR was studied by Solomon (20). He compared the GFR in animals from reduced litters and the GFR from intact litters. At the low weight ranges, animals from the former had higher filtration rates than animals from the latter. It must be stated that in human beings, Calcagno and Lowe (21) as well as

Edelmann and Wolfich (22) were unable to show an effect of high protein diet on GFR in PAH clearance in preterm infants.

One of the more fascinating aspects of neonatal physiology has been the demonstration that very young birth weight preterm infants have a greater basal excretion of sodium than term infants or adults on a normal salt intake. This was initially reported by Sulyok et al in 1971 (23). Oh and associates (16) extended this observation, demonstrating that the preterm infant at 27 weeks gestation has a high basal excretion of sodium. This decreases with gestational age so that by 34-35 weeks basal fractional sodium excretion was similar to that of term infants. Similar results were obtained when the sodium excretion was expressed as a fraction of the filtered load. It is also worthwhile to note that high basal fractional sodium excretion in these very low birth weight infants decreased with postnatal age so that by 10-30 days basal fractional sodium excretion was similar to term infants. The mechanism for the high basal fractional sodium excretion in preterm infants is not well understood. However, some insight may be gained from a study done by Solomon (24). He looked at the influence of the length of the proximal tubule on the ability to maintain a plasma to tubular fluid sodium gradient. In the adult, maximal plasma to tubular fluid sodium gradient was achieved when the proximal tubular length was greater than 1500 uM. In young rats less than 120 grams, as in the adult rats, absolute proximal tubular concentration gradients were achieved when the proximal tubular length was greater than 1500 uM. Since smaller animals had more proximal tubules with lengths less than 1500 uM, maximal gradients could not be achieved as often as in adults. It is possible that in the human preterm infant, proximal tubules behave in a similar fashion. If these studies could be extrapolated to preterm infants, the relatively higher distal sodium load would result in a greater sodium excretion. During saline loading, however, the preterm as well as the term infant have a limited ability to excrete an acute saline load.

While anatomical factors may be involved, and changes in GFR may be a factor in the limited ability of the newborn to excrete an acute salt load (25, 26), it now seems clear that an increase in the avidity of the distal tubule for sodium is responsible for this limitation. The latter may, in turn, be due to increased activity of salt retaining

hormones (ex. mineralocorticoid), or decreased level or activity of
natriuretic hormones (ex. oxytocin and kallikrein) (27, 28, 29).
Recently, Solhaug et al (30) from our laboratory reported that the
sodium diuresis associated with an acute saline load in neonatal puppies
could be improved if the puppies received an infusion of substance P.
While substance P had no effect on urinary sodium or kallikrein in the
hydropenic state, the concurrent imposition of an acute salt load
resulted in a greater increase in sodium excretion than following an
acute salt load alone. The urinary sodium excretion was positively
correlated with urinary kallikrein excretion when substance P was given
in conjunction with the saline load.

What are the clinical implications of these developmental changes
just described? Do they have any role in the development of acute
reual failure that is seen in about 5% of infants (31). Clinically, it
has been suspected that the newborn infant is relatively resistant to
the nephrotoxic effects of aminoglycosides. This was recently demonstrated in the puppy by Arant et al (32). They studied effects of gentamicin on GFR in neonatal puppies. Renal gentamicin levels were also measured.
Histopathology was evaluated by E.M.   They suggested that the
lower GFR and blood flow to the outer cortex in very young puppies had
a protective effect on the toxicity of gentamycin. We have recently
completed his studies on the renal effects of uranyl nitrate in
puppies of different age groups (34). Table I depicts 3-4 week old
puppies and 1-2 week old puppies. Two hours after uranyl nitrate
insignificant decreases in CFR occurred in both groups. Twenty-four
hours after uranyl nitrate the GFR was significantly decreased in both
groups of puppies. Note that only a 50% reduction in GFR occurred in
very young puppies while GFR was almost completely abolished in the
older puppies. Two hours after uranyl nitrate, the fractional sodium
excretion was lower in 3-5 week old puppies. Twenty-four hours after
uranyl nitrate, fractional sodium excretion was significantly greater
in the older puppies, $36.1 \pm 18.63\%$. The functional changes induced by
uranyl nitrate correlated with the observed structural changes. The
glomeruli and distal tubules seem to be be spared but the vacuoles in
proximal convoluted tubules were increased in number. These structural
abnormalities were more prominent in juxtamedullary than outer cortical
nephrons, particularly in the older puppies. Twenty-four hours after

uranyl nitrate no apparent structural abnormalities could be demonstrated
in either light or electron microscopy in either group of puppies. It
is also worthwhile to recall that structural changes persist in the adult
dog 24 hours after uranyl nitrate.

In summary: The rise in GFR with age is due to changes in intrarenal
factors including glomerular membrane characteristics, glomerular hydrostatic pressure gradients and plasma flow. The extrarenal factors include
the effects of gestational age hormones and possibly food intake. A few
days of extrauterine life markedly increases GFR. The high sodium
excretion in very premature infants may be related to short length of
proximal tubules. The inability to excrete a salt load in the term or
preterm infant may be due to the inability of the distal tubule to
excrete the increased delivery of salt and may be related to other
intrinsic factors. The low GFR is also a factor, particularly in the
outer cortex, and may afford a protective effect from some nephrotoxic
agents. Thank you.

Table I. The effect of uranyl nitrate on glomerular filtration rate (GFR),
renal plasma flow (RPF), urine flow (V) and fractional sodium
excretion (FeNa%) in puppies before (B), 2 hours and 24 hours
after intravenous uranyl nitrate (10 mg/kg).

1-2 wk old	B n=5	2 hrs n=5	24 hrs n=5
GFR[a]	0.29+0.05	0.24+0.05	0.16+0.04*
RPF[a]	1.73+0.09	1.37+0.16	2.00+0.17
V µl/min	16.60+3.50	26.66+0.16	11.80+4.56
FENa %	1.05+0.40	1.56+5.56	4.60+2.49
3-5 wk old	B n=5	2 hrs n=5	24 hrs n=5
GFR[a]	0.31+0.05	0.24+0.06	0.00+0.00*#
RPF[a]	1.73+0.14	1.96+0.20	1.83+0.09
V µl/min	36.15+11.85	29.49+8.19	1.23+0.52*#
FENa %	0.49+0.18	0.58+0.12	36.17+18.63*#

a=ml/min/100 g body wt. *=<.05 24 hrs vs 2 hrs or B. #=<.05 I vs. II.

REFERENCES

1. Robillard JE, Weismann DN and Smith FG. 1980. Development of glomerular perfusion rate (GPR) in fetal and newborn lambs. (Abs)
   Pediatr Res 14:987.
2. Tucker BJ and Blantz RC. 1977. Factors determining superficial nephron
   filtration in the mature growing rat. Am J Physiol 232:F97.

3. Ichikawa I and Brenner BM. 1979. Factors limiting glomerular filtration rate in the immature rat. Am J Physiol 236:F465.
4. Jose PA, Slotkoff LM, Lilienfield LS, Calcagno PL and Eisner GM. 1974. Sensitivity of neonatal renal vasculature to epinephrine. Am J Physiol 226:796.
5. Jose PA, Slotkoff LM, Montgomery S, Calcagno PL and Eisner GM. 1975. Autoregulation of renal blood flow in the puppy. Am. J. Physiol. 229:983.
6. Aperia A and Herin P. 1975. Development of glomerular perfusion rate and nephron filtration rate in rats 17-60 days old. Am J Physiol 228:1319.
7. Tavani N, Calcagno P, Zimmit S, Flamenbaum W, Eisner G and Jose P. 1980. Ontogeny of single nephron filtration distribution. Pediatr Res 14:779.
8. Jose PA, Logan AG, Slotkoff LM, Lilienfield LS, Calcagno PL and Eisner GM. 1971. Intrarenal blood flow distribution in canine puppies. Pediatr Res 5:335.
9. Olbing H, Blaufox MD, Aschinberg LA, Silkalns GI, Bernstein J, Spitzer A and Edelmann CM. 1973. Postnatal changes in renal glomerular blood flow distribution in puppies. J Clin Invest 52:2885.
10. Kleinman LI and Reuter JH. 1973. Maturation of glomerular blood flow distribution in the newborn dog. J Physiol (Lond.)228:91.
11. Aschinberg LC, Goldsmith DI, Olbing H, Hardy M, Spitzer A, Edelmann CM and Blaufox MD. 1975. Neonatal changes in renal blood flow distribution in puppies. 228:1453.
12. Aperia A, Broberger O, Herin P and Joelsson I. 1977. Renal hemodynamics in the prenatal period: a study in lambs. Acta Physiol Scand 99:261.
13. Spitzer A. 1980. The factors underlying the increase in glomerular filtration rate during postnatal development. Proc 1st Int Workshop on Devel Renal Physiol (in press).
14. Reeves W. 1980. Differentiation of anionic sites in glomerular capillaries of the newborn rat kidney. Proc 1st Int Workshop on Devel Renal Physiol (in press).
15. Arant BS. 1979. Developmental patterns of renal functional maturation compared in the human neonate. J Pediatr 92:705.
16. Ross B, Cowett R, Oh W. 1977. Renal function and low birth weight infants during the first two months of life. Pediatr Res 11:1162.
17. Leake RD and Trygstad CW. 1977. Glomerular filtration rate during the period of adaptation to extrauterine life. Pediatr Res 11:959.
18. Faver CL, Torrodo A and Guignord JP. 1979. Maturation of renal function in full term and premature neonates. Helv Pediatr Acta 34:11.
19. Aperia A (personal communication).
20. Solomon S and Capek K. 1972. Increased food availability and renal development of neonatal rats. Biol Neonate 21:9.
21. Calcagno PL and Lowe CU. 1963. Substrate induced renal tubular maturation. J Pediatr 63:851.
22. Edelmann EM and Wolfish NM. 1968. Dietary influence on renal maturation in preterm infants. Pediatr Res 2:421.
23. Sulyok E. 1971. The relationship between electrolyte and acid base balance in the premature infant during early postnatal life. Biol Neonate 17:227.
24. Solomon S. 1974. Maximal gradients of sodium and potassium across proximal tubules of kidneys and immature rats. Biol Neonate 25:327.

25. Aperia A, Broberger O, Thodenius K and Zetterstrom R. 1975. Development of renal control of salt and fluid homeostasis during the first year of life. Acta Paediatr Scand 64:393.

26. Kleinman LI. 1975. Renal sodium reabsorption during saline loading and distal blockade in newborn dog. Am J Physiol 228:1403.

27. Spitzer A and Schoeneman M. 1976. Sodium reabsorption during maturation. (Abs). Kidney Int. 10:598.

28. Solomon S, Hathaway S and Curb D. 1979. Evidence that the renal response to volume expansion involves a blood borne factor. Biol Neonate 35:113.

29. Kleinman LI, Banks RQ, and Garewitt K. 1979. Role of oxytocin in the natriuretic response to saline expansion in newborn dogs. (Abs). Pediatr Res 13:515.

30. Solhaug M, Eisner GM, Calcagno PL and Jose PA. 1979. Kinins, modulators of sodium excretion in the canine puppy (Abs). Pediatr 13:521.

31. Norman M and Asadi F. A prospective study of acute renal failure. Pediatr 63:475.

32. Cowan RH, Jakkola AF and Arant BS. 1980. Pathophysiologic evidence of gentamycin nephrotoxicity in neonatal puppies. Peds Res 11:1204.

33. Zink H and Horster M. 1977. Maturation of diluting capacity in loop of Henle of rat superficial nephrons. Am J Physiol 233:F519.

34. Pelayo JC, Andrews PM, Calcagno PL, Eisner GM and Jose PA. 1980. The influence of age on uranyl nitrate nephrotoxicity. Proc 13th Ann Meet Amer Soc Nephrol p 104A.

RENAL FUNCTION IN FETAL LIFE

Eddie S. Moore and Bruce A. Kaiser

1.   INTRODUCTION

Prior to 1958, study of renal function in the fetus was limited to analysis of bladder urine obtained from the fetus. In 1958, Alexander and Dixon[1] developed exteriorization techniques that allowed investigation of renal clearances in fetal laboratory animals without onset of fetal respiration ("intact fetal preparation"). The techniques for acute study of renal function in the fetus were subsequently expanded and improved by Alexander and Dixon[2] and by Smith et al.[3] In 1972, Gresham et al[4] reported their results of chronic studies of fetal lambs in utero for as long as 18 days. Since that time, there have been many investigations related to renal function in the developing fetus. In this chapter, we will present a review of the major work related to renal function in utero.

2.   RENAL PERFUSION - RENAL BLOOD FLOW

Although the fetal kidney does not directly participate in fetal homeostasis, knowledge of fetal circulation and fetal renal blood flow (RBF) is necessary for complete understanding of renal function in utero. One of the first major studies of changes in circulation in utero was reported in an acute fetal lamb preparation by Rudolph et al.[5] Umbilical blood flow increased throughout gestation in proportion to fetal weight, whereas umbilical pH, PO_2, and P_{CO_2} remained constant. Combined biventricular cardiac output increased steadily from age 60 days gestation to term. The placenta, which is the major organ regulating fetal homeostasis, received 40-65 percent of cardiac output. In contrast, the percentage of cardiac output received by the fetal kidneys at 60 days gestation was 2.9±0.4. This remained relatively constant until it decreased to 1.8±0.2 percent at 121 days gestation and remained at this level until term (140 days). In fetuses age 60 days gestation, mean RBF was 122 ml/100 gm/min. This decreased to 85 ml/100 gm/min at fetal age 100 days and thereafter rose gradually to 173 ml/100 gm/min at term.

Similar studies were done in nonhuman primates by Paton et al.[6] These investigators studied baboon fetuses at 116 to 124 days of gestation (term 184 days). Cardiac output in these studies represented systemic flow in contrast to the biventricular output studies in fetal lambs mentioned above. In younger fetuses, the percentage of cardiac output perfusing the kidneys was 4.90±2.05 and decreased with increasing gestational age to 3.17±1.76 in the older fetuses. Fetal arterial blood pressure and heart rate in the younger fetuses was 30±6 mmHg and 167±11 beats per minute. In the older fetuses, these values were 56±7 and 178±18, respectively. RBF (ml/min/gm) was 1.73±0.42 and 1.54±.60, respectively.

Studies of the circulation in previable human fetuses obtained by hysterotomy during performance of legal abortions were reported by Rudolph et al.[7] Cardiac output was determined as systemic flow as mentioned above. There was a significant decrease in percentage of cardiac output perfusing the kidneys as fetal weight increased. Mean percentage of cardiac output perfusing the kidneys in fetuses weighing less than 50 gm was 6.5 and decreased to 3.7 in fetuses weighing more than 151 gm. In smaller fetuses, fetal mean heart rate and mean arterial blood pressure was 126 per minute and 28 mmHg and 130 per minute and 34 mmHg in the larger fetuses. Mean RBF in fetuses weighing 104-225 gm was 155 ml/100 gm/min and ranged from 56 to 249 ml/100 gm/min.

The intrarenal distribution of RBF may significantly relate to renal function.[8] We studied the intrarenal blood flow distribution in primate fetuses.[9] RBF and intrarenal blood flow distribution were determined by injection of radiolabelled carbonized microspheres into the exteriorized fetus. The results are shown in Table 1. In early gestation there is a preponderance of

Table 1. Intrarenal blood flow distribution in fetal baboons.

	RBF ml/min/gm	Outer cortex ml/min/gm	Inner cortex ml/min/gm	Outer cortex/ Inner cortex
Mid-term	2.00	3.15	3.84	0.82
Term	3.11	6.96	6.75	1.03
Acidosis	3.26	6.10	6.98	0.97

inner cortical flow where growth of kidney tissue is most rapid. In late gestation, when outer cortical growth accelerates, there is a redistribution of blood flow to this area. In late gestation, physiologic stimuli such as an acute acidosis results in redistribution of fetal intrarenal blood flow. Similar studies in fetal lambs was also reported by our group.[10] Intrarenal blood flow distribution was determined in the outer (zone 1), mid (zone 2), and inner cortex (zone 3) in fetal lambs age 90-150 days gestation (Table 2).

Table 2. Intrarenal blood flow distribution in fetal lambs, age 90-150 days.

Cortical blood flow (ml/min/gm)

	Zone 1 (outer)	Zone 2 (mid)	Zone 3 (inner)
Mean	3.69	3.33	1.25
S.E.	0.65	0.51	0.25

Cortical blood flow, ml/min/gm, was 3.69±0.65 in zone 1, 3.33±0.51 in zone 2, and 1.25±0.25 in zone 3. The difference between intrarenal blood flow distribution in lamb and primate fetuses may be related to species differences in rates of kidney growth. In the fetal lamb, nephrogenesis is complete by age

70-90 days gestation, whereas in the primate, nephrogenesis is not complete until approximately 120-135 days gestation.

Measurements of renal vascular resistance in the above experiments demonstrated that fetal renal vascular resistance is extremely high when compared tc young animals or adults and increases further with increasing gestational age. It is highly probable that the elevated renal vascular resistance is the major factor responsible for the low RBF in utero. Fetal renal vascular resistance is discussed further in the section on Renin - Angiotensin.

3. GLOMERULAR FILTRATION-RENAL PLASMA FLOW

Some of the earliest studies of renal plasma flow and glomerular filtration in fetuses were those of Alexander and Nixon.[2,11] These workers investigated renal plasma flow in acute fetal lamb preparations by infusing para-aminohippuric acid (PAH). In fetuses age 89-119 days gestation, C_{PAH} was 0.6 ml/min/kg body weight. This increased to 0.9 and to 1.3 ml/min/kg at 121 days gestation and at term, respectively. These results were confirmed by Assali et al[12] using electromagnetic flow meters. In similar acute fetal lamb preparations, glomerular filtration was measured using inulin or iothalamate,[3,4] or by infusing exogenous creatinine.[13] Glomerular filtration rate (GFR) in these studies ranged from 0.75 to 1.41 ml/min/kg of fetal body weight. Gresham et al[4] investigated glomerular filtration in unstressed fetuses using a chronic lamb preparation in whom determinations were made 5-8 days after initial surgical procedures. In six fetuses, mean inulin, creatinine, and urea clearances were 1.07±0.06, 1.58±0.10, and 0.59±0.04 ml/ min/kg body weight, respectively. These data were not different from that demonstrated in acute experiments. The major difference demonstrated in these chronic experiments was an erratic urine flow rate during the first 24-72 hours after surgery.

Many theories have been proposed to explain the low GFR and low renal plasma flow during development. These include a small filtration surface area and low glomerular permeability,[15] low systemic arterial pressure,[15] and low glomerular capillary hydrostatic pressure.[16] Investigators have recently begun study of maturational changes in glomerular filtration in utero. We studied the effect of gestational age and arterial pressure on GFR in 17 acute fetal lambs age 90-150 days gestation.[17] Mean aortic pressure increased with gestational age from a low of 33 mmHg at age 100 days to 80 mmHg at age 150 days (p<.001). Total RBF (ml/min/gm) did not increase with gestational age and renal vascular resistance rose from 18 mmHg/ml/min/gm in early gestation to 143 near term (Fig. 1).

FIGURE 1.

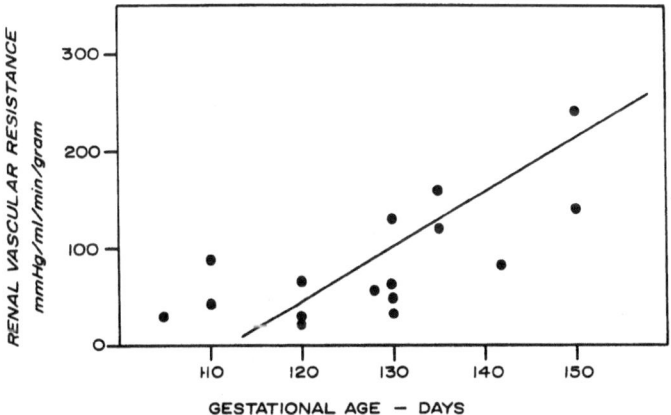

GFR (ml/min/gm of kidney) did not correlate with gestational age, mean aortic pressure, or with RBF. Robillard et al[18] reported similar findings in a chronic lamb preparation. In that study, absolute GFR (ml/min) increased with gestational age: since there was a greater increase in kidney weight, GFR/gm of kidney and GFR related to gestational age did not increase as demonstrated in our studies. These investigators did not correlate glomerular filtration with systemic arterial pressure or RBF as was done in our study.

4.   TUBULAR TRANSPORT

4.1 Sodium chloride

Early studies in human infants prior to birth demonstrated urine/plasma
Na$^+$ ratios of approximately 0.32 compared to 1.05 for the mother.[19] Corresponding urine/plasma Cl$^-$ ratios were 0.39 and 1.45, respectively. Studies of
fractional reabsorption of NaCl by the fetal kidney were reported by Alexander
et al.[1] In acute fetal lamb preparations, fractional reabsorption of filtered
Na$^+$ increased from 0.64 at fetal age 61 days to 0.95 at 142 days gestation.
Similar results were reported in a study of pig fetuses.[20] Using long-term
chronic fetal preparations, Robillard et al[21] demonstrated that fractional
reabsorption of Na$^+$ increased from 0.86 at 91-141 days gestation to 0.92 in
fetuses age 126-145 days gestation. Fractional reabsorption of Cl$^-$ was 0.90
and 0.98, respectively. The increase in fractional reabsorption of Na$^+$ and of
Cl$^-$ with gestational age was more rapid than the increase in GFR (ml/min) after
129 days gestation. However, the increase was not proportional to the rise in
absolute GFR (ml/min) for the same period. For fetuses up to age 129 days,
reabsorption of Na$^+$ was increased to 0.82 and that of Cl$^-$ to 0.91 when the
respective increase in GFR was 0.91 and 1.01, which is 10 percent greater than
the concomitant increase in tubular reabsorption of both electrolytes.

We studied interrelationships between renal Na$^+$ handling and various
stimuli known to effect tubular transport of Na$^+$ in the adult kidney in acute
fetal lamb preparations. The renal response to hypotonic volume expansion was
investigated in fetal lambs age 100-120 days.[22] Expansion of fetal ECF was
accomplished by infusing 0.45 N NaCl at 15-20 ml/min for at least 30 minutes.
The control GFR increased from a mean of 3.21 ml/min to 7.42 ml/min (p<.001)
at the height of diuresis. Initial mean fractional tubular reabsorption of Na$^+$
was 0.97 and decreased to a mean of 0.85 (p<.001) with maximal ECF expansion in
the fetus. Free water clearance increased significantly from a mean control

value of 5.1 ml/min to 15.4 ml/min (p<.001) at the height of diuresis. These data indicate the capacity of the distal tubule in the fetal lamb to markedly increase active reabsorption of NaCl.

Additional studies were performed in our laboratory using acute and chronic fetal preparations to study the effect of plasma concentration of Na^+ on fetal renal handling of filtered Na^+.[23] Plasma Na^+ concentration was significantly increased by infusing hypertonic NaCl (3%). An increase in GFR was minimized by acute removal of whole blood (10 ml/kg). Fractional tubular reabsorption of Na^+ increased and fractional Na^+ excretion also increased significantly from a mean control value of 0.14 to 0.25 (p<0.01). In additional studies, 9-α fluro-hydrocortisone was administered intravenously to the fetus. Fractional Na^+ excretion decreased after 60 minutes from the control value of 0.17 to 0.15, and decreased further after 120 minutes to 0.09 (p<.005) (Table 3). These

Table 3. Renal Na^+ excretion in 8 fetal lambs after IM administration of 9-α flurohydrocortisone.

	GFR ml/min	UV ml/min	FT_{Na^+}	FE_{Na^+}	$U_K V$ mEq/min
Control	2.95	0.69	0.82	0.18	6.61
S.E.	0.39	0.16	0.01	0.01	2.40
60 min	2.80	0.61	0.84	0.15	6.76
S.E.	0.41	0.13	0.01	0.01	2.11
120 min	2.35*	0.30*	0.91*	0.09*	12.87*
S.E.	0.15	0.04	0.01	0.01	1.71

*Statistically significant from control

studies indicate that fetal fractional excretion of Na^+ changes in response to stimuli such as an increase in plasma concentration of Na^+ and expansion of ECF volume, and that distal tubular reabsorption is operational by midgestation. These studies were confirmed by Robillard et al,[24] who studied the role of aldosterone on renal Na^+ and K^+ excretion in fetal and newborn lambs.

4.2 Potassium

Fetal renal tubular handling of K^+ has not been studied as extensively as have Na, Cl, Pi, and glucose. Alexander and associates[2] demonstrated that the concentration of K^+ in fetal urine decreased as the fetus matured. In a study of human fetuses reported by McCance and Widdowson,[19] the urine/plasma K^+ concentration ratio was 0.69 compared to a simultaneous value of 19.6 for the mother. In acute fetal lamb studies, Smith et al[3] demonstrated urine K^+ concentrations ranging from 4-22 mEq/l, mean 5.9 mEq/l. Gresham et al[4] demonstrated a total urinary excretion of 33 mEq of potassium during 18 days of continuous drainage of urine from chronically catheterized fetal lambs. This amounts to a K^+ excretion rate of 1.8 mEq/day or an extremely low absolute K^+ excretion of 1.25 µEq/min. In the study by Robillard et al,[24] fractional excretion of K^+ was 0.44 in fetuses age 100-125 days and increased to 0.92 in fetuses age 126-145 days gestation. Simultaneous urine/plasma Na^+ and K^+ concentration ratios were 0.67 and 0.17, respectively. The decrease in Na^+ and in K^+ concentration ratios with gestational age significantly correlated with an increase in fetal plasma aldosterone concentration.

4.3 Glucose

Among the first studies of glucose handling by the fetal kidney were those of Alexander and Nixon.[13] In three of eight fetuses (59-135 days gestation) studied, urine excretion of glucose was zero. In the remaining fetuses, urinary glucose excretion ranged from 0.002 to 0.055 mg/min. In a 77-day-old fetus, experimental elevation of plasma glucose concentration demonstrated a Tm glucose of 1.2 mg/min. In three fetuses, intravenous infusion of phlorrhizin resulted in a significant reduction in tubular reabsorption of glucose. Similar rates of fetal tubular transport of glucose were also reported for fetal pigs[20] and for rat fetuses.[25]

More recent studies of the maturation of glucose transport by the fetal kidney were reported by Robillard et al.[26] The mean value for blood glucose threshold in the fetuses was 200±13 mg/dl compared to 177±2.8 mg/dl in the ewes. Renal plasma threshold in the fetus correlated significantly to fetal body weight and to absolute GFR. A Tm glucose of 4.73 mg/min was demonstrated in only one of nine fetuses studied. Since plasma threshold values for glucose reabsorption by the fetal kidney increased with fetal absolute GFR, the authors concluded that glomerulo-tubular balance for glucose is present by midgestation in the fetal lamb kidney and is maintained throughout intrauterine life.

4.4 Phosphate

Low renal clearance of phosphate is associated with hyperphosphatemia in the human newborn as well as in sheep[19,32] and primate[27] fetuses. Studies by Smith et al[28] demonstrated that the fetal lamb kidney responds to exogenous parathyroid extract with a significant increase in urinary phosphate excretion. We studied the response of the fetal kidney to certain stimuli known to influence renal phosphate clearance by the adult kidney in 17 fetuses at age 85-100 days gestation.[29] In one group of fetuses, fetal ECF volume was expanded by infusing Ringer's lactate without added Ca^{++}. Fractional clearance of phosphate increased 3-fold (p<.001) and was linearly correlated with an increase in Na^+ clearance (p<.001) (Fig. 2). In a second group of fetuses, ECF volume expansion with added Ca^{++} did not produce a change in serum phosphate; however, fractional phosphate excretion increased 2-fold (p<.01), and again correlated significantly with Na^+ clearance. Plasma levels of immunoreactive parathyroid hormone (iPTH) remained stable in both groups of fetuses. In a third group of fetuses, exogenous bovine PTH was infused and produced a significant decrease in fractional tubular reabsorption of phosphate (p<.001) from the mean control value of 0.96 to a mean of 0.78. In a fourth group of fetuses, the response to

FIGURE 2.

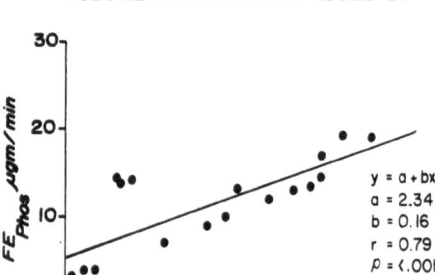

endogenous fetal PTH was studied by infusing EDTA into the fetuses to produce hypocalcemia. In this group, plasma Ca^{++} fell from a mean control value of 12.8 to 5.6 mg/dl (p<.001) and plasma iPTH increased from 0.071 to 0.723 ng/dl (Fig. 3). Fractional phosphate excretion increased 10-fold (p<.001) and was

FIGURE 3.

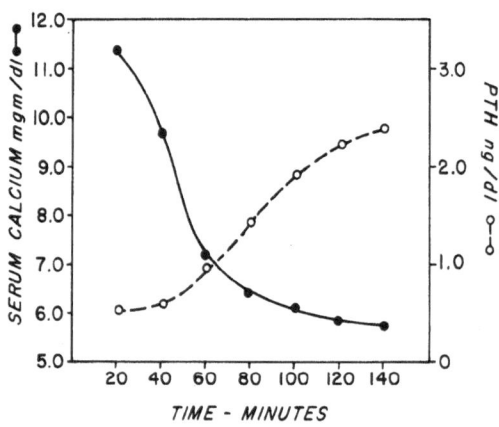

independent of the increase in urinary Na^+ excretion. The above studies demonstrated that acute ECF volume expansion in the fetal lamb produces a significant increase in urinary phosphate excretion which is independent of plasma Ca^{++} and iPTH, but is related to renal Na^+ clearance. These studies also confirmed the response of the fetal kidney to exogenous PTH and demonstrated for the first time that fetal kidney can respond to endogenous fetal-produced PTH.

4.5 Urea

Studies in human fetuses by McCance and Widdowson[19] showed identical mean plasma urea values for the term fetus compared to the mother. However, the urine urea concentration in the fetus averaged 17 mg/dl compared to 194 mg/dl for the mother. Gresham et al[30] investigated the production and excretion of urea by the fetal lamb. They demonstrated that urea is excreted by the sheep fetus via the placenta at a rate of approximately 0.54 mg/min/kg of fetal body weight, whereas in previous studies,[4] they demonstrated a mean fetal urea clearance of 0.6 ml/min/kg body weight. Thus, when the concentration of fetal urea is 40 mg/dl, the excretion rate by the fetal kidney is only one-half ($\sim$0.24 mg/min/kg) the excretion rate by the placenta. Additional studies of fetal renal tubular transport of urea are discussed in the section on fetal urinary concentrating and diluting capacity.

5. ACID-BASE EXCRETION

5.1 Bicarbonate reabsorption

The first detailed study of bicarbonate reabsorption by the fetal kidney was reported by Robillard et al.[31] The renal plasma bicarbonate threshold in control fetuses in an acute preparation varied from 12.0 to 23.5 mM/l with a mean value of 17.7±1.37 mM/liter. This value was significantly lower than the mean value of 28.7±1.68 mM in adult sheep. There was a significant positive correlation between the fetal plasma bicarbonate threshold and fetal body weight and fetal gestational age. These investigators also studied the relationship of bicarbonate excretion to Na^+ excretion in the fetus by producing fetal hydropenia via peritoneal dialysis. During fetal hydropenia, there was a significant decrease in urinary pH, bicarbonate excretion, and fractional Na^+ excretion, and a significant increase in bicarbonate reabsorption. Intravenous infusion of glucose had no effect on bicarbonate reabsorption. These studies indicate that the low threshold for bicarbonate by the fetal kidney is not due to a limited capacity to increase bicarbonate or Na^+ reabsorption. The capacity of the fetal renal carbonic anhydrase enzyme to facilitate bicarbonate reabsorption was also studied by Robillard et al.[32] These investigators infused acetazolamide into fetal lambs age 103-124 days gestation and demonstrated a significant increase in urinary excretion of bicarbonate, K^+, and urine pH. The authors concluded that renal carbonic anhydrase is present and active in utero and does not limit the capacity of the fetal kidney to reabsorb bicarbonate.

5.2 Hydrogen ion excretion

The ability of the fetal kidney to excrete fixed acids was studied by Vaughn et al[33] and by Smith and Schwartz.[34] Vaughn et al[33] infused HCl acid into near-term fetal lambs to produce a decrease in blood pH, bicarbonate, and base excess. Urine pH and acid excretion did not change significantly until the dose of acid given per unit weight was three times that required to lower urine pH significantly in adult animals. In nine fetuses studied, urine pH fell from 5.85 to 5.80 in one fetus, but did not fall below 6.0 in the remaining eight fetuses. Smith and Schwartz[34] reported similar studies in fetal lambs after infusing 0.1 to 0.3 M hydrochloric acid to reduce blood pH to a range of 7.11 to 6.94. In five of nine fetuses, urine pH fell to less than

6.0. These investigators concluded that a prolonged and severe systemic acidosis is necessary to demonstrate an increase in fetal excretion of H^+ ion.
Our group investigated the response of fetal primates to infused acid.   In
eight fetal baboons age 160-180 days gestation, systemic acidosis was produced
by infusing lactic acid over a 15-minute period. Fetal arterial blood pH
decreased to a mean of 7.16 (p<.05); however, fetal urine pH and excretion of
titratable acid did not change significantly from control values. The infused
lactic acid was distributed as follows: placental clearance - 82.3%, fetal
blood - 8.1%, amniotic fluid - 4.5%, and fetal urine - 0.2%. We concluded that
fetal acid-base balance is maintained primarily by placental clearance of H^+,
which is the major explanation for the results demonstrated with infusion of
HCl acid into fetal lambs.[33,34]

     In order to fully investigate the capacity of the fetal kidney to excrete
H^+, we studied the effect of infusion of Na_2SO_4 on urinary acidification in
fetal lambs.[35] Since urinary acidification occurs by a process of ion exchange
of Na^+ for H^+,[36] intense acidification of the urine will occur when there is a
stimulus for increased tubular reabsorption of Na^+.[37] In these studies, fetal
renal tubular avidity for Na^+ was increased by prior treatment of the ewes with
DOCA and subsequently infusing Na_2SO_4, a poorly reabsorbable Na^+ salt. Although
fetal blood pH remained normal, mean fetal urine pH fell to 5.2 and ranged from
4.7 to 5.7 (Table 4). Mean maximal fetal excretion of titratable acid and NH_4

Table 4. Effect of Na_2SO_4 on blood and urine pH in fetal lambs.

	Blood pH	Urine pH
Control	7.352	7.075
Na_2SO_4	7.362	5.20
ΔpH	0.010	-1.875
p	NS	< .001

was 5.29 and 6.93 mEq/min/kg body weight, respectively. The maternal urine pH

was unaffected by infusing Na_2SO_4 into the fetus. These studies demonstrated

that the fetal kidney is able to produce a clear-cut gradient between blood and

urine pH by increased excretion of H^+ similar to the adult.

6. URINARY CONCENTRATING-DILUTING MECHANISMS

6.1 Urine flow

Quantitative measurements of urine flow rates were first reported for

fetal lambs.[1,38] At 61 days gestation, urine flow ranged from 0.1 to 0.26

ml/min, mean 0.14 ml/min. Urine flow rate then steadily rose to a mean high of

0.64 ml/min (range 0.2-1.2) at fetal age 117 days. After fetal age 117 days,

the urine flow rate gradually decreased to a mean of 0.14 ml/min (range 0.09-

0.83) at 142 days gestation. Urine flow rates in chronic fetal lamb studies

was reported by Gresham et al.[4] In fetuses 117-134 days gestation, urine flow

was erratic for the first 24-72 hours postoperatively. Thereafter, urine flows

were stable between 0.25-0.4 ml/min. These values after stabilization appear

to be similar to those demonstrated for acute preparations.

6.2 Intrarenal solute and osmolar gradient

Stanier[39] demonstrated a steep intrarenal gradient for Na^+ in near-term

fetal lambs. However, intrarenal urea concentration increased only slightly

from cortex to papilla. Urea was given intraperitoneally to these fetuses

which produced no appreciable increase in intrarenal urea concentration. A

similar intrarenal solute gradient in near-term fetuses was demonstrated for

cows and pigs,[20] in the guinea pig,[40] and the rat.[25]

We studied the development of intrarenal solute and osmolar gradients in

fetal lambs age 70-100 days.[41] There was a steep intrarenal sodium as well as

urea gradient from cortex to papilla. The intrarenal urea concentrations were much higher than those previously reported in near-term fetal lambs. In those studies, the intraluminal-interstitial gradient for urea and Na^+ was increased by infusing hypertonic mannitol, urea, or NaCl. There was no significant change in the intrarenal solute gradient after infusing mannitol despite a significant increase in urine flow and sodium excretion. Intrarenal urea concentration increased significantly after infusing hypertonic urea. These data indicate that an intrarenal solute gradient is present in the fetal kidney by midgestation. The gradient is not limited by low tubular permeability to urea or low tubular capacity to reabsorb filtered NaCl.

6.3 Vasopressin release and tubular responsiveness

Robillard et al[42] investigated maturational aspects of renal tubular reabsorption of water in chronically catheterized fetal lambs 101-142 days gestation. In fetuses less than age 120 days, urinary flow rate increased compared to those greater than age 120 days. The increase was associated with a parallel increase in urine/plasma osmolar ratios. The percent of filtered water excreted was high before 120 to 130 days gestation, and then decreased significantly thereafter. The decrease in water excretion after 130 days gestation was not associated with a decrease in osmolar clearance. The authors concluded that the increase in urine osmolality at term results from an increase in free water reabsorption by the fetal kidney. Fetal production of vasopressin was investigated in chronic lamb fetuses.[43] Following controlled fetal hemorrhage, there was a significant increase in fetal plasma arginine vasopressin and fetal peripheral renin activity. The response of the fetal kidney to infusion of exogenous arginine vasopressin was also investigated in a chronic fetal lamb preparation.[44] In fetuses over 112 days gestation, free water reabsorption was demonstrated after infusing vasopressin. Urine osmolality was correlated with varying plasma concentrations of arginine vasopressin.

However, the slope of the regression line for the fetuses was less steep than that for adults, and the authors speculated that vasopressor receptors are not fully functional in fetuses age 112-142 days gestation.

7. RENAL HORMONES

7.1 Renin - angiotensin

Trimper and Lumbers[45] investigated the response of the fetal lamb kidney to infusion of furosemide. There was a significant increase in fetal-produced peripheral renin activity after infusing furosemide into fetuses 112 days gestation and older. Similar studies by Siegal et al[46] demonstrated a significant increase in fetal plasma renin activity as well as an increase in circulating levels of arginine vasopressin in fetal lambs after acutely administering 2 mg/kg of furosemide to fetal lambs. Smith et al[47] demonstrated high peripheral renin activity in fetal lambs when compared to the ewe at all gestational ages. These workers also demonstrated a significant increase in fetal peripheral renin activity after fetal hemorrhage and after constriction of the aorta. Fleishman et al[48] and Pipkin et al[49] demonstrated that fetal-produced renin does not cross the placenta and fetal peripheral renin activity is independent of that produced by the ewe. Pipkin and co-workers[50] also demonstrated that hypoxemia and removal of small volumes of blood produced a significant increase in renin and angiotensin II concentration in the plasma of fetal lambs. We studied the effect of changes in maternal and dietary Na^+ intake on fetal peripheral renin activity in near-term fetal lambs.[51] Maternal low dietary Na^+ intake resulted in a significant increase in peripheral renin activity and a decrease in urine Na^+ concentration in the fetus as well as in the ewe.

7.2 Prostaglandins

Pace-Asciak[52] demonstrated the presence of prostaglandin $F_2\alpha$ at 40 days gestation, and prostaglandin E_2 at 77 days gestation in fetal lambs. Walker and Mitchell[53] demonstrated high concentrations of PGE, PGF and 13,14-dihydro-15-keto-prostaglandin F (PGFM) in fetal lambs between 115-120 days gestation. In this study, the excretion of prostaglandins was related to urine flow rate. The excretion of PGF and PGFM was correlated with osmolar, Na^+, and free water clearances. The excretion of PGE, however, was correlated only with free water clearance.

8. SUMMARY

A major factor modulating renal function in utero is the fact that fetal renal blood flow does not increase with gestational age despite an increase in fetal cardiac output. The failure of an increase in renal blood flow to occur is related to a markedly elevated renal vascular resistance due in the main to the high levels of renin-angiotensin-prostaglandin produced by the fetal kidney. However, failure of the renal blood flow to rise throughout gestation will impart only a quantitative rather than a qualitative limitation on fetal renal function. Absolute GFR increases with gestational age but GFR/gm of kidney weight does not. The capacity of the fetal renal tubule to increase reabsorption and thereby decrease urinary excretion of electrolytes increases with gestational age. Glomerulo-tubular balance for glucose is present by mid-gestation and is maintained throughout gestation. Renal plasma HCO_3^- threshold is low in the fetus but it is not fixed, and responds appropriately to stimuli that changes fetal proximal tubular reabsorption of Na^+. The fetal kidney can increase excretion of H^+ and significantly lower fetal urine pH. By midgestation, the fetal kidney can establish a steep intrarenal solute gradient from cortex to papilla. However, urine passed in utero is hypotonic to plasma as a

result of distal tubular reabsorption of solute without water. Urine flow rate
in the fetus decreases with gestational age as a result of an increase in
response of the distal tubule to endogenous vasopressin. The fetal kidney
produces renin, angiotensin II, and prostaglandins by midgestation.

REFERENCES

1. Alexander DP, Nixon DA, Widdar WF and Wholzogen FX: Renal function in the
   sheep foetus. J Physiol 140:14, 1958.
2. Alexander DP and Nixon DA: The foetal kidney. Br Med Bull 17:112, 1961.
3. Smith FG, Adams FH, Borden M and Hilburn J: Studies of renal function in
   the intact fetal lamb. Am J Obstet Gynecol 96:240, 1966.
4. Gresham EL, Rankin JH, Makowski EL, Meschin G and Battaglia FC: An evaluation of fetal renal function in a chronic sheep preparation. J Clin Invest 51:149, 1972.
5. Rudolph AM and Heymann MA: Circulatory changes during growth in the fetal
   lamb. Circ Res 26:289, 1970.
6. Paton JB, Fisher DE, de Lannoy CW and Behrman RE: Umbilical blood flow,
   cardiac output, and organ blood flow in the immature baboon fetus. Am J
   Obstet Gynecol 117:560, 1973.
7. Rudolph AM, Heymann MA, Teramo KA, Barrett CT and Raiha NCR: Studies on
   the circulation of the previable human fetus. Pediatr Res 5:452, 1971.
8. Hollenberg AC and Herd JA: The renal circulation. N Engl J Med 47:455, 1968
9. Moore ES, Galvez, MB, Paton JB, Fisher DE and Behrman RE: Intrarenal blood
   flow in the baboon fetus. Pediatr Res 9:377, 1975.
10. Chung EE, Moore ES, Cevallos EE, Ocampo M and Lyons EC: The effect of
    gestational age and arterial pressure on renal function in utero. Pediatr
    Res 10:437, 1976.
11. Alexander DP and Nixon DA: Plasma clearance of p-aminohippuric acid by the
    kidneys of foetal, neonatal and adult sheep. Nature 194:483, 1962.
12. Assali NS, Bekey FA and Morrisson LW: Fetal and neonatal circulation. In
    Assali NS, (ed), Biology of Gestation, Vol. II, New York: Academic Press,
    1968, p. 51.
13. Alexander DP and Nixon DA: Reabsorption of glucose, fructose and meso-
    inositol by the foetal and postnatal sheep kidney. J Physiol 167:480, 1963.
14. Arturson G, Groth T and Grotte M: Human glomerular membrane porosity and
    filtration pressure: Dextran clearance data analyzed by theoretical models.
    Clin Sci 40:137, 1971.
15. Edelmann CM Jr and Spitzer A: The maturing kidney. J Pediatr 75:509, 1969.
16. Spitzer A and Edelmann CM Jr: Maturational changes in pressure gradients
    for glomerular filtration. Am J Physiol 221:1431, 1971.
17. Chung EE, Moore ES, Cevallos EE, Ocampo M and Lyons E: The effect of ges-
    tational age and arterial pressure on renal function in utero. Pediatr Res
    10:437, 1976.
18. Robillard JE, Kulvinskas C, Sessious C, Burmeister L and Smith FG Jr:
    Maturational changes in the fetal glomerular filtration rate. Am J Obstet
    Gynecol 122:601, 1975.
19. McCance RA and Widdowson EM: Renal function before birth. Proc R Soc Lond
    B141:488, 1953.

20. Perry JS and Stanier MW: The rate of flow of urine of foetal pigs. J Physiol 166:344, 1962.
21. Robillard JE, Sessious C, Kennedy RL, Hamel-Robillard L and Smith FG Jr: Interrelationships between glomerular filtration rate and renal transport of sodium and chloride during fetal life. Am J Obstet Gynecol 128:727, 1977.
22. Moore ES, Chung EE, Cevallos EE, McMann BJ, Ocampo M and Lyons E: Renal phosphate clearance in fetal lambs. Pediatr Res 11:554, 1977.
23. Moore ES, McMann BJ, Weiss LS, Ocampo M and Francisco F: Renal handling of sodium in utero: interrelationship of physical and hormonal factors (submitted for publication).
24. Robillard JE, Ramberg E, Sessious C, Consamus B, Van Orden D, Weismann D and Smith FG Jr: Role of aldosterone on renal sodium and potassium excretion during fetal life and newborn period. Dev Pharmacol Ther 1:201, 1980.
25. Daly H, Wells LJ and Evans G: Experimental evidence of the secretion of urine by the fetal kidneys. Proc Soc Exp Biol Med 64:78, 1974.
26. Robillard JE, Sessious CE, Kennedy RL and Smith FG Jr: Maturation of the glucose transport process by the fetal kidney. Pediatr Res 12:680, 1978.
27. Vernier RC and Smith FG Jr: Fetal and neonatal kidney. In Assali NS (ed.) Biology of Gestation, Vol. II, New York: Academic Press, 1968, p. 245.
28. Smith FG Jr, Tingloff B, Meuli J and Borden M: Fetal response to parathyroid hormone in sheep. Am J Physiol 27:276, 1969.
29. Moore ES, Chung EE, Cevallos EE and McMann BJ: Renal phosphate clearance in fetal lambs. Pediatr Res 12:1066, 1978.
30. Gresham EL, James EJ, Raye JR, Battaglia FC, Makowski ER and Meschia G: Production and excretion of urea by the fetal lamb. Pediatrics 50:372, 1972.
31. Robillard JE, Sessious C, Burmeister L and Smith FG Jr: Influence of fetal extracellular volume contraction on renal reabsorption of bicarbonate in fetal lambs. Pediatr Res 11:649, 1977.
32. Robillard JE, Sessious C and Smith FG Jr: In vivo demonstration of renal carbonic anhydrase activity in the fetal lamb. Biol Neonate 34:253, 1978.
33. Vaughn D, Kirschbaum H, Bersenka T, Dilts PV Jr and Assali NS: Fetal and neonatal response to acid loading in the sheep. J Appl Physiol 24:135, 1968.
34. Smith FG Jr and Schwartz A: Response of the intact lamb fetus to acidosis. Am J Obstet Gynecol 106:52, 1970.
35. Moore ES, de Lannoy CW, Paton JB and Ocampo M: Effect of Na_2SO_4 on urinary acidification in the fetal lamb. Am J Physiol 223:167, 1972.
36. Pitts RF: Physiology of the Kidney and Body Fluids (2d ed.). Chicago: Yearbook Publications, 1968, p. 179.
37. Bank NB and Schwartz WB: The influence of anion penetrating ability on urinary acidification and the excretion of titrable acid. J Clin Invest 39:1516, 1960.
38. Alexander DP, Nixon DA, Widden WF and Wohlzogen FX: Gestational variations in the composition of the foetal fluids and foetal urine in the sheep. J Physiol (Lond) 140:1, 1958.
39. Stanier MW: Development of intra-renal solute gradients in foetal and and postnatal life. Pflugers Arch 336:263, 1972.
40. Merlet-Benicham C and de Rouffignac C: Renal clearance studies in fetal and young guinea pigs: effect of salt loading. Am J Physiol 232:F178, 1977
41. Moore ES, Ocampo M, Galvez MB, McMann BJ and Simpson EH: Ontogeny of intra renal solute gradients (ISG) in fetal and postnatal life. Soc Pediatr Res, 1979.

42. Robillard JE, Matson JB, Sessious CE and Smith FG Jr: Developmental aspects of renal tubular reabsorption of water in the lamb fetus. Pediatr Res 13:1172, 1979.

43. Robillard JE, Weitzman RE, Fisher DE and Smith FG Jr: The dynamics of vaso-pressin release and blood volume regulation during fetal hemorrhage in the lamb fetus. Pediatr Res 13:606, 1979.

44. Robillard JE and Weitzman RE: Developmental aspects of the fetal renal response to exogenous arginine vasopressin. Am J Physiol 7:F407, 1980.

45. Trimper CE and Lumbers ER: The renin-angiotensin system in foetal lambs. Pflugers Arch 336:1, 1973.

46. Siegel SR, Leake RD, Weitzman RE and Fisher DA: Effects of furosemide and acute salt loading on vasopressin and renin secretion in the fetal lamb. Pediatr Res 14:869, 1980.

47. Smith FG Jr, Lupn AN and Barajas L: The renin-angiotensin system in the fetal lamb. Pediatr Res 8:611, 1974.

48. Fleishman AR, Oakes GF and Epstein MF: Plasma renin activity during ovine pregnancy. Am J Physiol 228:901, 1971.

49. Pipkin FB, Kirkpatrick SML, Lumbers ER and Mott JC: Renin and angiotensin-like levels in foetal, newborn, and adult sheep. J Physiol 241:575, 1974.

50. Pipkin FB, Lumbers ER and Mott JC: Factors influencing plasma renin and angiotensin II in the conscious pregnant ewe and its foetus. J Physiol 243:619, 1974.

51. Moore ES, Paton JB, de Lannoy CW, Ocampo M and Lyons EC: The effect of maternal dietary Na^+ and ECF on fetal plasma renin activity. Pediatr Res 8:184, 1974.

52. Pace-Asciak CR: Prostaglandin biosynthesis and catabolism in the developing fetal sheep kidney. Prostaglandins 13:661, 1977.

53. Walker DW and Mitchell MD: Prostaglandins in urine of foetal lambs. Nature 271:161, 1978.

ADAPTATION OF THE INFANT TO AN EXTERNAL MILIEU

BILLY S. ARANT, JR., M.D.

A statement attributed to Widdowson is, "In some respects we can regard birth as an incident in chemical development, which pursues the same steady course if all goes well from conception to maturity, and it matters little whether the organism spends the last few weeks of normal gestation inside or outside the uterus" (1). Between eight and 40 weeks gestation the sodium content of the human fetus decreases from 120 to 80 mEq/kg body weight, and the water content decreases from 95% to 78% (2). This reduction in salt and water in the human fetus is accomplished in part by high rates of fractional sodium excretion (FE_{Na}) of 8-15% (3) and high urine flow rates (V) that increase during gestation to 25 ml/hr at term (4). Following birth a more abrupt loss of salt and water results in a further decrease in body weight by 5% in the term infant and by nearly 15% in the infant whose birth weight is less than 1000 grams (5). In order for an infant whose birth weight is 1230 grams to have the same chemical composition as an infant whose birth weight is 2500 grams, according to Metcoff, a net loss of salt and water must occur; the osmotic activity of that solution lost from the skin would be 235 mOsm/l. We have studied infants during the first six hours of life and found that V decreases from 4 ml/kg/hr in infants born at 28 weeks gestation to 1 ml/kg/hr in infants born at term, while FE_{Na} decreased from 7% to <1%. Hansen and Smith (6) studied newborn infants that were fasted or thirsted for 72 hours from birth and demonstrated a negative sodium balance for the more premature infants that was not observed in term infants; neither group of infants became hyponatremic or hypernatremic. Studies performed more recently by Siegel and Oh (7) in infants receiving both calories and fluids during the same postnatal period reported FE_{Na} of 1-6% and a negative sodium balance in infants whose gestational ages were <32 weeks. It would appear, therefore, that reduction of salt and water in the term fetus in utero must continue during postnatal life in the infant born prematurely. The mechanisms to explain the high FE_{Na} in the fetus, the negative sodium balance of the premature infant and the failure of the term infant to excrete a sodium load are poorly understood. One conclusion should be, however, that the ability of the neonatal kidney to regulate sodium homeostasis in the neonate may be determined by factors other than "immaturity" of the kidney.

Most reports have characterized tubular function in the developing kidney as immature and have popularized the concept of glomerulotubular imbalance with glomerular preponderance (8); this hypothesis was used interpret studies of renal function during development for the past decade. Until recently no consideration has been given to the possibility that the developing kidney is not only responsive to volume expansion in a manner similar to the adult, but also that it may be this mechanism which permits the kidney to reduce the salt and water content of the fetus or infant following birth. Extracellular fluid volume (ECFV) decreases from 60% of body weight at 20 weeks gestation to 45% by 40 weeks, as compared with 39% at the end of the week of postnatal life (2). Following birth there are shifts in body fluids that occur between fluid spaces in the human neonate. As body weight decreases during the first three days of life, plasma volume increases from 42 to 46 ml/kg between birth and 24 hours, and ECFV increases from 330 to 380 ml/kg 3-5 days of age (9). The normal state of the fetus and the neonate, therefore, is one of an expanded ECFV. Tubular function measured while the neonatal kidney is responding to the stimulus of ECFV expansion would, if like the adult kidney, reflect a level of function that would be less than that observed during normovolemia or hydropenia. If the normal physiological state of the fetus and neonate could be reproduced in the adult animal, ECFV would be doubled, and one would expect to observe increased urinary losses of water, sodium, phosphate, glucose and bicarbonate--observations that have been used to support "immaturity" of renal function in the neonate.

The neonatal kidney, however, has been shown to respond appropriately to antidiuretic hormone following thirsting (10) and vasopression administration (11). Studies in puppies (12) and fetal lambs (13) demonstrated bicarbonate thresholds to increase during contraction of ECFV as bicarbonate excretion and urine pH decreased. Glomerulotubular balance for glucose was reported for human premature infants by us (14) and Brodehl (15). Moreover, we have demonstrated in puppies that glomerulotubular balance obtains from birth when volume expansion is avoided (16). Following saline loading, glucose reabsorption in the puppies decreased, and splay in the glucose titration curve was increased. Our studies of human infants at birth and during postnatal life (14) have documented that glucosuria is a frequent observation in normoglycemic infants whose conceptional ages (gestational age plus postnatal age) are <30 weeks and decreases with conceptional age when plasma volume and ECFV have been shown by others (2,9) to be decreasing.

We have demonstrated that tubular reabsorption of phosphate in infants following birth increased with conceptional age and that phosphate excretion during spontaneous diuresis in premature infants increases with distal delivery of sodium $(C_{H_2O} + C_{Na})$, suggesting decreased proximal tubular reabsorption of both sodium and phosphate (17). Spitzer and Brandis (18) reported that glomerulotubular balance for proximal tubular reabsorption of sodium and water obtains from birth in the guinea pig, but in the same animal model FE_{Na} in the proximal nephron is increased compared to the adult (19). The hypothesis that the neonatal kidney does not excrete a saline load as does the adult supposes that the sodium arrives to the glomerulus, is filtered, and that it is the unique capability of the distal nephron to reabsorb up to 50% of the filtered sodium load (20), perhaps under the influence of aldosterone, that results in the salt and water retention by the neonate. This unique capability appears to be impaired in the fetus and preterm infant whose plasma aldosterone concentrations are at least as high, if not higher than the full-term infant. We have demonstrated that saline loading in neonatal puppies produced a dilution of plasma protein, a decrease in plasma volume and blood pressure (BP) that resulted in a decrease in glomerular filtration rate (GFR) and sodium excretion (21). When the same saline load was given as a 5% albumin solution, plasma volume increased, but BP decreased in an age-related response that was greatest on the first day and least at 60 days of life. Changes in BP were directly related to changes in GFR and to sodium excretion. Although this BP response to plasma volume expansion appeared age-related, any puppy that increased its BP during saline loading, regardless of age, excreted the saline load like an adult animal. Whether the change in BP actually determined sodium excretion or rather the same factors that produced the fall in BP also affected renal sodium handling directly is unknown.

No study to date has described the physiologic mechanisms which determine renal vascular resistance and renal function during the period of transition from fetal to postnatal life. We have reported that GFR is low at birth in premature infants <34 weeks gestational age and does not increase significantly even in infants 4-6 weeks old until conceptional age approaches 34 weeks (14); similar findings were reported by Siegel and Oh (7). In the canine puppy GFR remains low for 10-14 days following birth and increases rapidly during the third week of life (16) when renal blood flow increases and is redistributed in a centrifugal fashion (22). There appears to be control of GFR until a critical time in development has been reached that corresponds to the time nephrogenesis is completed at least in the human and the dog; the control of this developmental change is likely the result of an interplay among vasoactive factors. Fawer et al (23) have observed a direct relationship between blood pressure and GFR in newborn infants, and Kleinman and Lubbe have observed the same relationship in newborn puppies (24).

The renin-angiotensin system has been demonstrated to be intact in most fetal and neonatal studies. Kotchen et al (25) observed that plasma renin activity (PRA) in newborn infants was greater than that of maternal blood and increased during the first three days of life. This increase in PRA may have been the effect of volume depletion associated with the weight loss most infants exhibit following birth; however, previous investigators have demonstrated that plasma volume and ECFV increase during this period of life (2,9). The major product of prostaglandin biosynthesis in fetal vascular tissues is prostacyclin (26) which, although similar in many respects to the actions of PGE_2 is a more potent vasodilator that is not metabolized in the lung, and when infused into the circulation of the dog lowers BP, increases in cardiac output and decreases in GFR and FE_{Na}. We have measured levels of PGE_2 and 6-keto $PGF_{1\alpha}$, a metabolite of prostacyclin, in arterial blood of puppies and found both to be higher at birth than at 60 days of life or the adult dog (27). It is possible that the production of prostacyclin accounts for the low vascular resistance of the fetal circulation. Following plasma volume expansion with 5% albumin/0.9% NaCl (10 mg/kg), we demonstrated PGE_2 to increase five-fold and 6-keto $PGF_{1\alpha}$ seven-fold as PRA increased (28).

Physiologic closure of the ductus arteriosus has been associated traditionally with increased oxygen tension in arterial blood following birth; however, constriction of the ductus when oxygen tension is high can be prevented by prostaglandins (29). Stevenson (30) has reported that ductal closure in premature infants can be reversed by increasing the volume of intravenous fluids administered to the infant. Inhibition of prostaglandin synthesis with indomethacin to effect non-surgical closure of the patent ductus arteriosus in premature infants, and the infusion of PGE_2 to maintain the ductus patent in some forms of congenital heart disease are used widely in the management of newborn infants. We have demonstrated that the physiologic closure of the ductus arteriosus in a three-day-old puppy can be reversed by the administration of 10 ml/kg of 5% albumin/saline intravenously over 5 minutes and is associated with increased concentrations of PGE_2 and 6-keto $PGF_{1\alpha}$ in arterial blood; indomethacin given prior to the study prevented the reopening of the closed ductus (17). Vascular resistance and BP regulation in the neonatal puppy, therefore, can be related at least in part to the endogenous synthesis of vasodilator prostaglandins and inversely to changes in blood volume.

Although mechanisms whereby the fetus adapts to postnatal life are poorly defined, this transitional process does take place in an orderly fashion under normal circumstances. Transitional physiology in the human neonate is difficult to study not only because of the ethical questions that are raised by such studies, but also because it is nearly impossible to separate normal transitional changes from pathophysiologic changes induced by clinical management. Our studies of the newborn puppy have integrated changes in body composition, renal function and blood pressure with changes in blood concentrations of vasoactive substances. It can be seen from the data given in the Figure that the pattern of changes in the newborn puppy is very similar to that reported by various authors for human neonates, providing a suitable animal model for further studies of adpatational responses.

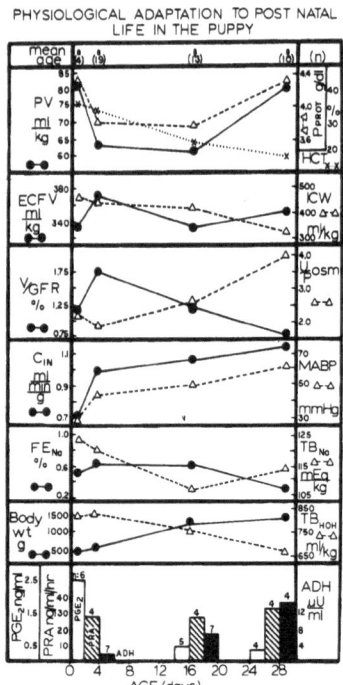

PHYSIOLOGICAL ADAPTATION TO POST NATAL
LIFE IN THE PUPPY

Figure--Changes in plasma volume (PV), extracellular fluid volume (ECFV), intracellular water (ICW), total body water (TB$_{HOH}$) and sodium (TB$_{Na}$) contents, plasma protein concentration (P$_{PROT}$), hematocrit (HCT) are compared with changes in urine flow rate (V/GFR), inulin clearance (C$_{IN}$), fractional sodium excretion (FE$_{Na}$), the ratio of urine:plasma osmolality (U/P osm) and mean aortic blood pressure (MABP) and related to changes in blood concentrations of prostaglandin E$_2$ (PGE$_2$), plasma renin activity (PRA) and antidiuretic hormone (ADH) during the first month of life in the puppy. Each point represents a mean value for that age group.

REFERENCES

1. Schafer, A.J. and Avery, M.E. Diseases of the Newborn, Chapter 1, p.19, (W.B. Saunders Co., Philadelphia), 1977.
2. Friis-Hansen, B. Body water compartments in children: changes during growth and related changes in body composition. Pediatrics 28:169, 1961.
3. Zeis, P.M. and Houston, I.B. Intrauterine renal function and the amniotic fluid. Third International Symposium of Pediatric Nephrology, Washington, D.C., 1974.
4. Wladimiroff, J.W. and Campbell, S. Fetal-urine production rates in normal and complicated pregnancy. Lancet L:151, 1974.
5. Metcoff, J. Synchrony of organ development contributing to water and electrolyte regulation in early life. Clinical Nephrology 1:107, 1973.

6. Hansen, J.D.L. and Smith C.A. Effects of withholding fluid in the immediate postnatal period. Pediatrics 12:99, 1953.
7. Siegel, S.R. and Oh, W. Renal function as a marker of human fetal maturation. Acta Paediatr Scand 65:481, 1976.
8. Edelmann, C.M., Jr. and Spitzer, A. The maturing kidney. J Pediatr 75:509, 1969.
9. MacLaurin, J.C. Changes in body water distribution during the first two weeks of life. Arch Dis Childhood 41:286, 1963.
10. Fisher, D.A., Pyle, H.R., Jr., Porter, J.C., Beard, A.G. and Panos, T.C. Control of water balance in the newborn. Amer J Dis Child 106:137, 1963.
11. Edelmann, C.M., Jr., Barnett, H.L. and Troupkou, V. Renal concentrating mechanisms in newborn infants. Effect of dietary protein and water content, role of urea and responsiveness to antidiuretic hormone. J Clin Invest 39:1062, 1960.
12. Moore, E.S., Fine, B.P., Satrosook, S.S., Vergel, Z.M. and Edelmann, C.M., Jr. Renal bicarbonate reabsorption in puppies. Effect of extra-cellular volume contraction on the renal threshold for bicarbonate. Pediatr Res 6:859, 1972.
13. Robillard, J.E., Sessions, C., Burmeister, L. and Smith, F.G., Jr. Influence of fetal extracellular volume contraction on renal reabsorption of bicarbonate in fetal lambs. Pediatr Res 11:649, 1977.
14. Arant, B.S., Jr. Developmental patterns of renal functional maturation compared in the neonate. J Pediatr 92:705, 1978.
15. Brodehl, J., Franken, A. and Gellissen, K. Maximal tubular reabsorption of glucose in infants and children. Acta Paediatr Scand 61:413, 1972.
16. Arant, B.S., Jr. Glomerulo-tubular balance following saline loading in the developing canine kidney. Amer J Physiol 235:F417, 1978.
17. Arant, B.S., Jr. Unpublished observations.
18. Spitzer, A. and Brandis, M. Functional and morphologic maturation of the superficial nephrons. J Clin Invest 53:279, 1974.
19. Spitzer, A. Renal physiology and functional development, in Pediatric Kidney Disease, C.M. Edelmann, Jr., editor, Little, Brown and Co., Boston, 1978, p. 54.
20. Kleinman, L.I. Renal sodium reabsorption during saline loading and distal blockade in newborn dogs. Amer J Physiol 228:1403, 1975.
21. Arant, B.S., Jr. Effects of changing plasma volume on sodium excretion by the neonatal kidney. Pediatr Res 12:538, 1978.
22. Aschinberg, L.C., Goldsmith, D.I., Olbing, H., Spitzer, A., Edelmann, C.M., Jr. and Blaufox, M.D. Neonatal changes in renal blood flow distribution in puppies. Amer J Physiol 228:1453, 1975.
23. Fawer, C.L., Torrado, A. and Guignard, J.P. Maturation of renal function in full-term and premature neonates. Helv Paediat Acta 34:11, 1979.
24. Kleinman, L.I. and Lubbe, R.J. Factors affecting the maturation of glomerular filtration rate and renal plasma flow in the new-born dog. J Physiol 223:395, 1972.
25. Kotchen, T.A., Strickland, A.L., Rice, T.W. and Walter, D.R. A study of the renin-angiotensin system in newborn infants. J Pediatr 80:938, 1972.
26. Terragno, N.A., McGiff, J.C., Smigel, M. and Terragno, A. Prostacyclin (PGI_2); the most abundant prostaglandin (PG) in the fetal vasculature. Fed Proc 37:732, 1978.
27. Arant, B.S., Jr. The relationship between blood volume, prostaglandin synthesis and arterial blood pressure in neonatal puppies. Proc of the First International Workshop on Developmental Renal Physiology, October 1-4, 1980.

28. Arant, B.S., Jr., Terragno, N. and Terragno, D.A. Effect of changing plasma volume on blood pressure and prostaglandins in neonatal puppies. Fed Proc 38:359, 1979.
29. Clyman, R.I., Mauray, F., Heymann, M.A. and Rudolph, A.M. Ductus arteriosus: Developmental response to oxygen and indomethacin. Prostaglandins 15:993, 1978.
30. Stevenson, J.G. Fluid administration in the association of patent ductus arteriosus complicating respiratory distress syndrome. J Pediatr 90:257, 1977.

FACTORS GOVERNING THE DEVELOPMENT OF RENAL CONTROL OF Na HOMEO_
STASIS.

A. APERIA, O. BROBERGER, G. ELINDER, P. HERIN, L. LARSSON and
R. ZETTERSTRÖM

During the last ten years we have performed a series of studies
on urinary Na excretion in newborn pre-term and full-term infants
during normal, low or high salt intake. The results from those
studies have given us a descriptive view of the development of the
Na excretory capacity. Pre-term infants (born before the 34th
gestational week) have at all levels of salt intake a higher Na
excretion than full-term infants (1,2,4,6). Normally, breastmilk
is higher in salt content during the first two to three weeks
after delivery (around 15 mmol/l) than later during lactation
(around 6 mmol/l) (3). If newborn pre-term infants are given
breastmilk or formula with the salt content of 6 mmol/l, they
continue to have a high Na excretion (4). The Na excretion then
exceeds Na intake during the first ten days of life. As a result,
newborn pre-term infants are prone to develop negative Na balance
and hyponatremia is a commonly reported complication of pre-term
birth (12,16). Hyponatremia can be avoided if extra salt is
supplemented to the food (16). High Na excretion in pre-term
infants is due to a high fractional Na excretion i.e. an inability of the tubules to reabsorb Na (2). Thus, there is in pre-
term infants an imbalance between glomerular and tubular function
with regard to the capacity to handle salt. A similar imbalance
has also been shown to exsist for Beta-2-microglobulin, a small
peptide which is exclusively reabsorbed in the proximal tubule
(2,8). This might imply that the inability of the immature kidney
to retain Na is due mainly to an inability of the more proximal
parts of the nephron to reabsorb Na. Active Na reabsorption in
the kidney is to a large extent monitored by Na-K-ATPase. The
low Na reabsorptive capacity implies a low activity of Na-K-

ATPase. Na-K-ATPase links the transport of Na and K across the
basal and lateral membrane at the proximal tubular cell (14).
Pre-term infants have significantly lower K/Na quotient in the
urine than full-term infants (4).

Newborn full-term infants have a low basal Na excretion (2)
and are able to retain Na when in negative Na balance. When,
however, an oral salt load is given to newborn full-term infants, the natriuretic response normally observed in older
children and adults is almost nonexsistant (5). The capacity
to excrete a salt load develops linearly during the first year
of life (7). Although pre-term infants have a higher basal Na
excretion than full-term infants, they are also unable to rapidly
increase Na excretion following an oral salt load (6). This
blunted natriuretic response to salt loading is due to an inability to reduce the net Na reabsorption. A well developed
diluting capacity present both in pre-term and full-term infants, implies that the high fractional Na reabsorption which
is evident in infants following a salt load, is present in the
more distal part of the nephron.

In summary those clinical studies have shown
a) that the Na reabsorptive capacity is low in the immature
kidney as revealed in pre-term infants where the glomerular
tubular balance for Na is not yet established.
b) that there is a less efficient homeostatic control in the
immature kidney as manifested by an inability to increase Na
excretion following an oral salt and fluid load.

To examine the mechanisms behind those manifestations of renal
immaturity we have performed studies on the development of Na
transport in the proximal and distal tubule of the superficial

rat nephron. We have also attempted to relate those findings
to ultrastructural and enzymatic development. In the proximal
tubule of the superficial rat nephron we have found that the
capacity to reabsorb Na develops linearly until full structural
maturation of the proximal tubular cells is obtained (10). In
the rat this does not occur until the postnatal age of fourty
days. An increase in Na-K-ATPase activity also parallels the
development of the Na reabsorptive capacity (11). The importance
of steroid hormones for the enzymatic differentiation is well
established from studies of other tissues such as liver (17) and
retina (15). We have found that glucocorticosteroid as well as
mineralcorticosteroid hormones can induce a premature increase
in the enzymatic activity of proximal tubular cells (11). The
increase was found already following doses as small as 10 µg/
100 g bw/12 h which suggests that both mineralcorticoid and
glucocorticoid hormones can be of physiological importance for
the postnatal increase of Na-K-ATPase activity in proximal
tubular cells. The sensitivity for hormonal induction was much
more pronounced in the immature than in the mature kidney. Eight
times higher doses of hormones were needed in the mature kidney
to induce significant increase of the enzyme. A comparison
between rats aged 10 and 20 days showed that the later stages
of proximal tubular differentiation represented by the 20-day-
old rats, were more sensitive to the enzymatic inductive effect
of steroid hormones than the earlier stages represented by the
10-day-old rats. This difference might explain the differences
in Na reabsorption observed between pre-term and full-term
infants.

In order to examine the reason for the blunted natriuretic
response to salt loading we have quantitated the Na reabsorption
in different segments of the nephron during hydropenia and during
isotonic volume expansion corresponding to 5% of the bw (13,9).
Rats aged 24 and 40 days have been studied. During hydropenia
the fractional Na reabsorption in the end of the proximal tubule
is approximately the same in the 24- and 40-day-old rats.
Fractional reabsorption along the distal tubule is however more

efficient in the 24- than in the 40-day-old rats. During volume expansion the fractional delivery of Na to the early distal tubule increases significantly both in the 24- and in the 40-day-old rats, but the 24-day-old rats still have a significantly higher reabsorption along the distal tubule which results in a lower delivery of Na to collecting tubule in the 24- than in the 40-day-old rats. The results strongly suggest that a relative overcapacity of the distal tubule in the developing nephron contributes to the difficulties to induce natriuresis in infants.

REFERENCES

1. Aperia A, Broberger O, Broberger U, Larsson L, Thodenius K, Zetterström R. 1979. Sodium and fluid homeostasis in normal and diseased newborns. Leo Stern: Intensive Care in the Newborns, II. Masson Publ. Inc. New York.
2. Aperia A, Broberger O, Elinder G, Herin P, Zetterström R. 1981, in press. Postnatal development of renal function in pre-term and full-term infants. Acta Paediatr Scand 70.
3. Aperia A, Broberger O, Herin P, Zetterström R. 1979. Salt-content in human breastmilk during the three first weeks after delivery. Acta Paediatr Scand 68:441-442.
4. Aperia A, Broberger O, Herin P, Zetterström R. 1979. Sodium excretion in relation to sodium intake and aldosterone excretion in newborn pre-term and full-term infants. Acta Paediatr Scand 68:813-817.
5. Aperia A, Broberger O, Thodenius K, Zetterström R. 1972. Renal response to an oral sodium load in newborn full-term infants. Acta Paediatr Scand 61:670-676.
6. Aperia A, Broberger O, Thodenius K, Zetterström R. 1974. Developmental study of the renal response to an oral salt load in pre-term infants. Acta Paediatr Scand 63:517-524.
7. Aperia A, Broberger O, Thodenius K, Zetterström R. 1975. Development of renal control of salt and fluid homeostasis during the first year of life. Acta Paediatr Scand 64:393-398.
8. Aperia A, Broberger U. 1979. Beta-2-microglobulin, an indicator of renal tubular maturation and dysfunction in the newborn. Acta Paediatr Scand 68:669-676.
9. Aperia A, Elinder G. Distal tubular Na reabsorption in the developing rat kidney. Submitted to Am J Physiol: Renal, Fluid and Electrolyte Physiology, 1980.
10. Aperia A, Larsson L. 1979. Correlation between fluid reabsorption and proximal tubule ultrastructure during development of the rat kidney. Acta Phys Scand 105:11-22.
11. Aperia A, Larsson L, Zetterström R. Hormonal induction of Na-K-ATPase in developing proximal tubular cells. Submitted to Am J Physiol, 1980.
12. Day G M, Radde I C, Balfe J W, Chance G W. 1976. Electrolyte abnormalities in very low birth weight infants. Pediatr Res 10:522-526.

13. Elinder G. 1981, in press. Effect of isotonic volume expansion on proximal tubular Na and fluid reabsorption in the developing rat kidney. Acta Phys Scand.
14. Jørgensen P L. 1980. Sodium and potassium ion pump in kidney tubules. Phys Rev 60:864-917.
15. Reit-Lehrer L, Amos H. 1968. Hydrocortisone requirement for the induction of glutamine synthetase in chick-embryo retinas. Biochem J 106:425-430.
16. Roy R N, Chance G W, Radde I C, Hill D E, Willis D M, Shephers J. 1976. Late hyponatremia in very low birth weight infants. Pediat Res 10:526-531.
17. Sanchez-Urretia L, Greengard O. 1977. Phenylalanine-pyruvate aminotransferase in immature and adult mammalian tissues. Biochim Biophys Acta 497:682-689.

THE KIDNEY FOLLOWING CARDIAC SURGERY

T.M. BARRATT AND S.P.A. RIGDEN

1. INTRODUCTION

The kidneys receive one quarter of the cardiac output: it is therefore hardly surprising that impairment of renal function is a major complication of cardiopulmonary by-pass surgery (CPBS) with a high mortality, both in adults and children (1). The principal cause is undoubtedly renal hypoperfusion resulting from a low cardiac output, but other factors may be additive: before surgery there is to consider the physiological characteristics of the neonatal kidney and the questions of congenital renal abnormality, cyanotic nephropathy and the nephrotoxicity of radiological contrast media; during CPBS there is the possible effect of haemolysis; and subsequently there may be septicaemia or drug nephrotoxicity (particularly antibiotics).

2. THE NEONATAL KIDNEY

The kidney in the first few weeks of life is particularly vulnerable to poor perfusion. On the basis of body surface area or kidney weight, glomerular filtration rate and renal plasma flow are low, and renal vascular resistance high (2). There is a preferential distribution of the renal blood flow to the juxta-medullary glomeruli and outer cortical perfusion is low. There is diminished fractional reabsorption of sodium by the proximal tubule, plasma renin activity and aldosterone concentration are high, and the infant is more dependent than the older child on renin-aldosterone stimulated distal sodium reabsorption for the maintenance of sodium balance. Low cortical perfusion and high plasma renin activity also characterise vasomotor nephropathy, and in some respects the neonatal kidney appears to be already halfway towards acute tubular necrosis.

3. INCIDENCE OF ARF POST-CPBS

In a group of patients as heterogeneous as children under-going CPBS, it is to be expected that there would be considerable variation in the frequency of acute renal failure (ARF), but discussions amongst colleagues point to a much greater disparity between units in the incidence (or awareness?) of the problem than can be accounted for by case selection alone. There are two difficulties of definition which are responsible for some of these discrepancies: first, what constitutes ARF, and second, if ARF is manifestly an epiphenomenon of a cardiac disaster, does it "count"? In some published series ARF does not feature at all as a cause of death, and one can only presume that the problem is subsumed into the general category labelled myocardial failure.

4. DEFINITION AND PATTERNS OF ARF

Two patterns of ARF can be discerned. In the first there is oligo-anuria, defined as a urine flow rate less than 0.5ml/kg body weight/hour. It has been our experience that such a situation is dangerous in the post-CPBS state because of the sensitivity to hyperkalaemia and the rapidity with which it develops in these hypercatabolic children: we therefore advise dialysis whatever the plasma urea concentration if oliguria persists for more than 4 hours and is resistant to volume repletion, dopaminergic support and intravenous frusemide 5mg/kg body weight, particularly if the urine is of poor quality (urine/plasma urea concentration ratio less than 5) and if there is already volume overload. We have also dialysed some infants with slightly higher urine flow rates in whom there was severe intractable volume overload. The decision to embark on dialysis on these criteria can also serve as the definition of ARF, and it has been our practise to dialyse virtually all such children, even if the cardiac prognosis appears very grave.

There are few children who develop progressive uraemia
in spite of an apparently adequate urine flow: urea excretion
is insufficient to match production in the hypercatabolic
state. The prognosis of this group is better than for the
oliguric patients as the threats of volume overload and
hyperkalaemia are less severe. We have advised dialysis if
the plasma urea concentration exceeds 40mMol/l and continues
to rise: as before the executive decision can also serve to
define polyuric ARF.

5. INCIDENCE AND MORTALITY OF ARF POST-CPBS

A prospective study was undertaken of the 456 children
who underwent CPBS at the Hospital for Sick Children during
1978-9 (1). Twenty four (5.3 per cent) of these children
developed ARF as defined above. Eleven (46 per cent) died
during the same hospital admission, but three of these were
late hospital deaths in the post-dialysis period. With simple
lesions the incidence of ARF was less than 1 per cent, but it
rose to 6 per cent with cyanotic lesions, and reached 21 per
cent in a group of 33 children with individually rare complex
cardiac anomalies. Six (29 per cent) of the 21 neonates
undergoing CPBS developed ARF, 10 (7.6 per cent) of the children
aged between one month and one year and 8 (2.6 per cent) of
the 304 older children. The association of ARF with younger
age is statistically significant. However, the mortality of
the different age groups was approximately the same.

There was a clear cut association between the incidence
of ARF and the duration of CPBS and cardiac arrest: 4 (1.6 per
cent) of the 237 children with a combined CPBS and arrest time
< 90 minutes developed ARF, in contrast to 17 (8.7 per cent)
of the 194 children in whom overall bypass and arrest time
exceeded 90 minutes.

Seventeen of the children were dialysed within 36 hours
of CPBS, and 10 (59 per cent) of these died, whereas there
was only 1 (14 per cent) death amongst the 7 patients who
presented later. It is not surprising that the group which
presented early had the highest mortality, as it contains

several cases with an unsatisfactory cardiac repair. Fifteen were dialysed for less than 2 days, and of these 8 (53 per cent) died, principally from cardiac causes. It is not clear whether any of the other 7 would have survived without dialysis, but it is noteworthy that they included 3 of the 7 children with pre-dialysis hyperkalaemia, and therefore it is probable that dialysis was a major factor in helping them over a difficult period.

For reasons described above it is difficult to compare the incidence and mortality figures of ARF post-CPBS between different units, but our current mortality rate of 46 per cent is better than the previous experience and that of other published series, probably reflecting in part our policy for early intervention.

6. ASPECTS OF MANAGEMENT OF ARF

Peritoneal dialysis is the technique of choice. It is safe, effective and easy to set up in the recovery room. Vascular access is not required, and there are no haemodynamic problems as may occasionally occur with haemodialysis. There are however occasional situations when haemodialysis is preferable, for example, when there are major communications between the peritoneal and pleural or pericardial cavities, in the older child with prolonged anuria when nutrition may be difficult to sustain, and peritoneal dialysis may be ineffective if gut perfusion is poor as may happen with coarctation.

Certain problems may be encountered with peritoneal dialysis. There may initially be some bleeding into the peritoneal cavity. Over-distension of the peritoneum causes respiratory or cardiac embarrassment. In sick poorly perfused infants lactic acidosis may develop, necessitating a bicarbonate dialysate instead. Assessment and control of the volume status of the child is the most demanding aspect of management, and a solution to the problem of regular accurate weighing of these children is eagerly awaited. Peritoneal infection is always a threat, and the late Candida peritonitis is particularly to be feared as it may lead to endocarditis. Peritoneal dialysis also provides a certain source of calories from glucose, but attention to nutrition is essential and parenteral aminoacids and vitamin supplements should be started as soon as possible.

7. RENAL FUNCTION AFTER UNCOMPLICATED CPBS

The vulnerability of the kidney to poor perfusion points to another interesting aspect of the problem which has so far not been sufficiently exploited: systematic study of post-operative renal function provides a sensitive assessment of the adequacy of bypass and surgical techniques. Rigden (3) studied 21 consecutive children undergoing CPBS at the Hospital for Sick Children. The plasma creatinine concentration rose on an average of 41 per cent above preoperative levels with a peak on the 1st post-operative day. The urinary excretion of N-acetylglucosaminidase (U_{NAG}: an enzyme from the brush border of the proximal tubule whose excretion rises with tubular damage), corrected for creatinine concentration, rose 6-fold in the immediate post-operative period, fell and then rose again on the 3rd and 4th post-operative days. The two phenomena are linked: there is a significant correlation between U_{NAG} in the first post-operative sample and the maximum percentage rise in plasma creatinine subsequently. The correlation may however be somewhat fortuitous, with the highest post-operative U_{NAG} values and plasma creatinine rises being in the youngest patients; within more homogeneous groups of patients the correlation was not observed. Nevertheless, the data do point to a major role of factors during or before CPBS in determining the outcome of renal function.

8. PREVENTION OF ARF POST-CPBS

If a change in surgical or bypass technique were to halve the incidence of post-CPBS ARF from 5 per cent to 2.5 per cent, it would be necessary to study about 500 cases before the effect could be rigorously established at the 95 per cent significance level. Thus studies comparing the incidence of ARF with different bypass regimes are unlikely to be fruitful, and more subtle depressions of renal function must be detected instead, assuming that they are the body of the iceberg which bears the tip of ARF.

No doubt the most important factor in preventing ARF is the perfection of surgical and bypass techniques. But other factors are amenable to investigation. It had, for example, been the practice at the Hospital for Sick Children to use gentamicin prophylaxis in infants and older children with complex lesions in whom surface prosthetic material was used. As described previously, this group has the highest incidence of ARF, and it was natural therefore to consider whether gentamicin nephrotoxicity was playing a role in this problem. We therefore embarked on a randomised prospective comparison of gentamicin and cephalexin as antibiotic prophylaxis. The result showed that U_{NAG} excretion was significantly greater in the gentamicin treated group from the 2nd day onwards, indeed the secondary rise in U_{NAG} described above could be entirely attributed to the effects of gentamicin. However, there was no difference in the plasma creatinine concentration in the two groups over the first 5 post-operative days, according with the clinical experience that gentamicin nephrotoxicity only becomes evident after one week of treatment. Incidentally, the study also showed that gentamicin prophylaxis was not superior to cephalexin, and therefore its routine use has now been discontinued.

Experimental evidence suggests that mannitol protects renal function in many models of ARF. There is suggestive evidence also in the clinical situation, but no randomised prospective trial has been undertaken, and therefore the use of mannitol during or after CPBS has not been based upon sound observational studies. We undertook a randomised prospective study of the addition of mannitol 0.5 G/kg body weight to the pump prime in children over one year of age. The data showed that there was no difference in U_{NAG}, but that the change in plasma creatinine concentration was significantly less in the mannitol treated group from the second post-operative day, and the proportion of patients in whom the plasma creatinine concentration rose more than 50 per cent was significantly less in the mannitol treated group than in the control series. The data therefore support the routine use of mannitol during CPBS.

9. SUMMARY

The incidence of ARF post-CPBS in children is 5 per cent, and is higher in young children, in those with complex lesions, and in those with overall bypass plus arrest time in excess of 90 minutes. Early peritoneal dialysis is indicated, and with vigorous treatment the mortality is less than 50 per cent. Studies on renal function after uncomplicated CPBS show that slight deterioration is usual, and that the urinary concentration of the renal tubular enzyme N-acetylglucosaminidase (U_{NAG}) reflects renal damage sustained during CPBS. Gentamicin prophylaxis in uncomplicated CPBS results in sustained high U_{NAG}, but no change in plasma creatinine concentration. The prophylactic administration of mannitol during CPBS abolishes the usual post-operative rise in plasma creatinine concentration. Measurement of renal function following CPBS is a sensitive method of assessing the adequacy of surgical and bypass techniques.

10. ACKNOWLEDGEMENTS

We thank our colleagues in the Thoracic Unit of the Hospital for Sick Children, Great Ormond Street, London for help and encouragement. Dr. Rigden was supported by grants from the National Kidney Research Fund and the Kidney Research Aid Fund.

11. REFERENCES

1. Rigden SPA, Barratt TM, Dillon MJ, de Leval M, Stark J. 1980. Acute renal failure complicating cardiopulmonary bypass surgery in children. Submitted for publication.
2. Spitzer A. 1978. Renal physiology and functional development. In: Edelmann CM (ed.) Pediatric Kidney Disease, pp. 25-127. Boston, Little, Brown and Company.
3. Rigden SPA. 1980. Renal function after cardiopulmonary bypass surgery. In preparation.

SICKLE CELL NEPHROPATHY

J. STRAUSS, V. PARDO, R. BAKER, M. KESSLER*, G. ZILLERUELO, H. GORMAN,
M. FREUNDLICH

Depts. Pediatr. and Pathol., Univ. Miami Sch. Med. Miami, Fla. 33101
USA; *Institut für Physiologie und Kardiologie, Univ. Erlangen-Nürnberg,
Erlangen, Germany

The pathophysiology of sickle cell nephropathy is still unclear (1,2);
until recently, even the histopathology, electronmicroscopy and immunofluorescence microscopy were uncertain (3,4). Therefore, means of
prevention and effective treatment have not yet been established. This
paper reviews the data of various experimental studies, mainly ours, and
relates them to findings already reported in patients with sickle cell
disease and trait. Finally, a hypothesis will be advanced for a pathophysiological explanation of sickle cell nephropathy, and based on this,
a rational approach to prevention, identification, and treatment will be
presented.

ANIMAL EXPERIMENTATION

Microcirculation

Simultaneous recordings of available oxygen (O_2a) were obtained from
cortex (C), outer medulla (OM), inner medulla (IM) and papilla (P) of
adult rabbit's left kidney (5,6). O_2 sensitive electrodes designed by us
and made of platinum (active) and Ag-AgCl wires (reference) were inserted
at pre-determined depths from the renal surface (Fig. 1) (5). Under normal
conditions, O_2a levels were higher in the outer (C and OM) than in the
inner renal areas (IM and P). In addition, the frequency of level fluctu-
ations ("slow waves") correlated with O_2a levels and decreased gradually
from C to P (Fig. 2) (5).

During hemorrhagic shock, O_2a levels decreased by about 50% in all areas,
and there was interference with microcirculation, as suggested by a
simultaneous decrease in the rate of slow waves. These changes were
reversed to normal after reinfusion of the shed blood (Fig. 3) (6).

286

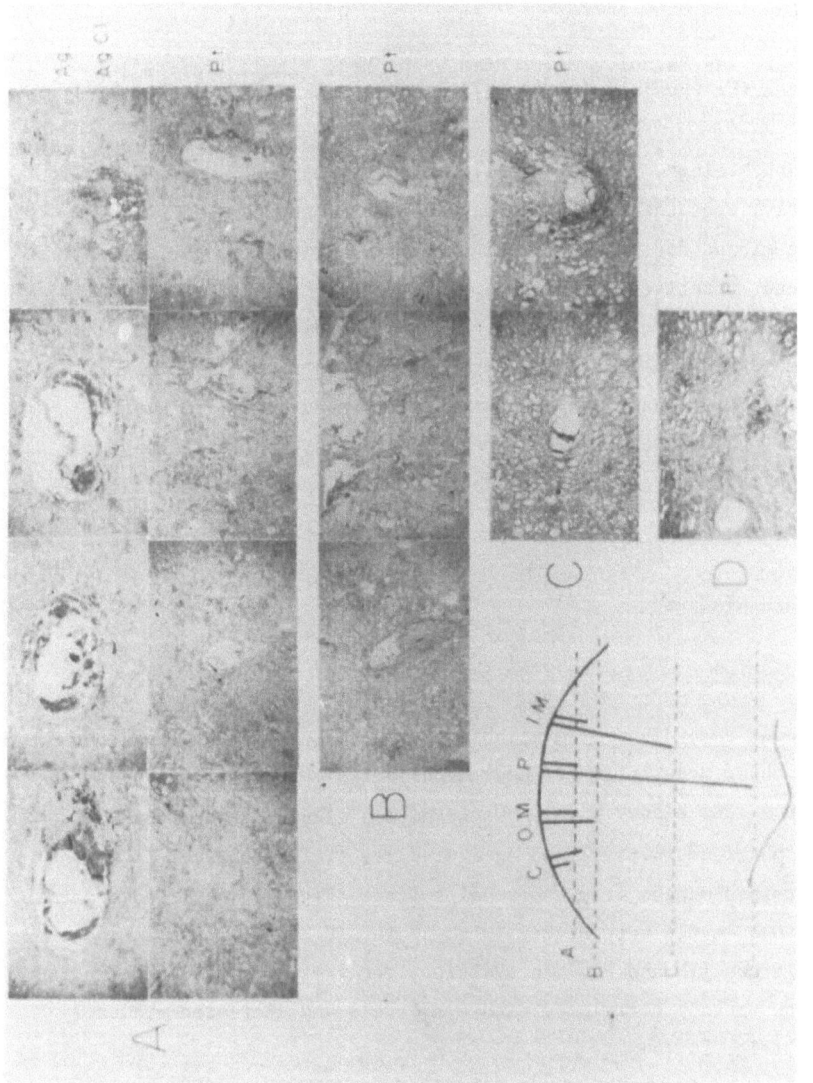

Fig. 1. Diagram of O_2 sensitive electrodes ÷ **rabbit's kidney and histological sections.** All reference (Ag-AgCl) wires were implanted in the cortex (C); active (platinum) wires were implanted in C., outer medulla (OM), inner medulla (IM) and papilla (P). Histological sections (A,B,C, and D) of renal areas revealed reaction only around reference electrodes (From Strauss, J. et al. Amer. J. Physiol. 215:1482, 1968).

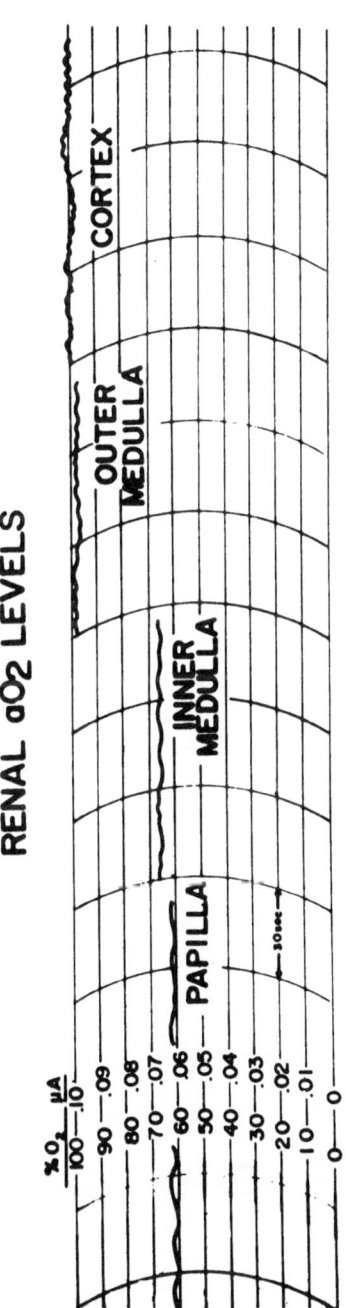

Fig. 2. Renal oxygen levels obtained from a rabbit under normal conditions. Original tracings from four areas (From Strauss, J. et al. Amer. J. Physiol. 215:1482, 1968).

288

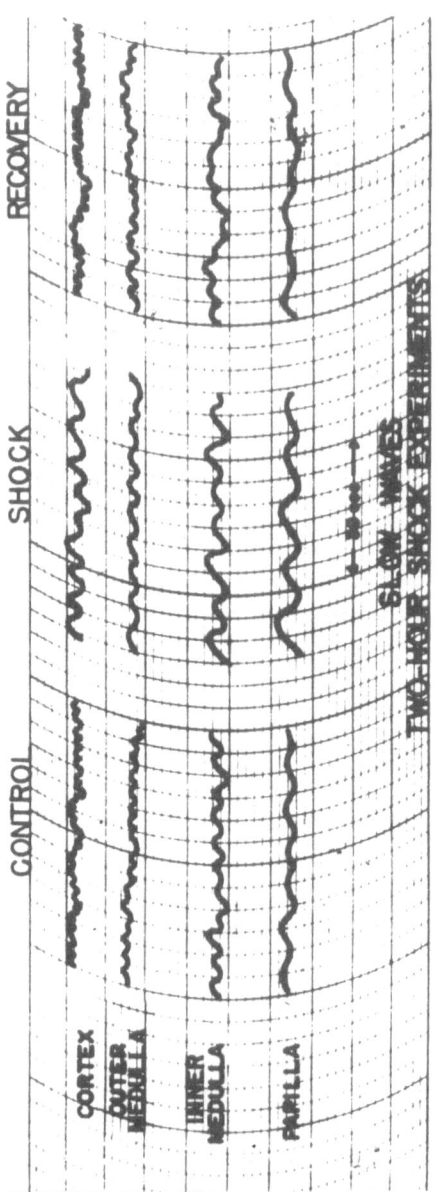

Fig. 3. Slow waves during control, hemorrhagic shock and after reinfusion of shed blood (recovery). Actual tracings from four renal areas during an experiment in an adult rabbit (From Strauss, J. et al. Amer. J. Physiol. 221:1545, 1971).

Due to the complex nature of physiological changes during hemorrhagic shock, further attempts to evaluate renal oxygenation and microcirculation were undertaken during more specific conditions such as hypoxic hypoxia and ischemia. In addition to the O_2 sensitive wire electrodes implanted in the four renal areas as described above, the surface multiwire electrode designed by Kessler and Lübbers (7) was placed over the renal cortex in order to obtain surface PO_2 histograms.

During both hypoxia and ischemia, there was a shift to the left in the histograms (more areas with lower PO_2 levels) in accordance with the accepted consequences of a disrupted microcirculation (8). The shift to the left was reversed by returning the animal to room air (hypoxic experiments) or by releasing the renal artery constriction (ischemic experiments).

Sodium excretion

Another aspect of hypoxic hypoxia was evaluated by quantitating fluid and electrolyte excretion when piglets were exposed to inspired gas with 10% O_2 content. A marked diuresis with increased sodium excretion promptly ensued, lasted for the duration of the hypoxic period, and returned to control levels once the animals were replaced in room air (9). It was postulated that natriuresis took place because there was not enough O_2 to support the sodium reabsorption process in the tubules; O_2 consumed for this function normally accounts for most of the O_2 consumed by the kidney (10).

Proximal tubule damage

Various substances have been used to selectively damage the surface (brush border) of the proximal tubule's epithelium (RTE) indicating a particular sensitivity of this portion of the nephron to various noxa. Membranous nephropathy was the most consistently demonstrated histological picture in animals with circulating immune complexes of RTE and its antibody (11).

CLINICAL STUDIES

Comparisons of the isolated physiological experiments described above will be made with the patient with sickle cell anemia (SS) or trait (SA).

Microcirculation

Sickle cell crises are characterized by the presence of severe hypoxia or ischemia of some organ of the body. In the kidney there is congestion-stasis (Fig. 4) (12) which must disrupt the microcirculation in a manner similar to that in the rabbit during hypoxia and ischemia (8).

Microcirculatory changes seem to be worsened by a high hematocrit since blood with more red cells has greater friction and difficulty in circulating than blood with fewer red cells (2, 13). Oxygenation of various organs is maintained or even increased in dogs as their blood hematocrit is gradually reduced up to 1/2 of the starting hematocrit level; from then on, surface tissue PO_2 decreases (14). Such a situation may in fact develop when sickle cell crises of patients with SSHb (usually anemic) are compared with those patients with SAHb (usually non-anemic).

The SS patient frequently has problems but usually survives crises while the SA patient may die during one of the extremely infrequent crises. The SS patient has crises more frequently and often without a readily identifiable cause while the SA patient's crisis usually has a clear cut association with an extreme situation (participation in a competitive sport in a high mountain area or flying in an unpressurized plane, e.g.).

Sodium excretion

The increased sodium excretion of piglets in a reduced O_2 environment (9) was also found in patients with SS disease in crisis (15).

Proximal tubular damage

In 1974 two patients with SS disease who were referred to us were found to have membrano-proliferative nephropathy. One of them expired and we eluted from her renal glomeruli, IgG and IgM antibodies which selectively stained proximal tubules (more markedly at the brush border) of normal kidney (Fig. 5) (16). After the glomerular eluate was absorbed with renal tubular antigen, tubular staining of normal kidney was no longer positive. The serum cryoprecipitate of this patient contained IgG and IgM, fixed to proximal tubular epithelium of normal kidney, and had anti-IgG properties (17). Subsequently, we evaluated black patients with renal failure at

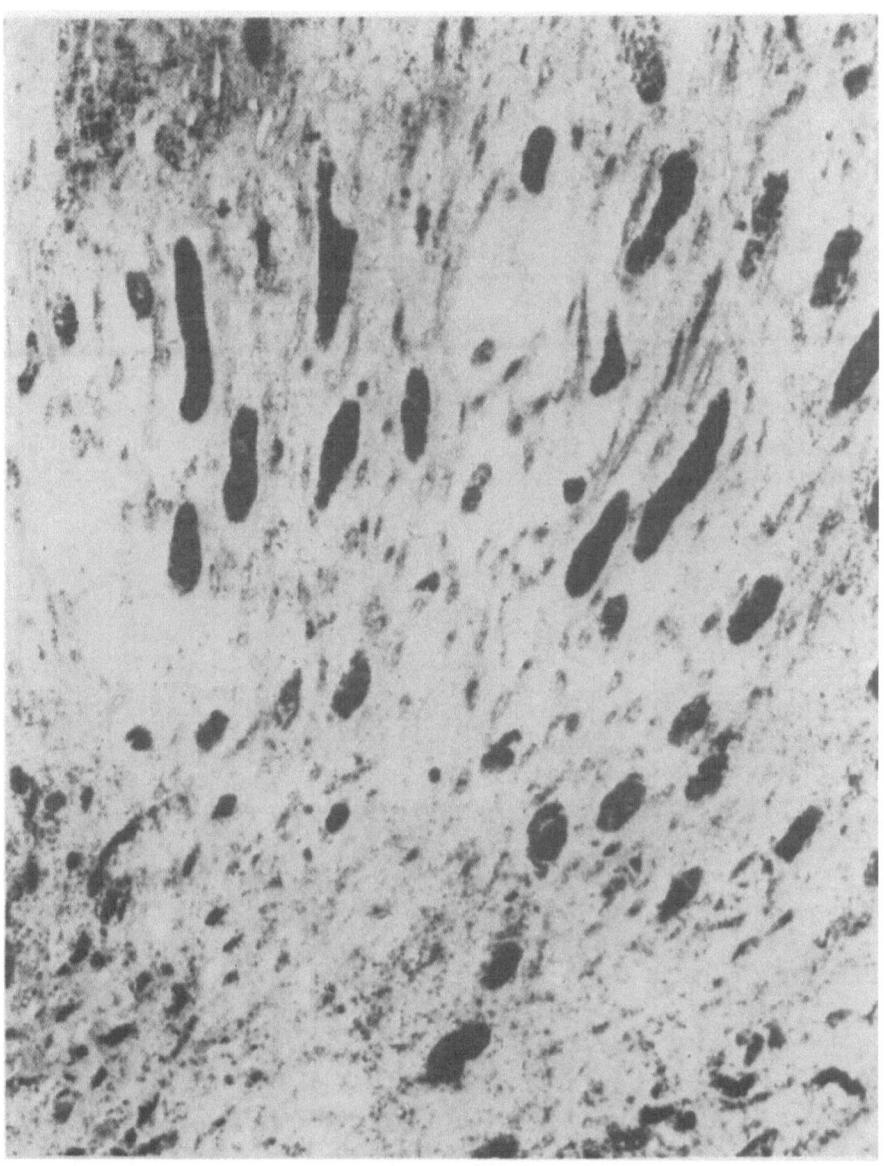

Fig. 4. Congestion of peritubular capillaries in renal medulla of a patient with sickle cell disease (From Buckalew, V.M. et al. Arch. Intern. Med. 133:660, 1974).

292

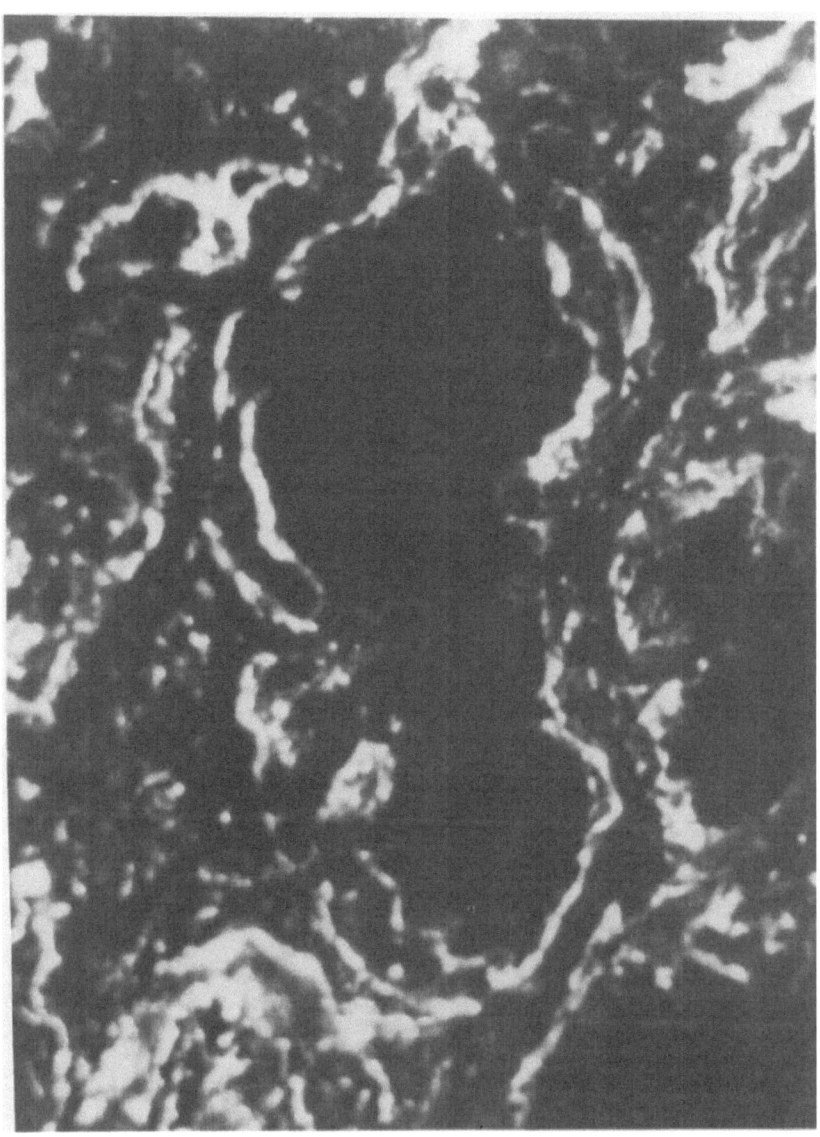

Fig. 5. Proximal tubular brush border of normal kidney stained by IgG eluted from kidney with sickle cell nephropathy, and rabbit antihuman IgG (From Strauss, J. et al. Amer. J. Med. 58:382, 1975).

Jackson Memorial Hospital in Miami. When only those with SS disease were studied, all had membrano-proliferative changes (18).

STATISTICAL DATA

Too little information is currently available on the incidence or prevalence of sickle cell (SS, SA) nephropathy. If all patients with a nephropathy were screened for a hemoglobinopathy, fewer patients would be labeled as having "idiopathic" (in the broad sense) renal disease. If all patients with a hemoglobinopathy were properly screened (arterial blood pressure, urinalysis, and blood chemistries), more patients would be identified early in the course of their nephropathy. The question as to whether or not a nephropathy present in a patient with a hemoglobinopathy may be a coincidental association rather than causally related, would be settled if statistical data were available. As it stands now, we rely on our impression that a nephropathy and hemoglobinopathy cannot occur in the same patient by chance alone.

PREVENTION

Prompt treatment of sickle cell crisis with the proper measures to restore microcirculation and oxygenation to normal as soon as possible, may be the best prophylaxis for the nephropathy found in these patients. Ideally, patients with hemoglobin SS or SA should not live under conditions limiting their tissue oxygenation, such as high altitude. They certainly should not be involved in sports or commercial flying in an unpressurized aircraft. They should not be allowed to become dehydrated and their SHb level should be maintained at a minimum ($<20\%$?).

IDENTIFICATION

A routine urine analysis (screening and microscopic) should be part of any physician encounter. Thus, time of onset of the nephropathy and other pertinent information would be available. Unfortunately, most times the renal status of these patients is not known. Referral patterns are haphazard; many general pediatric or hematology clinics are not aware of the nephropathy as a complication of SSHb or SAHb, and many nephrology services are not actively looking for the association of hemoglobinopathies with nephropathies. Every Black, Mediterranean or Latin patient seen by a nephrology service caring for pediatric and adult patients should be evaluated by sickle cell screening or by hemoglobin electrophoresis.

TREATMENT

The general approach to treatment which we recommend as rational is based on the hypothesis advanced above for a pathophysiological explanation of sickle cell nephropathy. Accordingly, all measures must attempt to restore microcirculation and oxygenation to normal as soon as possible. Prompt rehydration of a dehydrated patient should be instituted with slight overhydration as the final goal. Solutions used should be isotonic or only slightly hypertonic, and ideally contain glucose and sodium bicarbonate. The latter may be discontinued after proper documentation of a normal acid-base balance. Sodium (either as NaCl or as NaHCO$_3$, as indicated) should be administered in amounts sufficient to replace the excessive urinary losses frequently occurring during crises. Volume expanders of small molecular weight such as Dextran and efficient O$_2$ carrying solutions may be helpful (19). Preliminary results of a trial induction of hyponatremia by vasopressin and high fluid intake (20) are worthy of note, but need further evaluation since convulsions and coma were observed in one patient with hyponatremia in the absence of a cerebrovascular accident (15).

Treatment of a sickle cell occlusive crisis should include removal of sickled cells as well as administration of normal red blood cells (21). Desferoxamine must be used cautiously, only when deemed essential, and not in chronic renal failure (CRF) or end-stage renal disease (ESRD).

Treatment of the nephropathy should not include corticosteroids unless they are needed in small doses as part of a sophisticated immunological manipulation or after renal transplantation. Reduction in the edema from the accompanying nephrotic syndrome may be attained by the judicious intravenous administration of albumin and furosemide. When these patients reach CRF and ESRD levels of renal function deterioration, they should be worked up and made eligible for dialysis and transplantation. Almost all the dialysis experience reported with these patients consists of hemodialysis; no special arrangements are needed since they tolerate the usual procedure well. The use of chronic peritoneal dialysis in any of its variations may pose special infectious problems in patients so prone to overwhelming infections.

The question of kidney transplantation has not been resolved. Even more than for prophylaxis or treatment of a crisis, maintenance of a low SHb level ($\leqslant 10\%$) seems highly desirable or indispensable prior to and at all times after transplantation.

CONCLUSION

An attempt was made to review mainly pertinent work of our group which seems to point to a disruption of microcirculation and tissue oxygenation as the cause of sickle cell nephropathy. General guidelines for prophylaxis, identification and treatment were provided. A plea is made for actively seeking out these patients from the general pediatric, hematology and nephrology populations. Increased awareness that the nephropathy may be a complication, augmented research support and greater knowledge about effective treatment should result.

REFERENCES

1. Vaamonde, C.A., Oster, J.R., and Strauss, J.: The Kidney in Sickle Cell Disease. In Suki, W.N. and Eknoyan, G. (eds.): The Kidney in Systemic Diseases. New York: John Wiley & Sons, 1981, p. 86.
2. Strauss, J., Baker, R., Kessler, M., and McIntosh, R.M.: Renal Hemodynamics and Oxygenation. In: Strauss, J. (ed.): Pediatric Nephrology: Epidemiology, Evaluation, and Therapy. New York: Stratton Intercontinental Medical Book Corporation, 1976, vol. 2, p. 205.
3. Alleyne, G.A.O., Statius Van Eps, L.W., Addae, S.K., Nicholson, G.D., and Schouten, H.: The Kidney in sickle cell anemia. Kidney Int. 7:371, 1975.
4. Strauss, J., McIntosh, R.M.: Sickle Cell Nephropathy. In: Edelmann, C. M., Jr. (ed.): Pediatric Kidney Disease. Boston: Little, Brown and Company, 1978, p. 776.
5. Strauss, J., Beran, A.V., Brown, C.T., and Katurich, N.: Renal oxygenation under "normal" conditions. Am. J. Physiol. 215:1482, 1968.
6. Strauss, J., Beran, A.V., Baker, R., Boydston, L., and Reyes-Sanchez, J.L.: Effect of hemorrhagic shock on renal oxygenation. Am. J. Physiol. 221:1545, 1971.
7. Kessler, M. and Lübbers, D.W.: Aufbau und Verwendungsmöglichkeiten verschiedener PO_2 Elektroden. Pflügers Arch. 291:R 82, 1966.
8. Sinagowitz, E., Baker, R., Strauss, J., and Kessler, M.: Renal tissue oxygenation during hypoxic hypoxia. In Grote, J., Reneau, D., and Thews, G. (eds.): Oxygen Transport to Tissue - II. Advances in Experimental Medicine and Biology. New York: Plenum Press, 1976, vol. 75, p. 441.
9. Rowe, M.I., and Strauss, J.: The renal response of the newborn to hypoxia. Abstract, Pediat. Res. 7:411/183, 1973.

296

10. Kramer, K., and Deetjen, P.: Oxygen consumption and sodium reabsorption in the mammalian kidney. In Dickens, F., and Neil, E. (eds.): Oxygen in the Animal Organism. New York: Macmillan, 1964, p. 411.

11. Noble, B., and Andres, G.A.: Immunologically mediated tubular and interstitial nephritis. In Strauss, J. (ed.): Pediatric Nephrology: Current Concepts in Diagnosis and Management. New York: Plenum Press, 1981, vol. 6 (In press).

12. Buckalew, V.M., Jr., and Someren, A.: Renal manifestations of sickle cell disease. Arch. Intern. Med. 133:660, 1974.

13. Kessler, M., Bruley, D.F., Clark, L.C. et al. (eds.): Oxygen Supply: Theoretical and Practical Aspects of Oxygen Supply and Microcirculation of Tissue. Baltimore: University Park Press, 1973.

14. Messmer, K., Sunder-Plassmann, L., Jesch, F., et al: Oxygen supply to the tissues during limited normovolemic hemodilution. Res. Exp. Med. 159:152, 1972.

15. Radel, E., Kochen, J., and Finberg, L.: Hyponatremia in sickle cell disease. A renal salt-losing state. J. Pediatr. 88:800, 1976.

16. Strauss, J., Pardo, V., Koss, M.N., Griswold, W., and McIntosh, R.M.: Nephropathy associated with sickle cell anemia: An autologous immune complex nephritis. I. Studies on nature of the glomerular-bound antibody and antigen identification in a patient with sickle cell disease and immune deposit glomerulonephritis. Am. J. Med. 58:382, 1975.

17. Strauss, J., Koss, M., Griswold, W., Chernack, W., Pardo, V., and McIntosh, R.M.: Cryoprecipitable immune complexes, nephropathology, and sickle cell disease (Letter to the Editor). Ann. Intern. Med. 81:114, 1974.

18. Pardo, V., Strauss, J., Kramer, H., Ozawa, T., and McIntosh, R.M.: Nephropathy associated with sickle cell anemia. II. Clinicopathologic studies in seven patients. Am. J. Med. 59:650, 1975.

19. Strauss, J.: Clinical application of blood replacement solutions. Microvasc. Res. 8:341, 1974.

20. Rosa, R.M., Bierer, B.E., Thomas, R., Stoff, J.S., Kruskall, M., Robinson, S., Bunn, H.F., and Epstein, F.H.: A study of induced hyponatremia in the prevention and treatment of sickle-cell crisis. N. Engl. J. Med. 303:1139, 1980.

21. Elberg, A.J., Baker, R., Koch, K. et al: Transfusion requirement in patients with sickle cell disease on hemodialysis (Letter to the Editor). N. Engl. J. Med. 294:444, 1976.

CYSTINOSIS AND THE KIDNEY

John W. Foreman and Marc Yudkoff

Cystinosis is a recessively inherited metabolic disorder characterized
biochemically by a raised intracellular concentration of cystine. This
increased concentration of cystine, which appears to be stored in lysosomes,
leads to crystal deposition in the bone marrow, cornea, conjunctiva, and
internal organs, especially the kidney. In spite of this generalized
crystal deposition, the major symptomatology of cystinosis is limited to
the kidney. At birth and for the first six months of life these infants
appear normal, but with careful assessment of renal tubular function,
abnormalities, especially of amino acid handling, can be demonstrated (1).
Often the first signs of illness are polyuria and polydipsia because of
defective water handling which can also lead to dehydration and recurrent
unexplained fevers. By one year of age, growth retardation, acidosis, and
rickets are present and are paralleled by the appearance of the Fanconi
syndrome manifested by glucosuria, phosphaturia, bicarbonaturia and
generalized aminoaciduria. Cystine excretion by the kidney is increased
in proportion to the increase in the other amino acids which differs from
cystinuria where only cystine and dibasic amino acid excretion is increased.
In addition, these patients show a marked tendency to hypokalemia which can
be exacerbated with fatal consequences during glucose loading. On this
background of tubular dysfunction, there is superimposed a progressive
impairment of glomerular function. This impairment ultimately determines
the outcome since the tubular dysfunction can usually be managed with
supplemental alkali, potassium and vitamin D. As a general rule, the
glomerular dysfunction leads to uremia before the end of the first decade
of life.

The pathology of the kidney in cystinosis varies with the stage of the
disease (2). Early in the disease there is an interstitial edema and/or
round cell infiltration with granular fatty degeneration of the proximal
convoluted tubular epithelium. The "swan neck" deformity, which is atrophy

and shortening of the first portion of the proximal convoluted tubule, can
be demonstrated by microdissection. This deformity is not specific for
cystinosis since it can be seen in other forms of the Fanconi syndrome and
in congenital nephrosis. There is also a prominent epithelial cell proliferation in the glomeruli with the occasional formation of multi-nucleated
visceral epithelial cells. Further progression of the disease is characterized
by patchy glomerular and tubular necrosis, dilatation of tubules, loss of
proximal tubular brush border, further interstitial infiltration, and prominent
hypertrophy and thickening of interlobular arteries and afferent arterioles.
With advanced disease, there is a diffuse and conspicuous interstitial
fibrosis with atrophy or cystic dilatation of the tubules. The glomerular
changes vary from focal necrosis to complete hyalinization. Cystine crystals,
which can be found at any stage in the disorder, are usually evident in
interstitial cells and rarely in the glomerular mesangium and tubular cells.

The diagnosis of cystinosis can be made by demonstrating cystine crystals
in conjunctiva, bone marrow, or rectal mucosa cells. Slit lamp examination
of the cornea and conjunctiva showing the typical refractile bodies can also
be used to make the diagnosis. Laboratory confirmation of the diagnosis
can be made by finding an elevated non-protein cystine content in leukocytes
or cultured fibroblasts. Measurement of a raised intracellular cystine
content in cultured amniotic cells has permitted the prenatal diagnosis of
cystinosis (3,4).

In spite of this biochemical hallmark of raised intracellular cystine
content, the progressive renal failure remains enigmatic. In other lysosomal storage disorders, disease progression is correlated with increased
accumulation of stored material. This is not the case with cystinosis since
the cystine content in renal cells from aborted fetuses with cystinosis is
comparable to that found in kidneys removed at the time of transplantation
(3,4). Equally unexplained is the biochemical abnormality underlying the
raised cystine concentration. With the discovery that cultured fibroblasts
from patients with cystinosis express the biochemical phenotype of excessive
intracellular cystine content, a suitable in vitro model system has become
available. Although the primary biochemical abnormality remains undelineated,
several hypotheses have received experimental support. One hypothesis is
that the increased cystine content may be related to a defect in cystine
transport or the regulation of transport. Cystine uptake by cystinotic
fibroblasts is increased compared to normal fibroblasts with a third of the

transported cystine remaining unreduced (5). In contrast, only 1/5 of the transported cystine is unreduced in normal fibroblasts. Coincident with this increased uptake, there appears to be a more rapid turnover of glutathione in the cystinotic fibroblast which may play a role in the enhanced uptake and ultimately in the raised intracellular cystine concentration. A second hypothesis that has been proposed is that the source of the increased cystine is from protein degradation within lysosomes (6). Because of its molecular size, cystine cannot easily diffuse from this space and remains trapped inside the lysosome. Reducing agents which penetrate the lysosomal space have been shown to lower the cystine content of these fibroblasts. Presumably, these agents act by reducing cystine to cysteine which then can diffuse or be transported out of the lysosome into the cytosol for further degradation or use in protein synthesis.

Because the renal failure in cystinosis is not related to increasing intracellular cystine concentration, it would appear that other factors must be involved. Because of this assumption, an immunologic role in the patho-genesis of cystinosis was investigated in 5 patients with cystinosis (7).

TABLE

Patient	Age (yrs)	Creatinine Clearance (ml/min/1.73m^2)	Protein Excretion (mg/m^2/hr)	Cryoglobulin* (mg/dl)			
				IgG	IgM	IgA	C$_3$
M.	8	31	48	ND†	0.22	0.15	0.46
L.	8	21	252	0.06	0.10	ND	0.09
C.	7	59	50	ND	5.88	ND	ND
F.	5	58	12	0.11	9.46	0.32	0.55
B.	3	33	51	ND	9.79	0.86	0.77

* Significant amounts of cryoglobulin in our laboratory are:
  IgG > 0.38, IgM > 0.40, C$_3$ > 0.30, and any detectable IgA
† ND - Not detectable

As can be seen in the Table, 3 of the 5 patients had significant amounts of cryoprecipitable complement and immunoglobulins, especially IgM. Serum values of the third component of complement and immunoglobulins were normal except for a slightly low IgG in one patient. The raised intracellular cystine concentration may in some manner give rise to the formation of these circulating cryoglobulins. This in turn could lead to the progressive decline in glomerular function, similar to the course of events described for the progressive renal failure of sickle cell anemia (8) which is associated with circulating cryoglobulins containing antibody to and antigen of renal tubular epithelium. We have not characterized the antigen(s) in these cryoglobulins, but their presence raises the possibility that an immunologic mechanism(s) may play a role in the renal dysfunction of cystinosis. Cryoglobulinemia may, however, be only one of several mechanisms leading to the progressive renal failure that characterizes cystinosis since only 3 of the 5 patients studied had cryoglobulinemia. One of the 2 patients without cryoglobulinemia had the most severely compromised glomerular function of the group. The possibility arises that if cryoglobulins had been measured earlier in the disease, they would have been present since the disappearance of previously detectable cryoglobulinemia with the onset of end-stage renal failure has been noted (9).

Treatment of cystinosis has been limited to correcting the chemical abnormalities related to the tubular and glomerular dysfunction without halting the progression of renal failure. Agents which can reduce disulfide bonds, such as dithiothreitol and ascorbic acid, are effective in lowering intracellular cystine in cultured cystinotic fibroblasts. These reducing agents have been used to treat cystinosis, but without success because of toxicity and possibly the inability to lower adequately the intracellular cystine content in vivo. Recently, Thoene et al demonstrated that the aminothiol, cysteamine, was quite effective in lowering the intracellular cystine in both cultured fibroblasts and circulating leukocytes from a patient with cystinosis (10). However, cysteamine did not appear to have a beneficial effect on the renal function of this patient.

We have studied the effect of cysteamine on the renal function and growth in 5 patients with cystinosis (11). The children ranged in age from 2 to 7 years at the initiation of the study with creatinine clearances that ranged from 21 to 58 ml/min/1.73M^2. They were treated with 90 mg/kg/day of cysteamine for 20 months. Leukocyte cystine content fell from 7.9 nmoles 1/2 cystine/mg protein to 0.7 nmoles 1/2 cystine/mg protein with therapy. Because all of the children had a progressive decrease in creatinine clearance over the 20 to 40 months prior to the start of the study, a plot of 1/serum creatinine versus age was used to provide an index of the rate of compromise of glomerular function. In each patient this plot gave a straight line of negative slope indicating a constant rate of decline in glomerular function. In two of the patients this plot was no longer linear after treatment with cysteamine. The values for 1/serum creatinine were higher than would be predicted from the pretreatment line suggesting a stabilization of the progressive decline in glomerular function. The other patients showed

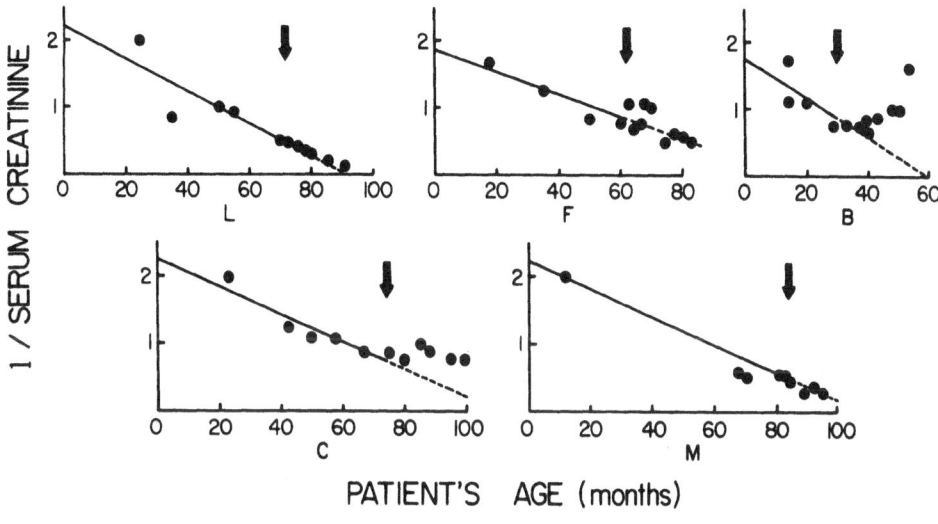

CYSTEAMINE THERAPY
STARTED

FIGURE.   Relation between Reciprocal of Serum Creatinine and Age in Each of
          the Five Patients. Reprinted by permission of the New England Journal
          of Medicine, 304:143, 1981.

no deviation from the pretreatment line indicating that cysteamine had neither
a beneficial nor a detrimental effect on their glomerular function. Of the
two patients who responded, one was the youngest patient on entry into the
study, and the other had the highest creatinine clearance on entry. All of the
patients had renal glucosuria and marked phosphaturia on entry into the study
that was not significantly altered with cysteamine treatment. The growth retar
dation that was evident prior to the start of the study was also not chnaged
with cysteamine treatment.

     In conclusion, cysteamine appears to be the best hope thus far for a speci-
fic therapy for cystinosis, although only 2 of 5 patients had a positive response and then only in respect to glomerular function. Cystinosis is an
enigmatic disease in which work remains to be done to elucidate the biochemical
basis of this inherited disorder and to formulate rational, effective therapy.

REFERENCES

1. Schneider, J.A., Wong, V. and Seegmiller, J.E. The early diagnosis of
    cystinosis. J.Pediat. 74, 114, 1969.
2. Spear, G.S. The pathology of the kidney. In Schulman, J.D., editor:
    Cystinosis, DHEW Publication no. (NIH) 72-249, 1973.
3. Schneider, J.A., Verroust, F.M., Kroll, W.A. et al. Prenatal diagnosis
    of cystinosis. N. Engl. J. Med. 290, 878, 1974.

4. States, B., Blazer, B., Harris, D., et al. Prenatal diagnosis of cystinosis. J. Pediat. 87, 558, 1975

5. States, B., Harris, D. and Segal, S. Uptake and utilization of exogenous cystine by cystinotic and normal fibroblasts. J. Clin. Invest. 513, 1003, 1974

6. Thoene, J.G., Oshima, R.G., Ritchie, D.G., et al. Cystinotic fibroblasts accumulate cystine from intracellular protein degradation. Proc. Natl. Acad. Sci. U.S.A., 74, 4505, 1977

7. Foreman, J.W., Yudkoff, M. and Segal, S. Circulating cryoglobulins in nephropathic cystinosis. J. Pediat., in press

8. Pardo, V., Strauss, J., Kramer, H., et al. Nephropathy associated with sickle cell anemia: An autologous immune complex nephritis. Amer. J. Med. 59, 650, 1975

9. McIntosh, R.M., Griswold, W.R., Chernack, W.B., et al. Cryoglobulin III: Further studies on the nature, incidence, diagnostic, prognostic and immunopathologic significance of cryoproteins in renal disease. Q. J. Med. 44, 285, 1975

10. Thoene, J.G., Oshima, R.G., Crawhall, J.C., et al. Cystinosis: Intracellular cystine depletion by aminothiols in vitro and in vivo. J. Clin. Invest. 58, 180, 1976

11. Yudkoff, M., Foreman, J.W. and Segal, S. Effects of cysteamine therapy in nephropathic cystinosis. N. Engl. J. Med. 304, 141, 1981

PERITONEAL NUTRITION IN CHILDREN - PRELIMINARY RESULTS IN RENAL FAILURE

C.Giordano,N.G.De Santo,G.Capodicasa,Chair of Nephrology,1st Medical
Faculty,University of Naples,Naples,Italy

INTRODUCTION

Recent data from this laboratory have demonstrated the feasibility
of total nutrition through the peritoneal route(1).Furthermore our
data indicate that the peritoneal route of feeding nutrients is adequate
for therapeutic purposes.

The present paper reports our preliminary results in children and
also indicates that for this age group of patients peritoneal nutrition
is feasible and adequate even under condition of stress.

PATIENTS AND METHODS

Patients

Patient no.1 was a female,aged 13 and weighing 30 kg.She was on hemodialysis since January 1976.She was anuric and dialyzed thrice a week.
On June 16,1980 she was dialyzed and on returning home she underwent a
severe car-accident.Both legs and left humerus were broken.There was
hemorrhagic pleural effusion.Shock supervened and the a-v fistula was
closed.She was treated in the emergency unit of a city hospital.Two days
later she was sent back to our unit.On admission plasma urea was 4 g/l.
It was decided to treat her with peritoneal nutrition.The subsequent
course will be described later on.

Patient no.2 was a male,15 year old middle class student,weighing
45 kg.He had developed renal cortical necrosis after an episode of gastro-
enteritis with dehydration.Two days later,July 10,1980 the patient was
anuric.BP was 80/50,pulse 110/min,plasma urea 5 g/l,plasma creatinine
12 mg/dl.Also for this patient peritoneal nutrition was chosen for
treatment.

Technique of peritoneal nutrition

The patients were implanted with TWH,acute type permanent catheters with 1 felt-cuff.The catheters,kindly provided by Mr.G.Zellerman,Bio-Engineer,Accurate Surgical Instruments,Toronto,Canada,were positioned with a trocar.

The dialysate composition was the following:Sodium 132 mEq/L,Potassium 4 mEq/L,Chloride 101.5 mEq/L,Acetate 35 mEq/L,Magnesium 1.5 mEq/L,Calcium 3.5 mEq/L.The dextrose concentration was 42.5 g/L.Both patients underwent 8-3-hours exchanges.Patient no.1 exchanged daily 8 liters(1 L/exchange) while patient no.2 exchanged 12 liters(1.5 L/exchange).

Amino acids were added to the dialysate.Amino acid preparations were in 250 ml bottles.Their composition was the following:L-Isoleucine 1.40 g L-Leucine 2.20 g,L-Lysine(acetate) 2.25 g,L-Methionine 2.20 g, L-Phenyl-alanine 2.20 g,L-Threonine 1.00 g,L-Tryptophan 0.50 g, L-Valine 1.60 g, L-Histidine 0.62 g, L-Cysteine 0.08 g.In total each unit cotained 14.05 g of amino acids.For patient no.1 only one unit of amino acid was used(30 ml for each L of dialyzate) while for patient no.2 40 ml/L dialyzate were used(2 units).

Lipids cannot be given intraperitoneally(1) so that patient no.1 received 83 ml of a 10% preparation(Lipiphysan,Egic,Amilly,France) every 6 hours intravenously by drip infusion while patient no.2 received 125 ml of the same preparation every 6 hours.

Protein-energy input is outlined in Table I and is of 1,765 cal for patient no.1(28% as lipids- 59 cal/kg) and of 2,203 cal for patient no.2(34% from lipidis - 49 cal/kg).

Table I: Nitrogen and energy input during peritoneal nutrition

	Patient no.1	Patient no.2
Amino acids	1 unit:50 cal	2 units:100 cal
Lipids	50 g:495 cal	75 g: 743 cal
Dextrose from dialyzate	300 g: 1,020 cal	400 g:1,360 cal
Total calories	1,765(59/kg)	2,203(49/kg)

Control of peritoneal nutrition

We have measured urea generation rates after Walser and Bodenlos(2). This method is accurate and gives also information on urea synthesis and urea breakdown.In addition we have also measured the levels of 3-methyl-histidine in plasma which is an indicator of muscle breakdown (3).Glucose utilization from dialyzate was measured as usually in our laboratory(4).

RESULTS

Figure 1 depicts the time course of plasma urea and 3-methyl-histidine levels.Both were elevated after the crush-injury.During treatment both were controlled.Corresponding data for urea pool,urea removal via dialyzate are to be found in Table II.

Figure 2 reports all pertinent data of the 15 year old boy with ARF. Plasma urea which was very high 48 hours after the onset of anuria was under control 7 days after starting treatment.On this day for the first time the patient passed 400 ml of urine.Table III gives all data on urea pool and urea removal via dialyzate,and gives an insight on the catabolism of this patient.

DISCUSSION

Our interest in peritoneal nutrition was prompted by the dramatic need of easing the difficult task of total parenteral nutrition.At the present status of knowledge this technique requires a team approach of specialized people and a set up of facilities either not available everywhere or insufficient to cover the need of all patients requiring treatment.

A significant contribution to the present approach derived from our experience with Continous Ambulatory Peritoneal Dialysis(CAPD).These patients usually receive a daily load of dextrose via dialyzate which averages 200 g and may be increased up to 400-700 g/day by working with dialyzate containing only 42.5 g/L of dextrose and by exchanging 2 L

306

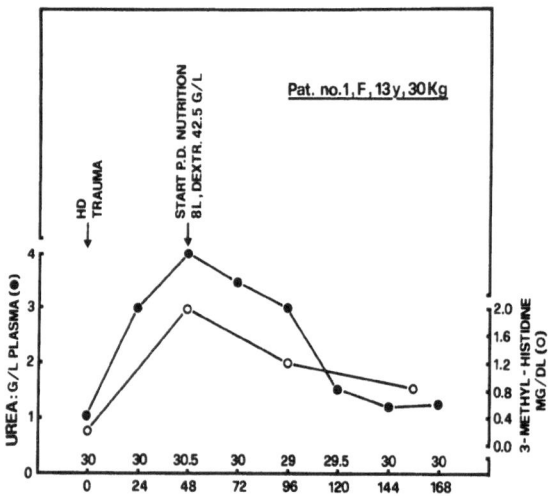

Figure 1: time course of urea and 3-methyl-histidine in
          patient no.1

Table II: data on urea pool, urea removal via dialyzate, urea from the
          diet in patient no.1

Time	Urea Pool	Urea Removal	Urea in the diet
hrs	g	g/day	g/day
0			
24			
48	84		4.85
72	73.5	33.7	4.85
96	63	29.3	4.85
120	45	22.5	4.85
144	26.3	11.7	4.85
168	26.2	12.0	4.85

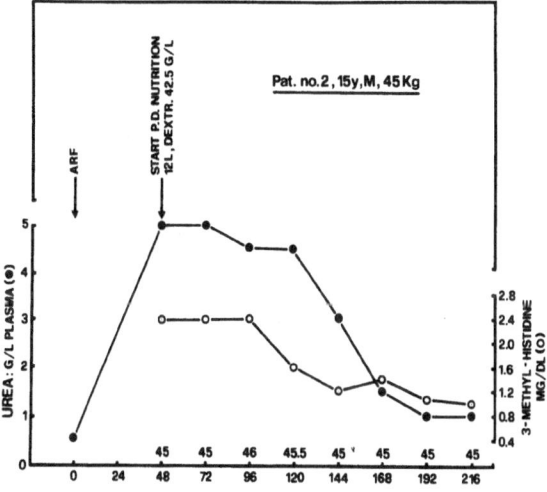

Figure 2: time course of urea and 3-methyl-histidine in

patient no.2

Table III:Data on urea pool,urea removal via dialyzate,urea from the

diet in patient no.2

Time	Urea Pool	Urea removal	Urea in the diet
hrs	g	g/day	g/day
O	15.3		
24			
48	153		9.7
72	153	55	9.7
96	138	50	9.7
120	138	51	9.7
144	92	44.7	9.7
168	45.9	24	9.7
192	30.6	12	9.7
216	30.6	10	9.7

every 3 hours.

Furthermore we have been longly aware of the fact that amino acids may be added to the dialysate of patients on intermittent peritoneal dialysis with significant improvement of the nutritional status(5).

The preliminary data here and those reported elsewhere(1) indicate that peritoneal nutrition is possible and adequate for therapeutical purposes for every age.Furthermore it is available at every bed-side, it works without the support of machines,without the intervention of an ad hoc team of specialists.

In our previous experience we have shown that lipids given intravenously are better utilized than by the intraperitoneal route.There is a need to study lipid transport through the peritoneal membrane,but this will not prevent widespread use of this approach.

This experience has to be regarded as preliminary but the methodology used in controlling the efficacy as well as the catabolis status of our patients at start of peritoneal nutrition are indicative of adequacy. Both urea generation rates and 3-methyl-Histidine levels were under control indicating that energy-nutrients feeding was utilized for plastic purposes and that muscle breakdown was also under control.

ACKNOWLEDGEMENTS

Supported in part by NIH,Bethesda,USA,Contract no.1-AM-9-0066,National Institute of Arthritis,Metabolism and Digestive diseases and by Consiglio Nazionale delle Ricerche,Rome,Italy

REFERENCES

1.Giordano C,Capdocasa G,De Santo NG.Feasibility and adequacy of nutrition through the peritoneal route.Int J Artif Organs 1980,in press
2.Walser M and Bodenlos LJ.Urea metabolism in man.J Clin Invest 38:1617, 1959
3.Young VR,Alexis SD,Baliga BS,Munro HN.Metabolism of administered 3-methyl-histidine. J Biol Chem 247:3592,1972

4.De Santo NG,Capodicasa G,Senatore R,Cicchetti T,Cirillo D,Damiano M,
   Torella R,Giugliano D,Improta C and Giordano C.Glucose utilization
   from dialyzate in patients under Continous Ambulatory Peritoneal
   Dialysis(CAPD).Int J Artif Organs 2:119,1979
5.Kobayashi K,Maniji T,Hiramatsu S,Maeda K,Uemura J.Nitrogen metabolism
   in patients on peritoneal dialysis.In Today's art of peritoneal
   dialysis.Trevino-Becerra A and Boen FST,Editors.Karger,Basel 1979,p.93

AMINO ACID AND PROTEIN METABOLISM IN CHRONIC RENAL FAILURE

C. CHANTLER, R.W.A. JONES, N. DALTON

Evelina Department of Paediatrics,
Guy's Hospital,
London SE1 9RT

SUMMARY

Protein malnutrition is common in uraemia. Protein synthesis is probably reduced but protein breakdown is not increased at least under basal conditions. The reduction in protein synthesis may be due to a direct effect of an unidentified uraemic toxin(s) but, in addition, the adaptation to altered energy metabolism may reduce protein synthesis by increasing branch chain amino acid oxidation with a consequent reduction in the extracellular and intracellular pools of branch chain amino and keto acids. Lowering nitrogen toxicity by reducing nitrogen intake and supplementing with essential amino acids or keto acids may improve growth in some children.

INTRODUCTION

Clearly a positive balance between protein synthesis and protein breakdown is essential for growth and therefore an understanding of protein metabolism in uraemia is fundamental to the problem of poor growth in children with chronic renal failure (CRF).

PROTEIN MALNUTRITION IN URAEMIA

The major signs of protein malnutrition in uraemia are summarised in Table 1 and the evidence has recently been reviewed by Kopple (27).

Table 1.   EVIDENCE FOR PROTEIN MALNUTRITION IN URAEMIA

Anthropometric		Muscle
Body Height and Weight	- reduced	Mass, synthesis and
Skeletal Development	- retarded	turnover - reduced
Sexual Development	- retarded	Cellular concentration
Cell Mass	- reduced	of alkali soluable
		protein and valine - reduced

Plasma

Serum proteins, albumin synthesis
Transferrin, Clq, C_3, cholinesterase
Branch chain amino and keto acids
Tryptophan, tyrosine   - reduced

Twenty-seven of 46 children starting haemodialysis for chronic renal failure
at Guy's Hospital between 1975 and 1979 were below the 3rd centile for height
(22); the growth of children whose renal failure dated from early infancy
was significantly reduced compared to children with later onset of CRF.
Cell mass estimated from the intracellular volume measured as the difference
between the volume of distribution of tritiated water (total body water)
and sodium bromide (extra cellular fluid) was significantly reduced in
uraemic prepubertal children (7) and this reduction was especially pronounced
in infants less than 3 years old with CRF (23). Plasma transferrin concentration as an index of the adequacy of protein nutrition was reduced in
a proportion of children on regular haemodialysis and correlated with body
weight expressed as a ratio of height (7). We have found a similar relationship in infants with chronic renal failure (23) and a significant association
between plasma transferrin and the degree of growth retardation in these
infants. This suggested that the growth retardation was the result of
protein malnutrition. Dietary intakes for both energy and protein were
more reduced in infants than in older children with CRF when compared to
the intakes of normal children of the same height (23). Uraemia appears
to affect protein metabolism and growth more severely in the younger child
perhaps because of the rapidity of normal growth and the high food intakes
in this age group (6,7).

Low extra and intracellular pools of threonine, valine, tyrosine and
histidine are characteristic of CRF (14). Plasma valine, leucine and
isoleucine concentrations are frequently low in uraemic children (9) and
we have found a weak but significant correlation between plasma valine and
leucine concentrations and growth in children on regular haemodialysis(7).
There are notable similarities between uraemia and protein energy malnutrition (5) both in terms of growth and development (delayed bone and sexual
maturation) and biochemistry but differences are also apparent. Kopple (6)
found a decreased ratio of plasma valine to glycine concentration in uraemia
which was also found in normal individuals fed a low protein diet but for
any given level of protein intake the ratio was reduced more in uraemic
individuals. Furst et al (13) found that plasma and muscle valine concentrations were low in adults with CRF and failed to normalise on a low protein
diet adequate in energy and supplemented with essential amino acids (EAA),
given in proportions recommended by Rose as suitable for normal individuals
(34), even though nitrogen balance was positive and the tissue concentrations

of other EEA's increased. They later showed that a supplement of EAA's
designed for use in CRF with an increase in the proportions of valine and
threonine was more successful in sustaining positive nitrogen balance and
normalising tissue valine levels (14).

Muscle protein synthesis in uraemic rats measured by C14 leucine incorporation was low in fasted animals compared to controls (19) and although
carbohydrate gavage improved protein synthesis it did not restore it to
normal.

Muscle breakdown estimated by the excretion of 3 methyl histidine
did not appear to be increased in rats rendered uraemic by 5/6 nephrectomy
(31). Recently Conley et al (8) have demonstrated reduced protein turnover
in children with CRF. Protein flux in children on regular haemodialysis
was higher than in non dialysed children for a given level of protein energy
intake. Whilst some of the reduction in protein flux was probably due to
the reduced food intake, a direct effect of uraemia cannot be excluded and
a significant negative correlation of 0.78 is found if the data on protein
turnover is plotted against blood urea for the 6 children studied who had
protein intakes more than 100% of recommended daily allowances (RDA) and
energy intakes at least 60% of RDA. It seems likely that CRF is associated
with a reduction in protein synthesis rather than an increase in protein
breakdown though direct measurements of synthesis and breakdown in uraemic
children are not yet available. Changes in protein metabolism in uraemia,
after surgery, with malnutrition and with sepsis are compared in Table 11;
the similarities between protein energy malnutrition and uraemia are apparent
and it is likely that infection by increasing breakdown when synthesis is
already reduced will have a major impact on the uraemic child. It is possible
that a major effort to reduce breakdown during intercurrent infection in
the child with CRF by high energy feeding with insulin if necessary might
significantly improve the rehabilitation and even the growth of children
with CRF. Studies to support this speculation are however not yet available.

Table 11.   Protein metabolism in various conditions

	Protein Turnover	Protein Synthesis	Protein Degradation
Uraemia (see text)	↓	↓ ?	↓ or → ?
P.E.M. (18)	↓	↓	↓
Surgery (41)	→	↓	→
Sepsis (16)	↑	↑	↑↑

The reduction in protein synthesis in uraemia may be the consequence of protein energy malnutrition but a direct effect of uraemic toxins on protein synthesis cannot be excluded. Uraemic toxicity and protein synthesis was studied by Delaporte et al (12). They demonstrated inhibition of in vitro protein synthesis by a small molecular, heat labile constituent of uraemic plasma. Haemodialysis was associated with a reduction in the inhibitory effect.

ENERGY, AMINO ACID AND KETO ACID METABOLISM IN URAEMIA

There is no doubt that energy intake affects protein metabolism (30), that energy intake is often low in uraemia and that this is a major determinant of poor growth (7). Moreover glucose intolerance is prominent in uraemic children and is associated with resistance to the hypoglycaemic action of insulin (4) and to its action in stimulating amino acid transport in vitro (2). The hyperglycaemia of uraemia appears to be due mainly to a reduction in tissue utilisation of glucose (10), but there is evidence for increased glucose production from gluconeogenesis from alanine (15,35). Metcoff (29) has demonstrated abnormalities in glycolysis in leukocytes from uraemic patients with improvements in the activity of pyruvate kinase, phospho-fructokinase, and glucose 6 phosphate dehydrogenase and protein synthesis after dialysis. He has emphasised the link between abnormal glycolysis, glucose intolerance and protein synthesis. Brain cortex from rats and erythro-cytes from normal individuals in uraemic sera metabolised less glucose and lactate production was reduced with increased glucose metabolism via the hexose monophosphate shunt (33). This suggests that the hyperglycaemia in uraemia may be due to a failure to metabolise glucose normally rather than to the failure to transport glucose into the cell. Pyruvate turnover was decreased in kidney cortex incubated in uraemic sera with decreased pyruvate dehydrogenase complex activity (33).

Failure of normal glucose metabolism suggests inefficiency in energy metabolism and decreased growth and muscle nitrogen in uraemic rats compared to control pair fed rats has been found by Mehls et al (28). The derangement of energy metabolism in uraemia was emphasised by the tendency of children with CRF to become obese with high carbohydrate diets in spite of having low cell masses (7) presumably as a result of the hyperglycaemia and hyperinsulinaemia.

If glucose metabolism for energy is reduced then presumably other sources of energy may be utilised. The mobilisation of fat may be limited

in uraemia by the antilipolytic action of insulin and the plasma concentration
of free fatty acid and glycerol tended to be low in children on regular
haemodialysis (4). A considerable amount of energy metabolism in muscle
is derived from the oxidation of branch chain aminoacids after transamination
to their respective keto acids (fig 1). Branch chain α ketoacid oxidation
may be regulated by phosphorylation: dephosphorylation of the branch chain
ketoacid dehydrogenase complex (17, 32) in a reciprocal manner to the
regulation of the pyruvate dehydrogenase complex. The oxidation of leucine
provides acetyl COA and serves to preserve glucose and pyruvate by the
indirect transamination of pyruvate to alanine and the transfer of alanine
to the liver for gluconeogenesis (fig 1) (37). Valine oxidation provides
citric acid cycle intermediates and as well as stimulating the formation
of alanine from pyruvate aids gluconeogenesis by the formation of phosphoenol
pyruvate (fig 1). Clearly the formation of alanine in muscle for gluconeogenesis is dependant on the availability of pyruvate as well as the transamination of branch chain amino acids. Whether, and under what conditions,
alanine production in uraemia is increased is controversial (11), but there
is some evidence for increased oxidation of branch chain keto acids (BCKAA).
Reduced plasma concentrations of BCDAA have been found in uraemia with a
negative correlation between plasma creatinine and urea and plasma α ketoisocaproic acid (KICA: keto leucine) (36). We have found reduced plasma
concentrations of KICA, α keto β methyl-n-valeric acid (MEVA ketoisoleucine)
and α ketoisovaleric acid (KIVA: ketovaline) in adolescents on regular
haemolialysis. Fig 2,3,4,). The ratio of isoleucine to MEVA and leucine
to KICA was significantly higher in the uraemic patients compared to controls
indicating an altered equilibrium between the amino and ketoacid. This
change could be determined by an increase in ketoacid oxidation, a decrease
in availability of pyruvate or a reduction in protein breakdown. Jones
and Kopple (20) found decreased metabolism of valine in uraemia with no
evidence of increased oxidation in the post absorptive state but increased
oxidation of valine was found after intravenous infusion (21). It is
tempting to speculate that uraemic individuals are well adapted to the
consequence of diminished protein synthesis, with a reduction in protein
breakdown and a limitation on branch chain amino acid oxidation partly
controlled by the low pool of branch chain amino acids or a reduction in
pyruvate availability, unlike uncontrolled diabetes where both branch chain
amino and ketoacid concentrations in plasma rise considerably. Under

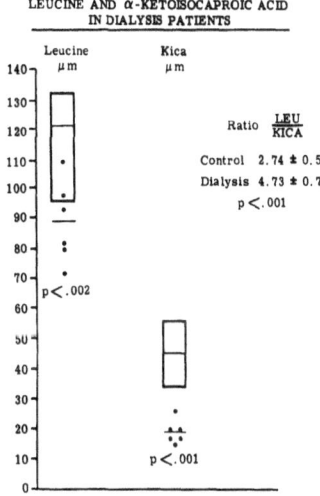

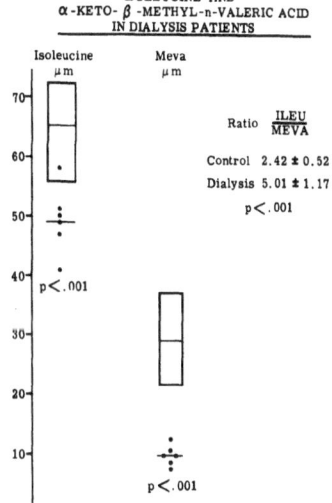

FIGURE 2. Plasma leucine and α ketoisocaproic acid (KICA) concentrations in adolescents on regular haemodialysis compared to normal range in young adults after 12 hour fast.

FIGURE 3. Plasma isoleucine and α Keto β methyl-n-valeric acid (MEVA) concentrations in adolescents on regular haemodialysis compared to normal range in young adults after 12 hour fast.

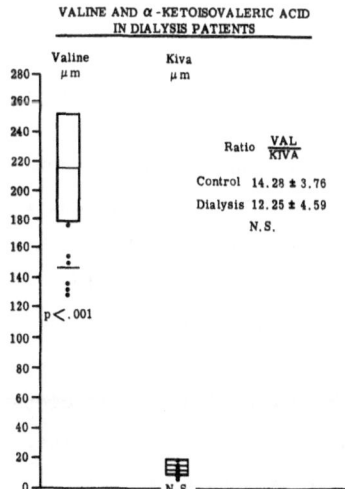

FIGURE 4. Plasma valine and α ketoisovaleric acid (KIVA) concentrations in adolescents on regular haemodialysis compared to normal range in young adults after 12 hour fast.

stresses such as a prolonged fast, infection or exercise it might be that this adaptation would be insufficient and lead to increased oxidation of keto acids, increased gluconeogenesis, increased protein breakdown, and perhaps further reduction in protein synthesis due to depletion of branch chain amino acids especially leucine which is a powerful stimulator of protein synthesis (1).

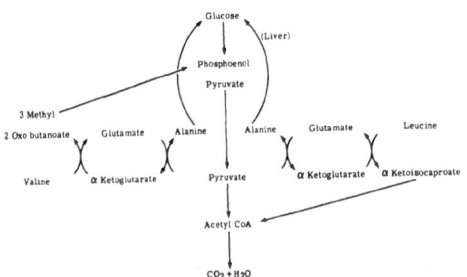

FIGURE 1.
Oxidation of Leucine and Valine

LOW PROTEIN HIGH ENERGY DIETS, ESSENTIAL AMINO ACIDS (EAA) AND KETO ACID (KAA) SUPPLEMENTS

There is more evidence for the effect of high energy diets rather than low protein diets in improving growth in uraemia (7). Nitrogen balance improved in 5 children on a low protein diet supplemented with EAA (25) but height velocity did not change significantly. Unfortunately most of the children were not able to reduce their protein intakes to the desired extent out of hospital so that the desired reduction in nitrogen toxicity was not maintained throughout the study period. It is easier to manipulate the diet of infants and a more normal growth velocity was achieved in 3 infants with a GFR less than 10 ml/min/1.73m^2 fed a low protein EAA supplemented diet (Fig 5). Height velocity fell in 2 and weight velocity fell in each of the 3 infants when the EAA supplement was discontinued. We have recently investigated the use of low protein diets supplemented with KAA (38, 39, 40, 3) in children with CRF (24). Walser (40) has suggested that KAA may stimulate protein synthesis as well as permit a reduction in nitrogen intake by their substitution for the appropriate EAA in the diet. In children this may provide a special advantage over EAA supplements by allowing a higher intake of non essential

nitrogen and therefore a more liberal and palatable diet.   We have been
able to demonstrate an improvement in nitrogen balance in children on KAA
and an improvement in growth (24).

FIGURE 5.   Growth Velocity in 3
infants less than 3 years of age
with GFR or less than 10ml/mm/1.73m²
treated with low protein diets
supplemented with essential amino
acids compared to growth velocity
in similar infants on a free diet.

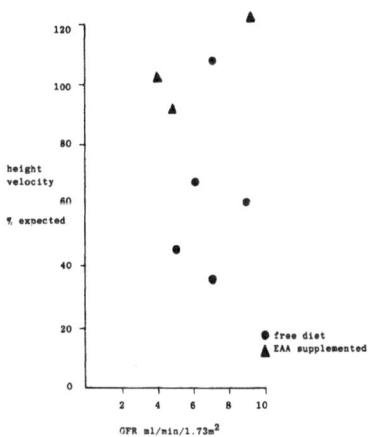

DIETARY POLICY

Clearly an adequate energy intake is of major importance in aiding
growth in uraemic children. Nonetheless reduction in nitrogen toxicity
by reducing protein intake down to minimal levels (6) when growth is poor
and as renal failure worsens, will in some cases improve growth and survival
If growth is still poor the child should be admitted to hospital, placed
on a high energy diet with little or no protein, administered if necessary
by nasogastric tube especially in infants and after a satisfactory reduct
ion in blood urea and urea appearance rate has been achieved supplementation
with EAA or KAA can be attempted. It must be emphasised that with current
knowledge dramatic success is rare and much research is still required.

REFERENCES

1. Adibi S.A. (1980 Roles of branched chain amino acids in metabolic
    regulation. J. Lab. Clin. Med. 95 475 - 484
2. Arnold, W.C., Holliday, M.A. (1979) Tissue resistance to insulin stim-
    ulation of amino acid uptake in acutely uraemic rats. Kidney Int.
    16 124 - 129
3. Bergstrom J., Ahlberg, M., Alvestand, A., Furst, P. (1978) Metabolic
    studies with ketoacids in uraemia. Amer. J. Clin Nutr. 31, 1761-1766
4. Bishti, M., Counahan, R., Bloom S.R., Chantler, C. (1978) Hormonal and
    metabolic responses to intravenous glucose in children on regular
    haemodialysis. Amer. J. Clin. Nutr. 31, 1865-1869
5. Chantler, C. and Holliday, M.A. (1973) Growth in children with renal
    disease with particular reference to the effects of caloric malnutrition.

6.   Chantler, C. 1979 1979 Renal failure in childhood in Renal Disease
        edited by Black D. and Jones N.F., 4th edition. Blackwells Scientific
        Publications, London. Paged 825-868

7.   Chantler, C., Bishti M.M., Counahan, R. (1980) Nurtritional therapy in
        children with cnronic renal failure. Amer. J. Clin Nutr. 33 1682-1689

8.   Conley S.B., Rose G.M., Robson A.M., Bier D.M. (1980) Effects of diet-
        ary intake and haemodialysis on protein turnover in uraemic children.
        Kid. Int. 17 837 - 846

9.   Counahan R., Bishti M., Cox B.D., Ogg C.S., Chantler C. (1976) Plasma
        aminoacids in children on haemodialysis. Kidney Int. 10 471 -477

10.   De Fronzo R.A., (1978) Pathogenesis of glucose intolerance in uraemia,
        Metabolism 27 Supp 2 1866 - 1879

11.   De Fronzo R.A., and Felig P. (1980) Aminoacid metabolism in uraemia;
        insights gained from normal and diabetic man. Amer. J. Clin. Nutr.
        33 1378 - 1386

12.   Delaporte C., Gros F, Anagnostopoulos T. (1980) Inhibitory effects of
        plasma dialysate on protein synthesis in vitro; influence of dialysis
        and transplantation. Amer. J. Clin. Nutr. 33 1407 - 1410

13.   Furst P., Ahlberg M., Alvestrand A., Bergstrom J., (1978) Principles
        of essential amino acid therapy in uraemic. Amer. J. Clin. Nutr.
        31, 1744 - 1745

14.   Furst P., Alvestrand A., Bergstrom J., (1980) Effects of nutrition
        and catabolic stress on intracellular muscle aminoacid pools in
        uraemia. Amer. J. Clin. Nutrition. 33 1387 - 1395

15.   Garber A.J. (1978) Skeletal muscle protein and amino acid metabolism
        in experimental chronic uraemia in the rat. J. Clin. Invest 62 623 - 632

16.   Garlick P.J., McNurlan M.A., Fern E.M., Tomkins A.M., Waterlow J.C.,
        (1980) Stimulation of protein synthesis and breakdown by vaccination
        B.M.J. 11 263 - 265

17.   Goldberg A.K., Chang T.W., (1978) Regulation and significance of
        amino acid metabolism in skeletal muscle. Federation Proc 37 2301-2307

18.   Golden M., Waterlow J.C., Picou D., (1977) The relationship between
        dietary intake, weight change, nitrogen balance and protein turnover
        in man. Amer. J. Clin. Nutr. 30 1345 - 1348

19.   Holliday M.A., Chantler C., MacDonell R. Keitges J. (1977) Effect
        of uraemia on nutritionally induced variations in protein metabolism.
        Kidney Int. 11 236 - 245

20.   Jones, M.R. and Kopple J.D. (1978) Valine metabolism in normal and
        chronically uremic man Amer. J. Clin. Nutrition 31 1660-1664.

21.   Jones, M.R. and Kopple J.D. (1979) Valine metabolism during saline
        and amino acid infusion in normal and uraemic man. Abstracts of 2nd
        International Cong of Nutrition in renal disease, Bologna 1979 pp76

22.   Jones, R.W.A., Bishti M.M., Chantler C. (1980) The promotion of
        anabolism in children with chronic renal failure in Topics in Paed-
        iatrics edited by Wharton B., Royal College of Physicians, published
        by Pitmans Medical, Tunbridge Wells UK paged 90 - 109

23.   Jones, R.W.A., Rigden S., Barratt T.M. and Chantler C., (1980) Body
        composition studies in infants with chronic renal failure. Abstracts
        3rd Int. Congress of Paediatric Nephrology Philadelphia

24.   Jones R.W.A., Dalton N., Start K., Chantler C., (1980) Keto-
        aminoacid therapy in uraemic children. Abstracts 3rd Int. Congress
        of Paediatric Nephrology, Philadelphia

25.   Jones R.W.A., Dalton N., Start K., Bishti M., Chantler C. (1980)
        Oral essential aminoacid supplements in children with advanced
        chronic renal failure. Amer. J. Clin. Nutr. 33 1696 - 1702

26. Kopple J.D., Swendseid, M.E. (1975) Protein and aminoacid metabolism in uraemic patients undergoing maintenance haemodialysis. Kid. Int. 7 S 64-S-72

27. Kopple J.D., (1978) Abnormal aminoacid and protein metabolism in uraemia. Kidney Int. 14 340 - 348

28. Mehls O., Ritz E., Gilli G., Bentholome K., Beibbarth H., Hohenegger M., Schnofnitzel W., (1980) Nitrogen Metabolism and growth in experimental uraemia. Int. J. of Paed. Nephrology 1 34 - 41

29. Metcoff J., Lindeman R., Baxter D., Pederson J. (1978) Cell metabolism in uraemia Amer. J. Clin. Nutrition 30 1627 - 1634

30. Munro H.W., (1978 Energy and protein intakes as determinatnts of nitrogen balance Kid. Int 14 313 - 316

31. Orloff S., Wassner S., Holliday, M.A., (1976) Effect of starvation on muscle protein catabolism in normal and uraemic rats. Kid. Int. 10 564

32. Randle P.J. (1980) Selection of respiratory fuels in symposium on regulation in cell metabolism. Biochemical Society Transactions (in press)

33. Renner D. and Heintz R. (1972) The inhibition of certain steps of glucose degradation in uraemia in 'Uraemia'. Edited by Khuthe R., Berlyne G. and Burton B. Verlag Stutthart pages 195-200

34. Rose, W.C. (1938) The nutritive significance of the aminoacids. Physiological Review 18 109-136

35. Rubenfield S., Garber A.J. (1978) Abnormal carbohydrate metabolism in chronic renal failure J. Clin. Invest. 62 20 - 28

36. Schauder P., Matthaei D., Scheler F., Mench-Hoinowski A., Langenbeck U., (1979) Blood levels of branched chain Ketoacids in uraemia: therapeutic implications Klin. Wochenschr 57 825 - 830

37. Snell K.(1980) Muscle alanine synthesis and hepatic gluconeogensis Biochemical Society Transactions 8 205-213

38. Walser M. (1975) Ketoacids in the treatment of uraemia. Clin. Neph. 3 180 - 186

39. Walser M. (1978) Ketoanalogues of essential aminoacids in the treatment of chronic renal failure. Kid. Int. 13 supp 8 S100 - S184

40. Walser M. (1978) Principles of ketoacid therapy in uraemic Amer. J. Clin. Nutr 31 1756 - 1760

41. Waterlow J.C., Golden M., Picou D., (1977) The measurement of rates of protein turnover, synthesis and breakdown in man and the effects of nutritional status and surgical injury. Amer. J. Clin. Nutr. 30 1333 - 1339

ENERGY METABOLISM IN CHRONIC RENAL FAILURE

MALCOLM A. HOLLIDAY, M.D. AND WATSON C. ARNOLD, M.D.

Energy metabolism encompasses the intake and expenditure of energy-
hence nutrition and physical activity and the metabolic controls of substrate use which lead to energy expenditure or storage. It is a large
subject.

Interest in energy metabolism in chronic renal failure or uremia has
many origins. Important among them is the presence of signs of protein-
energy malnutrition in a significant number of patients - particularly
children - with uremia including patients on dialysis (1,2). Evidence
for other metabolic disturbances affecting substrate use are common.
Resistance to insulin action (3) hyperlipidemia and early atheroclerosis
(4) are reported. Exaggerated catabolic response to fasting is described
(5,6). How much these different manifestations are integrated into a
common metabolic disorder or are interrelated is a subject of great interest. For example, in evaluating the effect of giving carbohydrate
supplement to improve energy intake the question of whether these supplements accelerate atherosclerosis must be considered. The value of increasing physical activity to lower plasma triglycerides is offset by the
question of whether it is possible in someone who is already showing signs
of dietary energy deficiency to increase energy demand.

This discussion focuses first on the evidence that a state of protein
energy malnutrition is a common but not unusual part of renal failure and
whether dietary supplements do have any effect. Evidence relating insulin sensitivity to plasma lipid levels is cited (7). In this matter, the
report of the effect of aerobic exercise training is provocative (8).
Evidence for an exaggerated catabolic response is reviewed. The clinical
implications of these findings are not clear-cut, but point to a need for
a carefully considered integrated approach to modify energy metabolism in
uremia and a careful evaluation of the results. The recent development

of continuous ambulatory peritoneal dialysis (CAPD) makes this subject all the more germane because CAPD provides gratuitously a carbohydrate supplement and the possibility for greater physical activity.

Protein energy malnutrition in the simplest forms, dietary deficiency of energy, or of protein and energy, has a range of clinical manifestations. On one extreme, marasmus typifies the state where dietary energy intake is insufficient and, on the other, Kwashiorkor where dietary protein and energy intake are insufficient. Marasmus is characterized by a loss of adipose tissue and muscle mass as these energy pools are used to meet expenditure. Plasma proteins are less affected and edema is slight. Physical inactivity and a reduction in basal metabolic rate are adaptive responses. A feature of marasmus is the reduction in muscle mass or muscle protein, even though the diet is not deficient in protein. There is just not sufficient food. Kwashiorkor, by contrast, includes development of edema, enlarged fatty liver, loss of hair and greater atrophy of the gastrointestinal mucosa. In both conditions muscle mass decreases and immune responses are diminished (9,10).

Signs typical of protein energy malnutrition, low weight for height ratio, decreased skin fold thickness, decreased muscle mass and muscle protein and some decrease in plasma proteins are well described in adults and children with uremia (11-14). The predominant findings are typical of mild marasmus or undernutrition, more than of Kwashiorkor. Growth failure is common in children with uremia and undernutrition contributes (15).

We reported the effects upon growth of giving dietary calorie supplements to children on chronic dialysis therapy. Total energy intake which was low correlated with growth rate. Growth rate improved in children who accepted a calorie supplement (16). We have completed a study in which 16 children were followed for 1 year in clinic without supplement and 1 year during which a supplement was given (17). Comparing intake and growth rate in each child during the unsupplemented (U) and supplemented (S) period we found intake increased from 75 to 100% and growth rate from 60 to 90% of normal. Since all of the children were growth retarded (average height-3.0 S.D.) the improved rate of growth did not improve the degree of growth retardation but kept it from worsening significantly. During the unsupplemented period, standard deviation scores worsened. Skin fold thickness which was below normal in the U period increased to normal levels during the S period. Plasma albumin increased slightly with supplementation.

Dietary intake of energy not only increased but the diet composition changed. With supplements, dietary intake of carbohydrates increased from 47 to 54%. Plasma cholesterol and triglycerides increased from values already above normal, similar to the findings of Sanfellippo and colleagues (18). We observed a similar change in plasma lipids in children on CAPD who derive a carbohydrate supplement from the glucose in dialysate (19). Patients with diabetes and hypertriglyceridemia have been given continuous insulin intraperitoneally and triglyceride levels have declined (20). It is possible that the hypertriglyceridemia in uremia is partly a consequence of insulin deficiency i.e. an output that is insufficient to compensate for the resistance.

Our present conclusions from these studies are that dietary energy deficiency or undernutrition does occur in patients with uremia and accounts for some of the clinical findings typical of simple undernutrition. Giving calorie supplements improves some of these indices - growth rate and adipose tissue mass - but does not restore stature or muscle mass to normal. Preliminary data on children undergoing CAPD are ambiguous. Growth may improve, skin fold thickness may increase; plasma lipids do increase (19).

Plasma triglyceride levels correlate with insulin resistance in patients with normal and increased levels of triglycerides (7). Resistance to insulin action accounts for the lowered glucose tolerance seen in obese patients with hypertriglyceridemia whereas insulin deficiency is associated with glucose intolerance in lean subjects (21). Patients with uremia show a correlation between plasma very low density lipoprotein (VLDL) levels and meal response to insulin and a corresponding correlation between VLDL-triglyceride secretion rate and rate and insulin response. Exchanging fat for carbohydrate in the diet lowers both VLDL levels and insulin response (22).

Both resistance to insulin and decreased insulin output may exist in uremia (23). Which of these, if either, contributes to the hypertriglycerdemia is not clear. Whether improving insulin sensitivity or giving insulin will improve the plasma triglyceride response to carbohydrate supplements either from food or dialysate sources needs to be explored.

Aerobic exercise training in normal sedentary subjects is associated with a decrease in plasma insulin responses to glucose loads with no change in glucose disposal rates (24). Plasma lipid levels also decline (25). Aerobic exercise training in patients on chronic dialysis therapy is associated with an improved glucose disposal rate and lower plasma lipid levels (8). These findings are very provocative. They raise the possibility that exercise in a population that has a tendency to energy deficiency can improve well being, insulin sensitivity and plasma lipids even though energy expenditure increases and, by inference, energy intake (cf-8).

The response to short fasting tests the adaptive response of the individual to a switch from exogenous to endogenous substrate use for energy. To the extent protein is spared, muscle mass is spared. The response to injury or infection as measured by nitrogen loss correlates with loss of tissue mass. Giving glucose reduces this response. We have reasoned that the nitrogen loss in response to a short fast might be modified in uremia. We measured urea nitrogen production in control and uremic rats fasted 36 hours in association with measuring muscle protein synthesis rates. We found urea nitrogen loss from 24-36 hours of fasting was increased in uremic rats. This correlated with a greater depression of muscle protein synthesis rates (5). Rubenfeld and Garber have found higher alanine turnover rates in uremic fasted subjects than in comparably fasted controls (6). These findings are consistent with an exaggerated catabolic response to infection in uremia (26). Whether insulin resistance at low insulin levels plays a role in this response is not clear. We have found resistance to insulin mediated muscle uptake of amino acids in uremic rats (23). However leg exchange of branch chain amino acids in response to high dose insulin infusions is not affected (29).

There is a general clinical impression that uremic patients sustain greater weight loss with infection and slower recovery rates. The experimental observations just cited generally fit with this impression. Whether we can take steps that effectively block an exaggerated catabolic response remains uncertain.

Energy metabolism in uremia is affected in several ways. Muscle wasting and poor growth are due in part to undernutrition. Calorie supplements help, but may increase hypertriglyceridemia. Physical inactivity may also contribute to insulin resistance and hypertriglycerdemia.

324

Aerobic training may ameliorate these changes. Both of these strategies
directly challenge a patient's living style, diet and activity. It is
certainly far from clear whether patients can be induced to adopt these
changes. The author feels that effort to gain "compliance" that accen-
tuate a dependent state are ill advised. Efforts in which information
assists a patient in deciding to make these changes is preferred. Studies
that characterize the relation between energy intake, physical activity,
insulin action, plasma lipids and muscle metabolism will give a clearer
picture of the metabolic derangement in uremia and may point to therapy
that will improve nutritional state in patients with uremia.

REFERENCES

1. Chantler C, Holliday MA. 1973. Growth in children with renal disease
   with particular reference to the effects of calorie malnutrition.
   Clin Neph 1, 288.
2. Blumenkrantz MJ, Kopple JD, Gilman RA et al. 1980. Methods for
   assessing nutritional status of patients with renal failure. Am Journ
   Clin Nutr, 33, 1567.
3. Hampers CL, Saeldner JS, Doak PB, Merrill JP. 1966. Effect of chronic
   renal failure and hemodialysis on carbohydrate metabolism. Journ Clin
   Invest 45, 1719.
4. Bagdade JD, Porte D, Bierman EL. 1968. Hypertriglyceridemia: A
   metabolic consequence of chronic renal failure. New Eng Journ Med
   279, 181.
5. Holliday MA, Chantler C, MacDonnell R, Kietges J. 1977. Effect of
   uremia on nutritionally induced variations in protein metabolism.
   Kidney Int 11:236.
6. Rubenfeld S, Garber AJ. 1978. Abnormal carbohydrate metabolism in
   chronic renal failure. Journ Clin Invest 62, 20.
7. Olefsky JM, Farquar W, Reavan GM. 1974. Reappraisal of the role of
   insulin in hypertriglyceridemia. Amer Journ Med 57, 551.
8. Goldberg AP, Hagberg J, Delmey JA et al. 1980. The metabolic and
   psychological effects of exercise training in hemodialysis patients.
   Amer Journ Clin Nutr 33, 1620.
9. Keys A, Brozek J, Henschel A, et al. 1950. The biology of human
   starvation. Minnesota University of Minnesota Press.
10. Waterlow JC, Alleyne GA. 1971. Protein malnutrition in children:
    Advances in knowledge in the last 10 years. Adv in Protein Chem 25,117.
11. Coles GA. 1972. Body composition in chronic renal failure. Quart
    Journ Med 41,25.
12. Holliday MA, Chantler C. 1978. Metabolism in children with renal in-
    sufficiency. Kidney Intl 14, 306.
13. Weber H, Michalk D, Raul W et al. 1980. Total body potassium in
    children with chronic renal failure. Int Journ Ped Neph 1, 42.
14. Delaporte C, Bergstrom J and Broyer M. 1976. Variations in muscle
    cell protein of uremic children. Kidney Int 10, 239.
15. Potter DE, Greifer I. 1978. Statural growth of children with renal
    disease. Kidney Int 14, 334.
16. Simmon JM, Wilson CJ, Potter DE, and Holliday MA. Relation of calorie
    deficiency to growth failure in children on hemodialysis and the growth
    response to calorie supplementation. New Eng Journ Med 285, 653. 1971.

17. Arnold WC, Holliday MA. 1979. Assessment of nutritional status in children with chronic renal failure (abst) Kidney Int 16, 950.
18. Sanfelippo ML, Swenson RS, Reavan GM. 1977. Reduction of plasma triglycerides by diet in subjects with chronic renal failure. Kidney Int 11, 54.
19. Potter DE, McDaid TK, Ramirez JA. 1981, in press. Peritoneal dialysis in children, in Proceedings of the Pan Pacific Symposium on Peritoneal Dialysis (R. Atkins, ed.), Churchill Livingstone.
20. Tamborlane WV, Sherwin RS, Genel M, Felig P. 1979. Restoration of normal lipid and amino acid metabolism in diabetic patients treated with a portable-infusion pump. Lancet, I, 1258.
21. Soffolo G, Bergman RN and Finegold DT et al. 1980. Quantitative estimation of beta cell sensitivity to glucose in the intact organism. Diabetes 20.
22. Reavan GM, Swenson RS, and Sanfelippo ML. 1980. An inquiry into the mechanism of hypertriglyceridemia in patients with chronic renal failure. Amer Journ Clin Nutr 33, 1476.
23. DeFronzo RA and Alvestrand A. 1980. Glucose intolerance in uremia: site and mechanism. Amer Journ Clin Nutr 33, 1438.
24. Winder WW, Hickson RC, Hagberg JM et al. 1979. Training induced changes in hormonal and metabolic responses to submaximal exercise. J Appl Physiol 46, 766.
25. Gyntelberg F, Brennan R, Hollaszy JO et al. 1977. Plasma triglyceride lowering by exercise despite increased food intake in patients with Type IV hyperlipoproteinemia. Amer Journ Clin Nutr 30, 716.
26. Grodstein GP, Glumenkrantz MJ, Kopple JD. 1980. Nutritional and metabolic response to catabolic stress in uremia. Amer Journ Clin Nutr 33, 1411.
27. Arnold WC, Holliday MA. Tissue resistance to insulin stimulation of amino acid uptake in acutely uremic rats. Kidney Int 16, 24.
28. DeFronzo RA, Felig P. 1980. Amino acid metabolism in uremia: insights gained from normal and diabetic man. Amer Journ Clin Nutr 33, 1378.

LIPID METABOLISM IN CHRONIC RENAL FAILURE

ALFRED DRUKKER, MD
Division of Pediatric Nephrology
Shaare Zedek Medical Center
Jerusalem, Israel

Disturbances of lipid metabolism in chronic renal disease have been known since the first half of the 19th century. In 1836, Bright[1] noticed that the serum of some patients with 'nephritis' appeared 'milky and opaque'. More than 75 years later, in 1913, Munck[2] first described the double refractile lipid bodies in the urine of patients suffering from 'lipoid nephrosis'.

The recognition of altered lipid metabolism in non-nephrotic chronic renal failure patients is, however, of a more recent date and goes back to the work of Bagdade and coworkers[3] who in the late 1960s called attention to the significant hypertriglyceridemia present in may dialysed and non-dialysed uremic patients. At the same time it also became evident that many adult patients with cronic renal failure age prematurely and have accelerated atherosclerosis with a high rate of cardiovascular morbidity and mortality. Hyperlipidemia, or more precisely hypertriglyceridemia, was at the time considered a major causal risk factor for atherosclerosis in the general population. In renal failure cause (hypertriglyceridemia) and effect (atherosclerosis) were widely accepted and few questioned at the time the validity of this causal relationship. Hence the interest and the research activity in the field following the publications of Bagdade and associates [3].

From the work of Ibels et al. [4], Heuck et al. [5], Huttünen et al. [6], Ponticelli et al. [7], Bagdade et al. [8] and many others it is now clear that uremic (non-dialysed), dialysis and transplant patients all tend to have high serum triglyceride (TG) levels in comparison with normolipemic control subjects. Serum cholesterol (CHOL) levels are generally normal and are significantly elevated only in renal transplant patients. (In this review we will not deal with the hyperlipidemia of renal transplant recipients.)

Hypertriglyceridemia with normal cholesterol levels is the characteristic finding of type IV hyperlipoproteinemia which is the major lipid abnormality in the adult chronic renal failure population. The incidence varies enormously in the reported series: from 30 to 75 percent [7,9]. The composition of the neutral lipids in these patients is also abnormal, apparently a universal finding in uremia irrespective of the presence of hypertrigliceridemia [8, 10]. The very low density lipoproteins (VLDL), the low density lipoproteins (LDL) and the high-density lipoproteins (HDL) all contain an increased percentage of TG, whereas the percentage of CHOL is reduced. Decreased levels of high-density lipoprotein cholesterol are found not only in dialysis patients but also in patients with moderately severe, stable uremia. Thus, the dialysis treatment cannot be responsible for these metabolic abnormalities. They are apparently part of the chronic uremic state.

All these data were obtained in adult renal failure patients. Relatively few studies are available on lipid metabolism in chronic renal failure in childhood. However, from the publications of Pennisi et al. [11], Berger et al. [12], El Bishti and Chantler [13], Broyer and coworkers [14] as well as from our own, unpublished, data it is clear that generally in children with chronic renal failure a pattern similar to that described in adults is observed.

The pathogenesis of the uremic hypertriglyceridemia is still not completely understood, despite a wealth of available experimental data. Elevated serum lipoprotein concentrations can be the result either of increased hepatic synthesis or of impaired peripheral catabolism. Hepatic VLDL synthesis is enhanced by insulin. Since in uremia circulating immunoreactive insulin levels are increased, a direct relationship between hyperinsulinemia and hypertriglyceridemia was assumed. Glucagon is also elevated in uremia. This promotes lipolysis and augments VLDL production. Parathyroid hormone (PTH) acts on adipose tissue adenylcyclase and promotes insulin secretion and/or peripheral glucose utilization by changes in the extra- and intracellular calcium concentration. Several lines of evidence, however, show that there is no increased hepatic VLDL production. The high immunoreactive insulin levels in uremia are probably caused by cross-reacting physiologic inactive pro-insulin. The active insulin levels in uremia are generally normal or even below normal. The same holds for glucagon and the role of PTH in this setting is not yet clear. Furthermore, hepatic triglyceride turnover and production rates have been measured in uremic rats by Heuck and coworkers [15] and Bagdade and associates [16]. These studies failed

to show a significant increase in the production of triglycerides by the
liver. The situation in humans may be different as shown in the work by
Verschoor et al. [17] who established an increased triglyceride synthesis
rate in twelve uremic patients. In summary, there are not many data to
support the concept of increased hepatic triglyceride production in uremia.

Even if this mechanism is operative, the burden of evidence now points
to decreased lipoprotein catabolism as the major lipid abnormality in
chronic uremia. It has been known for a long time that serum lipolytic
activity, measured after administration of heparin, is decreased in uremia
[3, 18]. Subsequently it has been shown that hepatic lipoprotein lipase
and adipose tissue lipoprotein lipase activity is also reduced [19,20].
Moreover, the serum of dialysed uremic patients appears to contain a
'middle molecule' toxin which in vitro inhibits lipoprotein lipase activity
and/or release. Finally, in uremia a normally present lipoprotein lipase
activator may be absent.

These findings can explain the phenomenon of high serum TG levels,
which is mainly due to defective peripheral clearing of lipoproteins. The
data fail, however, to throw light on the question of why serum CHOL-levels
are (relatively) low in uremia and why the levels of HDL-cholesterol are
reduced.

Brunzell et al. [21] offered the following explanation. They suggested
that when serum TG-levels are high, the protein fraction of the lipoproteins
(apoprotein) is saturated by the TG leading to a reduced affinity of the
apoprotein to CHOL. However, Rapoport et al. [22] could not confirm these
findings. Their studies show a reduction in apoprotein C-II in the HDL and
VLDL. This apoprotein is a major activator of lipoprotein lipase. A
deficiency of this substance and/or an abnormal composition of the involved
lipoprotein thus explains, at least in part, the TG clearing defect. The
high relative TG content of the VLDL is according to Rapoport et al. [22] a
secondary event. The abnormal HDL will also impair the transfer of CHOL
from the tissues to the liver.

Additional factors have been described which influence serum TG-levels
in uremic patients, such as hyperparathyroidism, treatment with androgens
and beta-blockers and the composition of the dialysis bath in particular
in regard to acetate and glucose [9]. It is not clear whether these
factors have any direct causal relationship with uremic hypertriglyceridemia.

Chronic renal failure is a state of generalized uremic toxicity in which many organ systems are affected. We have recently studied the abnormalities of the gastro-intestinal tract in uremia, and in particular the intestinal absorption of fat, with a relatively new technique: the acute oral fat loading test.   In the early morning hours 50 gram of fat of dairy origin is given in the form of a 'milkshake' (57% unsaturated and 43% saturated fats).   The absorption of fat from the gut is then followed by hourly determination of TG, CHOL and lipoprotein electrophoresis (LPEP) in peripheral venous blood.   The validity of this test for the study of fat absorption from the gut has been tested by other investigators as well as by us in control subjects and in patients with primary malabsorption syndromes[23,24].   With this technique we studied five adult dialysis patients (21-55 years of age) and five children who are on hemodialysis (2-14 years of age). The results of the test in these ten patients were compared with two control groups: C-1, ten healthy age-matched controls with normal fasting serum TG levels and C-2, ten healthy control subjects with normal renal function but with elevated fasting serum TG levels, comparable to those seen in the dialysis patients. The results are summarized in figure 1.

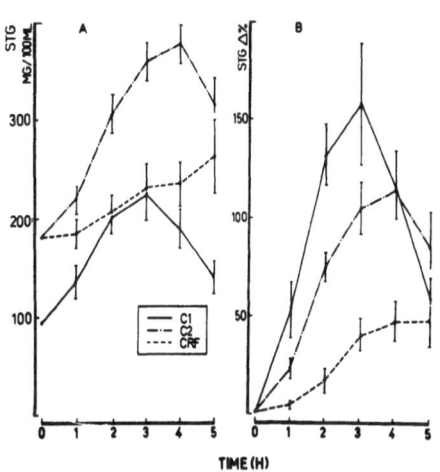

Figure 1. For explanation see text.

The slopes of the initial ascending part of the curve of serum TG ('absorption curve') in the ten chronic renal failure patients (CRF) are clearly less steep than the corresponding slopes of the curves of groups C-1 and C-2.   This indicates defective intestinal fat absorption.   The second, descending part of the curve ('clearance curve'), representing the disappearance of TG from the serum is, as expected, also pathologic in the CRF patients.

In figure 2 the data are considered separately for the adult and the pediatric CRF patients, each with their age-matched healthy controls. The slopes of the 'absorption curve' in the pediatric and adult CRF patients are not significantly different.   However, in the pediatric CRF patients serum TG-levels tend to fall during the last two hours of the fat loading

330

test, indicating reasonable TG clearing, whereas in the adult CRF patients
serum TG levels continue to rise during the entire period of the test.

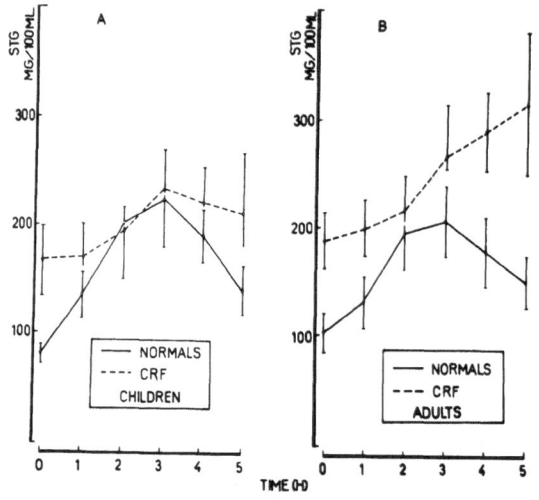

These results thus
point to an additional
abnormality of fat meta-
bolism in renal failure:
the malabsorption of fat
from the gut. Whether
this finding has any cli-
nical significance in
respect to the hypertri-
glyceridemia of uremia
or in regard to loss of
energy, in particular in
childhood, still has to
be evaluated.

Figure 2. For explanation see text.

The importance and
the implications of the uremic hypertriglyceridemia can at present only be
discussed within the framework of the relationship of hypertriglyceridemia
and atherosclerosis in general. Considerable doubt has been cast on the
notion that hypertriglyceridemia is indeed a significant risk factor for
cardiovascular disease in normal populations. This was once again stressed
recently in a stimulating article by Hulley and coworkers[25]. In uremia
the situation is probably similar. Several studies have shown that smoking
and hypertension are far more significant risk factors than hypertriglyceridemia in uremic (dialysis) patients[26,27]. Cholesterol though is
probably important. Decreased levels of HDL-cholesterol have a strong correlation with (the risk of) atherosclerosis in the general population.
Since in uremia this abnormality is a universal finding, the uremic patient
is prone to develop cardiovascular disease.

We can now envision a unifying picture with the abnormal lipoprotein
composition of uremia, placed centrally. This abnormality is responsible
for decreased serum TG clearing whereas this same abnormality can independently offer an explanation for the accelerated atherosclerosis of uremia.
This defect results in a decreased mobilization of cholesterol from the
periphery and in defective cholesterol transport to the liver. Cholesterol
will accumulate in the tissues and the vascular bed.

In addition, the response-injury theory of atherosclerosis may still play a part in uremia. A uremic toxin can cause a defect of the arteriolar wall, inducing smooth muscle proliferation and cholesterol deposition in the endothelium[9]. Smooth muscle cell proliferation has indeed been observed on post mortem examination in the coronary vessels of adults and even of pediatric dialysis patients[11]. At present we lack further information regarding the development of accelerated atherosclerosis in young uremic patients.

The treatment of the hypertriglyceridemia of the uremic state is still an enigma. It is a sound physiologic principle to strive for normalization of biochemical abnormalities. At the same time one should assess risks and benefits and above all adhere to the principle of *'primum non nocere'*. The treatment of the hypertriglyceridemia can be achieved by the administration of lipid-lowering drugs, all rather toxic, by absorbents, by a change in dialysis modality (hemodialysis versus hemofiltration, for example) or by increasing the efficiency of dialysis (type of dialyzer, of membrane, of surface, etc.)[9,28,29,30].

The most promising approach, however, is that of dietary restriction of carbohydrates. The studies by Sanfelippo *et al.*[31], Okubo and co-workers[32], Catran and associates[33], all show significant reduction in serum TG-levels induced by a carbohydrate-poor diet. This apparently easy diet restriction may, however, lead to a major nutritional upheaval in pediatric patients. The carbohydrates often constitute the all important 'goodies' in the life of the ill-fated youngsters. Quite apart from the psychological problems of additional diet restriction in these patients, the carbohydrate-poor diets may result in medical problems. In order to enhance growth and development in young chronic renal failure and dialysis patients, the carbohydrates form an important source of energy and thus an essential part of the dietary handling of these patients[34].

Given the difficulties of effectively treating uremic hypertriglyceridemia and taking into account the debatable importance of this abnormality, it appears to be advisable to concentrate our efforts at present on the clear cut risk factors of atherosclerosis in dialysis patients: control of hypertension, smoking and hyperparathyroidism. This is especially true for the pediatric patients.

332

REFERENCES

1. Bright R, 1936. Cases and observations illustrative of renal disease accompanied with the secretion of albuminous urine, Guy's Hosp Rep 1: 338-350.
2. Munck F, 1913. Klinische Diagnostik der degenerativen Nierenerkrankungen, Ztschr Klin Med 78:1-10.
3. Bagdade JD, Porte D jr, Bierman EL, 1968. Hypertriglyceridemia: a metabolic consequence of chronic renal failure, N Eng J Med 279:181-185.
4. Ibels LS, Simons LA, King JO et al., 1975. Studies on the nature and causes of hyperlipidemia in uremia, maintenance dialysis and renal transplantation, Quart J Med (new series) 44:601-614.
5. Heuck CC, Ritz, E, Liersch M et al., 1978. Serum lipids in renal insufficiency, Am J Clin Nutr 31:1547-1553.
6. Huttunen JK, Pasternack A, Vänttinen T et al., 1978. Lipoprotein metabolism in patients with chronic uremia, Acta Med Scand 204:211-218.
7. Ponticelli C, Barbi G, Cantaluppi A et al., 1978. Lipid abnormalities in maintenance dialysis patients and renal transplant recipients, Kidney Int 13:572-578.
8. Bagdade JD, Casaretto A, Albers J, 1976. Effects of chronic uremia, hemodialysis and renal transplantation on plasma lipids and lipoproteins in man, J Lab Clin Med 87:37-48.
9. Bagdade JD, 1979. Hyperlipidemia and atherosclerosis in chronic dialysis patients in Replacement of renal function by dialysis, Drukker W, Parsons FM and Mahler JF, eds,Martinus Nijhoff, the Hague, Chap 29, pp 538-545.
10. Bagdade JD, Albers JJ, 1977. Plasma high density lipoprotein concentrations in chronic hemodialysis and renal transplant patients. N Eng J Med 296:1436-1439.
11. Pennisi AJ, Heuser ET, Mickey MR et al., 1976. Hyperlipidemia in pediatric hemodialysis and renal transplant patients (associated with coronary artery disease), Am J Dis Child 130:957-961.
12. Berger M, James GP, Davis ER et al., 1978. Hyperlipidemia in uremic children: response to peritoneal dialysis and hemodialysis, Clin Nephrol 9:19-24.
13. El Bishti MM, Counahan R, Bloom SR et al., 1977. Abnormalities in plasma lipids in children on regular hemodialysis, Arch Dis Childh 52:932-939.
14. Broyer M, Czernichow P, Tete MJ et al., 1978. Insulin and growth hormone in dialyzed children: influence of dietary manipulation, Am J Clin Nutr 31:1876-1880.
15. Heuck CC, Liersch M, Ritz E et al., 1978. Hyperlipoproteinemia in experimental chronic renal insufficiency in the rat, Kidney Int 14:142-150.
16. Bagdade JD, Yee E, Shafrir E et al., 1978. Hyperlipidemia in renal failure: studies of plasma lipoproteins, hepatic triglyceride production and tissue lipoprotein lipase in a chronically uremic rat model, J Lab Clin Med 91:176-180.
17. Verschoor L, Lammers R, Birkenhäger JC, 1978. Triglyceride turnover in severe chronic non-nephrotic renal failure, Metabolism 27:879-883.
18. Ibels LS, Reardon MF, Nestel PJ, 1976. Plasma post-heparin lipolytic activity in triglyceride clearance in uremic and hemodialysis patients and renal allograft recipients, J Lab Clin Med 87:648-658.
19. Bolzano K, Krempler F, Sandhofer F, 1978. Hepatic and extrahepatic triglyceride lipase activity in uremic patients on chronic hemodialysis, Eur J Clin Invest 8:289-293.

20. Goldberg A,Sherrard D, Brunzell JD, 1976. Hypertriglyceridemia in hemo-
    dialysis patients: dual defect of adipose tissue lipoprotein lipase,
    Clin Res 24:361 A.
21. Brunzell JD, Albers JJ, Haas LB et al., 1977. Prevalence of serum lipid
    abnormalities in chronic hemodialysis, Metabolism 26:903-910.
22. Rapoport J, Aviram M, Chaimovitz C et al., 1978. Defective high-density
    lipoprotein composition in patients on chronic hemodialysis: a possible
    mechanism for accelerated atherosclerosis, N Eng J Med 299:1326-1329.
23. Goldstein R, Blondheim O, Bronza N et al., in press. The oral fat load-
    ing test; a measure of intestinal fat absorption.
24. Jonas A, Weiser S, Segal P et al, 1979. Oral fat loading test: a
    reliable procedure for the study of fat malabsorption in children,
    Arch Dis Childh 54: 770-772.
25. Hulley SB, Rosenman RH, Bawol RD et al, 1980. Epidemiology as a guide
    to clinical decisions; the association between triglycerides and
    coronary heart disease, N Eng J Med 302:1383-1386.
26. Manis T, Friedman, EA, 1979. Dialytic therapy for irreversible uremia,
    N Eng J Med 301:1321-1328.
27. Bonomini V, Feletti C, Scolari HP et al,1980. Atherosclerosis in
    uremia: a longitudinal study, Am J Clin Nutr 33:1493-1500.
28. Goldberg AP,Applebaum-Bowden DM, Bierman EL et al, 1979. Increase in
    lipoprotein lipase during clofibrate treatment of hypertriglyceridemia
    in patients on hemodialysis, N Eng J Med 301:1073-1076.
29. Friedman EA, Staltzman MJ, Delano BG et al, 1978. Reduction in hyper-
    lipidemia in hemodialysis patients treated with charcoal and oxidized
    starch (oxystarch), Am J Clin Nutr 31:1903-1914.
30. Sanfelippo MJ, Grundy S, Henderson L, 1979. Transport of very low-
    density lipoprotein triglyceride (VLDL-TG): comparison of hemodialysis
    (HD) and hemofiltration (HF), Kidney Int 16:868 (abstract).
31. Sanfelippo MJ, Swenson RS, Reaven GM, 1978. Response of plasma tri-
    glycerides to dietary change in patients on hemodialysis, Kidney Int
    14:180-186.
32. Okubo M, Tsukamoto Y, Yoneda T et al, 1980. Deranged fat metabolism
    and the lowering effect of carbohydrate-poor diet on serum triglycerides
    in patients with chronic renal failure, Nephron 25:8-14.
33. Catran DC, Steiner G, Fenton SSA et al, 1980. Dialysis hyperlipidemia:
    response to dietary manipulations, Clin Nephrol 13:177-182.
34. Chantler C, El Bishti M, Counahan R, 1980. Nutritional therapy in
    children with chronic renal failure, Am J Clin Nutr 33:1682-1689.

CURRENT ISSUES IN PEDIATRIC RENAL PATHOLOGY: SEGMENTAL HYPOPLASIA &
GLOMERULOCYSTIC DISEASE

J. BERNSTEIN

I have chosen to restrict my remarks at this symposium to several
problems in developmental renal pathology. The first is renal hypoplasia,
the second, glomerular cystic disease.

Renal Hypoplasia

The recognition in recent years that vesicoureteric reflux (VUR) is
associated with severe renal atrophy and very small kidneys (1,2) has prompted
a reevaluation of renal hypoplasia. The literature on renal hypoplasia
contains an odd mixture of small kidneys with uncertain histology (3,4).
Unilateral hypoplasia, in particular, is said to be a relatively common
occurrence with a postmortem frequency of approximately 1:500 (4). We
have always known the difficulty in differentiating the shrunken kidneys of
of atrophic pyelonephritis from the small kidneys of congenital hypoplasia (5).
To compound the difficulty, hypoplastic kidneys have commonly been regarded as
prone to infection, lithiasis, and vascular disease. I had always been
puzzled by the high prevalence of pyelocalyceal deformity in what was reported
as congenital hypoplasia (6). I somehow assumed that the pyelocalyceal
irregularities in hypoplastic kidneys might reflect maldevelopment, such as
renal dysplasia, but always had a lingering suspicion that not all of us were
talking about the same thing, despite our using the same terminology.

A great deal of my uncertainty has been resolved by the recognition that
renal segmental hypoplasia and parenchymal reduction are also associated with
VUR (7-9) and that segmental hypoplasia of this sort is likely to be a sort
of reflux nephropathy.

We have had the opportunity of studying a series of nephrectomy specimens
with segmental hypoplasia, a form of irregular renal atrophy that has been
known as the Ask-Upmark kidney (10,11). This abnormality is defined as a
small kidney, containing a decreased number of pyramids, with pyelocalyceal
distortion to form an elongated calyx that extends almost to the capsule

beneath an externally visible groove. Between calyx and capsule there is only a very thin band of parenchyma, containing some obsolete glomeruli or none at all, hyperplastic arterioles, and atrophic tubules with tubular microcysts. The medullary pyramid in the abnormal segment is ordinarily effaced or severely atrophic, grossly inapparent.

Because of the smallness of the kidneys and an apparently aglomerular, severely hypoplastic lobe(s), Ask-Upmark (12) and most subsequent writers regarded the lesion as developmental. Like Zollinger (13), I have long thought the lesion to be acquired (14). The abnormal areas correspond approximately to lobes or segments, and microscopic examination shows, even in the absence of an identifiable medullary pyramid, corticomedullary differentiation with intervening arcuate blood vessels. The cortical segment does contain tubules, and hyalinized glomeruli are often identifiable. The remnant of medulla usually contains collecting ducts. The evidence indicates that a lobar segment had developed through ductal branching and metanephric induction to at least a point and that the existing nephrons subsequently underwent regressive changes. It would be unlikely vertebrate embryology for metanephric tubules to have developed without glomeruli. There may also have been an inhibition of development or growth, as there is evidence in a few specimens that the process had intrauterine origins. On the other hand, the surviving segments frequently undergo compensatory hypertrophy. There is equally good evidence that the process goes on during infancy, and progressive changes have been demonstrated radiographically.

I suggested that the segmental lesion was more likely to be ischemic than developmental (14), although there was but little precedent for that view (15). It has now become clear, however, that a high proportion of patients with segmental hypoplasia have also had VUR (16,17). In our own study of 17 cases (18), we found evidence of VUR in 16. The frequency of VUR in the literature is approximately 60%.

All 17 kidneys were small, weighing less than 2 S.D. below the mean weight for age. We found the severity and extent of scarring, for which I will use the term "hypoplastic atrophy," to be highly variable. Lesions were usually multiple, and typical lesions coexisted with zones of less severe scarring. There was, in other words, a spectrum of renal damage, in which the typical hypoplastic scar represented the end of the process.

In what is now an expanded series of 21 cases, we found hypertension to be related to the severity of the renal injury. Hypertension was in general associated with bilaterality and multifocality. Hypertension was associated also with the presence of JG granules, which could be demonstrated in the areas of scarring within both sclerotic glomeruli and sclerotic blood vessels. The degree of granulation was, however, quite variable, much like reported measurements of plasma renin activity (19). We have not identified the cause of increased granules in what would ordinarily be regarded as a nonfunctioning segment of kidney, and we have not learned why one kidney contains more granules than the next.

Many questions remain, the biggest, of course, about the pathogenesis of segmental hypoplastic atrophy and about the means of preventing it. We need to define the limits of reflux nephropathy and of segmental hypoplastic atrophy, either to preserve the latter or to recognize its nonexistence. If hypoplastic renal atrophy is indeed part of reflux nephropathy and if most cases can be explained in this way, it becomes a little more understandable that segmental hypoplasia bears a high incidence of inflammation, medullary microlithiasis and pyelolithiasis (20).

The next big question is the pathogenesis of hypertension. Most children with this condition come to medical attention because of hypertension, a few because of renal insufficiency, and a few because of recurrent urinary tract infection.

There seems to be little doubt that other forms of renal hypoplasia remain unperturbed by these revelations. The small, unirenicular kidney, for example, must be regarded as primarily hypoplastic, even if it is associated with a dilated ureter or other urinary tract malformation. The necessary distinctions between developmental and acquired disease are usually easiest in very young children, when there is little renal inflammation and atrophy. Distinguishing between hypoplastic atrophy and congenital hypoplasia will be most difficult in older individuals, who are likely to have a mixture of inflammation, scarring, compensatory lobar hypertrophy, and reduced renal mass. The only way to know what they have is to know what has happened over a period of years.

Glomerular Cystic Disease

Renal glomerular cystic disease has been described as a potentially distinct entity (21-23). Localized glomerular cysts are, of course, found in several different syndromes, e.g., trisomy D and tuberous sclerosis, but a diffuse cystic disease that was responsible for renal impairment seemed to be something new. At about the same time, the literature contained an increasing number of reports of autosomal dominant, so-called adult polycystic disease

(APCD) in young children (24). The early infantile form of APCD was often dominated by glomerular cysts (25-27), and it was soon apparent that APCD of precocious onset must enter into the differential diagnosis of what has come to be known as glomerular cystic disease (28). Our own experience carries the argument a step further by showing that glomerular cysts are the typical pattern of APCD in infancy and conversely by suggesting that most examples of diffuse glomerular cystic disease are accounted for by APCD.

Our own morphologic studies have demonstrated few features in the cyst epithelium that are distinctive of APCD. The epithelium may sometimes be hyperplastic, but we have not been able to demonstrate intracystic polyps that could, as in adult-onset APCD, have caused ductal obstruction and have been responsible for the cysts (29). We have demonstrated a large number of smooth muscle cells surrounding the cysts, a feature common in lesser degree to all forms of APCD. The smooth muscle cells may represent a transformation of the metanephric mesenchyme in response to the tension of the cysts, and there is no evidence for their playing a primary role.

The importance of recognizing the association between glomerular cysts and APCD lies in clinical recognition and genetic counselling. The occurrence of APCD in a young infant may antedate its recognition in older members of the family; indeed, subsequent studies of the parents have on occasion turned up evidence of previously inapparent disease (30). The disease in infants appears to be genetically no different than the disease in adults. The reasons for a precocious onset in one member of a kindred are unknown; we suggested, but have not yet found evidence for double-dose dominant inheritance that might have accelerated the clinical onset.

Recognition of this association is important also because some specimens of glomerular cystic disease in young infants have been deficient in metanephric differentiation, suggesting that the heritable defect responsible for APCD interfered with normal nephrogenesis. We thought at first that these kidneys were examples of diffuse cystic dysplasia, a condition that is seldom familial. We have concluded tentatively that APCD, like several other heritable syndromes, can affect the kidney in several ways, depending upon the timing and severity of metabolic impairment. The variability of effect is best understood as continuing responses to metabolic abnormalities, rather than as a group of static malformations.

338

REFERENCES

1. Bialestock D. 1965. Studies of renal malformations and pyelonephritis in children, with and without associated vesico-ureteral reflux and obstruction. Aust NZ J Surg. 35:120.
2. Hodson J. 1978. Reflux nephropathy. Med Clin North Am. 62:1201.
3. Ekström T. 1955. Renal hypoplasia. A clinical study of 179 cases. Acta Chir Scand, Suppl 203.
4. Bengtsson C, Hood B. 1971. The unilateral small kidney with special reference to the hypoplastic kidney. Review of the literature and authors' points of view. Int Urol Nephrol 3:337.
5. Emmett JL, Alvarez-Ierena JJ, McDonald JR. 1952. Atrophic pyelonephritis versus congenital renal hypoplasia. J.A.M.A. 148:1470.
6. Boissonnat P. 1962. What to call hypoplastic kidney? Arch Dis Child 37:142.
7. Boccon-Gibod L, Gallian Ph, Boccon-Gibod L. 1972. Le petit rein unilatéral de l'adulte en dehors des obstructions de la voie excrétrice. Étude anatomo-clinique de 37 observations. Ann Urol. 6:1.
8. Andersen HJ, Jacobsson B, Larsson H, Winberg J: 1973. Hypertension, asymmetric renal parenchymal defect, sterile urine, and high E. coli antibody titre. Br Med J. 3:14.
9. Holland NH, Kotchen T, Bhathena D. 1975. Hypertension in children with chronic pyelonephritis. Kidney Int 8:S243.
10. Batzenschlager A, Blum E, Weill-Bousson M. 1962. Le petit rein unilatéral. I. Petit rein unilatéral acquis. Ann Anat Pathol (Paris). 7:427.
11. Habib R, Courtecuisse V, Ehrensperger J, Royer P. 1965. Hypoplasie segmentaire du rein avec hypertension arterielle chez l'enfant. Ann Pediatr (Paris). 12:262.
12. Ask-Upmark E. 1929. Über juvenile maligne Nephrosclerose und ihr Verhaltnis zu Störungen in der Nierenentwicklung. Acta Pathol Microbiol Scand. 6:383.
13. Zollinger HU. 1957. Pathogenese und Folgen einseitiger Zwergnieren bei Jugendlichen. Frühinfantile Pyelonephritis oder Hypogenese? Schweiz Med Wschr. 87:990.
14. Bernstein J. 1975. Developmental abnormalities of the renal parenchyma -- renal hypoplasia and dysplasia, in Sommers SC, ed. Kidney Pathology Dicennial 1966-75, New York, Appleton-Century-Crofts.
15. Abe K, Saito T, Otsuka Y et al: 1973. Seven cases of hypertension due to segmental renal ischemia. Jpn Heart J. 14:110.
16. Benz G, Willich E, Schärer K. 1976. Segmental renal hypoplasia in childhood. Pediatr Radiol 5:86.
17. Johnston JH, Mix LW. 1976. The Ask-Upmark kidney: A form of ascending pyelonephritis? Br J Urol. 48:393.
18. Arant BS Jr, Sotelo-Avila C, Bernstein J. 1979. Segmental "hypoplasia" of the kidney (Ask-Upmark). J Pediatr. 95:931.
19. Bailey RR, McRae CU, Maling TMJ et al: 1978. Renal vein renin concentration in the hypertension of unilateral reflux nephropathy. J Urol. 120:21.
20. Batzenschlager A, Weill-Bousson M, Guerbaoui M. 1974. L'hypoplasie segmentaire aglomérulaire du rein. I. Lésions rénales associées. Sem Hop Paris. 50:601.
21. Baxter T. 1965. Cysts arising in the renal corpuscle. Arch Dis Child. 40:455.
22. Vlachos J, Tsakraklidis V. 1967. Glomerular cysts. An unusual variety of "polycystic kidneys": report of two cases. Am J Dis Child. 114:379.

23. Taxy JB, Filmer RB. 1976. Glomerulocystic kidney. Report of a case. Arch Pathol Lab Med. 100:186.
24. Shokeir MHK. 1978. Expression of "adult" polycystic renal disease in the fetus and newborn. Clin Genet. 14:61.
25. Bengtsson U, Hedman L, Svalander C. 1975. Adult type of polycystic kidney disease in a new-born child. Acta Med Scand. 197:447.
26. Ross DG, Travers H. 1975. Infantile presentation of adult-type polycystic kidney disease in a large kindred. J Pediatr. 87:760.
27. Fellows RA, Leonidas JC, Beatty EC Jr. 1976. Radiologic features of "adult type" polycystic kidney disease in the neonate. Pediatr Radiol. 4:87.
28. Bernstein J. 1979. Hereditary renal disease. Kidney Disease-Present Status, IAP Monograph, Ch 13. Baltimore, Williams & Wilkins.
29. Evan AP, Gardner KD Jr, Bernstein J. 1979. Polypoid and papillary epithelial hyperplasia: a potential cause of ductal obstruction in adult polycystic disease. Kidney Int. 16:743.
30. Stickler GB, Kelalis PP. 1975. Polycystic kidney disease. Recognition of the "adult form" (autosomal dominant) in infancy. Mayo Clin Proc. 50:547.

The Glomerular Morphology of Membranoproliferative Glomerulonephritis (MPGN)

A. James McAdams, M.D.

Morphologically the lesion of MPGN is characterized by proliferative change of the glomerular tuft with alteration of the capillary wall and associated with glomerular deposits. Three types of MPGN have been described, each with distinctive features, often allowing correct assessment by standard light and immunohistologic techniques. Significant difficulty in correct diagnosis by these means is, however, frequent enough to justify confirmation by ultrastructure whenever possible.

Mesangial proliferation is usually conspicuous in all types but is the notable feature of type I MPGN. Consequently, due to the diffuse mesangial proliferation, glomerular enlargement and lobulation are greater and more frequently seen in type I than in the other types. Irregularity of proliferation within the tuft is characteristic of types II & III but in some instances of these types the severity and diffuseness of the process is such that the H&E appearance is indistinguishable from type I.

In all forms of MPGN, the thickening of the capillary wall is produced primarily by interposition of mesangial cytoplasm between the basement membrane and endothelial cells, and contributed to by subendothelial deposit. Although splitting of the basement membrane is popularly spoken of, this technically does not occur. The tram-tracking appearance often seen in PAS preparations is attributable to the non-staining of the mesangial cytoplasm interposed in the capillary wall. In some instances, new lamina densa, as demonstrated ultrastructurally may be seen between the interposed mesangial cytoplasm or deposit and the endothelial cell. This may give rise to a split appearance in the silver stained section. Since severe mesangial proliferation is more characteristic of type I MPGN, it is not surprising that mesangial interposition is also more severe in type I. This results in a severe reduction of apparent capillary lumens in the histologic preparation.

Identification of the subtypes of MPGN is accomplished by determining the relationship of the lamina densa to the deposits in the capillary loop. From the descriptive advances that have been made in MPGN utilizing electron microscopy, particularly the silver impregnated electron micrograph, it would be anticipated that proper distinction can be made using a silver stained histologic preparation. While this is often the case there have been sufficient occasions of error in our own hands in the case of type I & III to indicate that ultrastructure is essential for final classification.

Silver impregnated electron micrographs greatly simplify the task of identification. Lamina densa and the basement membrane-like material of the mesangial matrix are densely impregnated by the silver methenamine and collagen fibers, when present, have a distinct beaded appearance. Deposit material maintains essentially the same electron density seen in uranyl acetate-lead citrate stained preparation. In type I MPGN, the lamina densa is clearly intact with only occasional minor imperfections. In type II MPGN, the bulbous thickenings appreciated in the standard EM preparation as dense deposit, impregnate with silver in a manner not clearly distinguishable from normal lamina densa. Abrupt transitions from normal lamina densa are common and support the notion that the dense deposit is a form of basement membrane. In type III MPGN, the basement membrane alterations are complex. Deposit material is abundant and located both subendothelial and sub-epithelial. In addition there is much interruption of the lamina densa and elaboration of new lamina densa. This process leads to an appearance of duplication of the lamina densa and, in the advanced lesion, stretches of a fenestrated-like membrane may result.

Translating these observations to the Jones preparation, in type I MPGN the lamina densa should be observed as an intact black line producing a smooth outline of the lobules. In type II MPGN, the thickened lamina densa resists the gold toning of the procedure and appears as a brown icing of the capillary loop. In type III the lamina densa in many areas is impossible to define and there may be an appearance of grains of silver in its place.

Although the 3 types of MPGN cannot be reliable differentiated by immunohistology there are helpful observations to be made. A fringe pattern (outlining the perimeter of the tuft) is most often seen in type I MPGN. This appears to be a consequence of the severity of the mesangial proliferation since a similar pattern in seen in the severely proliferative forms of types II & III. A labeling pattern corresponding to the capillary loops is more characteristic of types II & III. While the incidence of labeling with antiserum to IgG is essentially invariable in the case of childhood type I MPGN, it is quite variable in type II and seldom occurs in type III. It should be noted that in the case of type II the anti IgG does not label the dense deposit. All types of MPGN label with antiserum to C_3. In the case of type II MPGN an unusually sharply defined extensive linear label of the capillary wall is most suggestive of this diagnosis.

Labeling of deposits with antiserum to C_3 in a mesangial distribution is common with all types of MPGN but the deposits are often unusually coarse and discrete in type II. Of importance is the fact that type II MPGN does not label with antiserum to properdin. Irregular label of scattered tubule basement membranes is often seen in type II but this can also occur in the presence of tubular atrophy in any form of renal disease.

REFERENCES
1. Appropriate references may be found in the review article. The Chronic Glomerulonephritis of Childhood, Part II. Clark D. West & A. James McAdams, M.D. J. Peds. 93: 167, 1978.

344

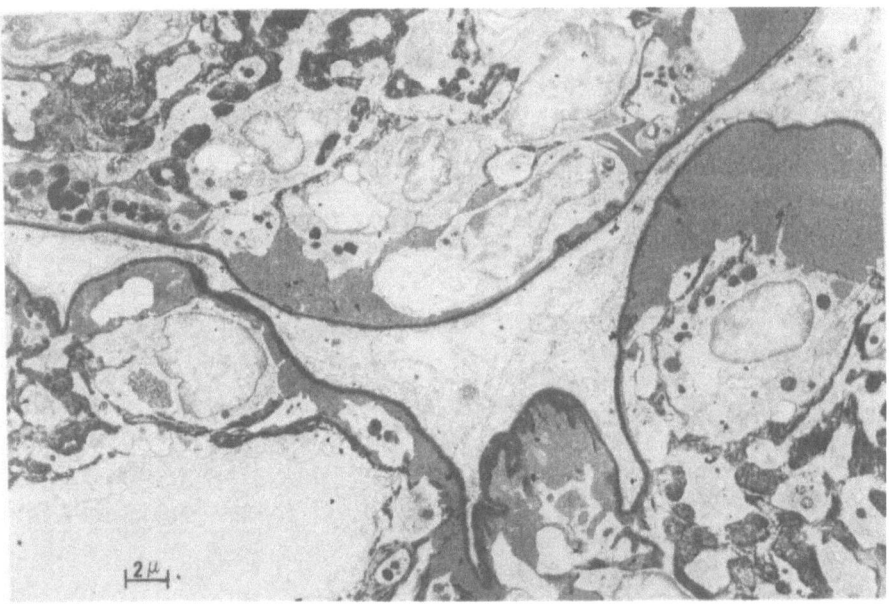

Figure 1 Silver impregnated electromicrograph of type I membranoproliferative glomerulonephritis. The silver blackened lamina densa of normal thickness is intact, delineating the outer limits of the capillary wall. Electron dense but not silver impregnated deposit material is seen extensively in a sub-endothelial location. Deposit material with proliferated mesangial matrix is also visualized, as seen in the left upper corner.

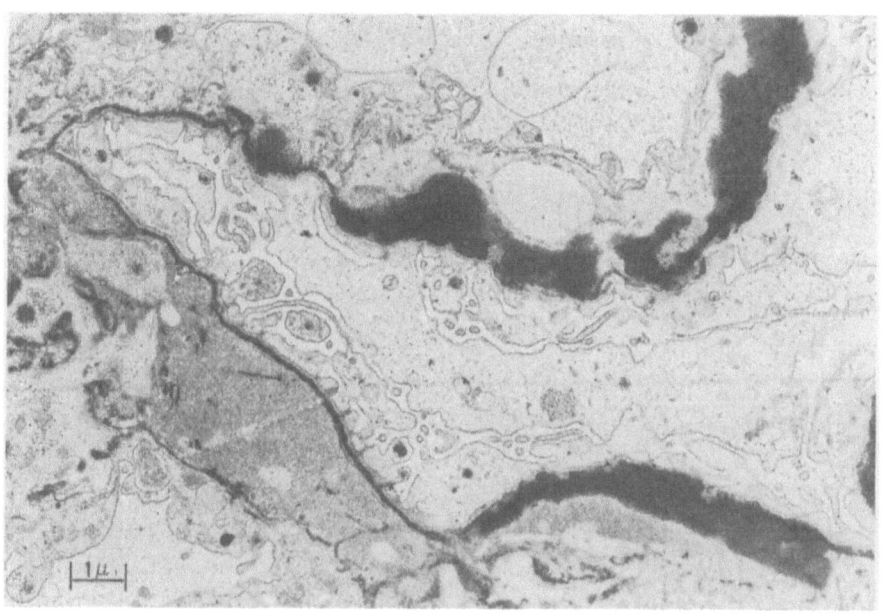

Figure 2   Silver impregnated electromicrograph of type II membranoproliferative glomerulonephritis. As one follows the normal lamina densa, seen in the left portion of the photograph, there are abrupt transitions to bulbous silver impregnated thickenings in the position of the lamina densa. This basement membrane-like substance is the dense deposit. Also shown are subendothelial electron dense deposits and in the lower left new lamina densa between the deposit and endothelial cell.

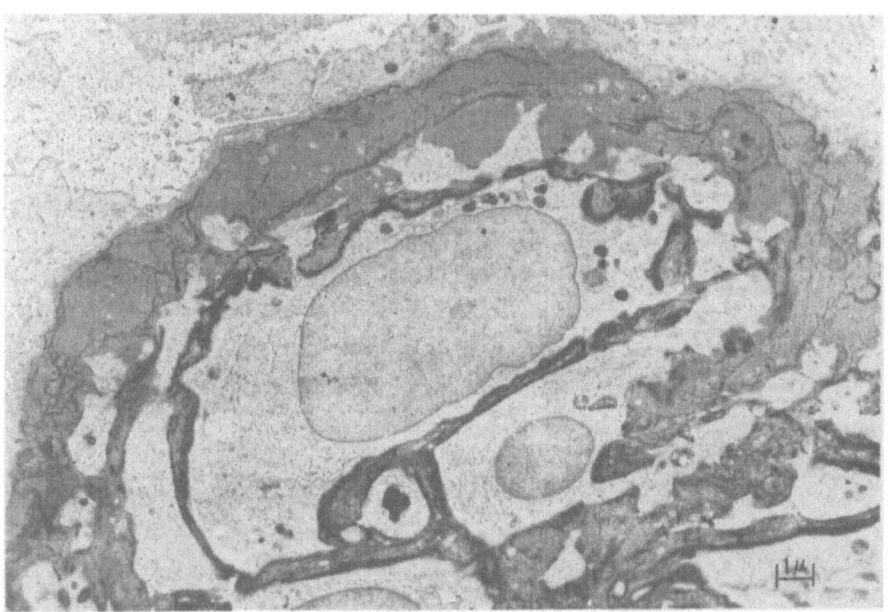

Figure 3   Silver impregnated electronmicrograph of type III membranoproliferative glomerulonephritis. Shown is massive alteration of the capillary wall by deposit material. Original lamina densa cannot be identified. Sub-endothelial and sub-epithelial deposits are in essence in continuity and this associated with extensive breaks and duplications of the lamina densa, produces this complex appearance of the wall. In the right lower portion of the photograph deposit material can be seen in the mesangial matrix.

CIRCULATING IMMUNE COMPLEXES AND SYSTEMIC LUPUS ERYTHEMATOSUS

EDMUND J. LEWIS, M.D. and JIMMY L. ROBERTS, M.D.

INTRODUCTION

The immunopathologic features of systemic lupus erythematosus appear analogous to the vascular lesions found in experimental serum sickness (1). Ultrastructural and immunopathologic studies reveal the deposition of immune aggregates not only in various renal structures, but also in the pulmonary alveolar capillary bed (2), myocardial vessels (3), choroid plexus (4) and the media of larger arteries (5). Because the development vascular lesions in experimental acute serum sickness appears at a time when there are circulating immune complexes, much attention has been centered around the role of these complexes in the pathogenesis of inflammatory diseases of small vessels.

Systemic lupus erythematosus provides an excellent model for the study of the role of immune complexes in the pathogenesis of renal diseases. Circulating immune complexes have been readily demonstrated in the serum of patients with this disease (6). In addition, the variability of histologic lesions found in lupus nephritis provides an interesting model for the investigation of qualitative and quantitative variations seen in circulating immune complexes in these patients.

Circulating Immune Complex Assays in Patients with Lupus

We have studied the serum of patients with proliferative lupus glomerulonephritis and membranous lupus glomerulonephritis in order to determine whether quantitative differences could be found in the levels of immune complexes seen in these patients (6). In addition, 10 patients with membranous glomerulonephritis of idiopathic nature, or associated with secondary causes other than lupus, were studied. The assays used were the Raji cell radioimmunoassay, the solid phase Clq binding assay and total serum cryoprecipitable immunoglobulins (cryoglobulins). In our laboratory the normal values are as follows: Raji cell assay 16.8 µG/ml ± 25.2 (2 SD); Clq binding assay upper limits of normal 10 µG/ml; cryoglobulin assay mean 14 µG/ml ± 7 (2 SD).

We found in the proliferative glomerulonephritis group that cryoglobulins were present in all 13 patients, Clq binding assay was positive in 11 and the Raji cell assay was positive in 10. Amongst patients with membranous lupus, the cryoglobulins were positive in 9 of 10 patients, Clq binding assay was positive in 8 and Raji cell assay in 5. The "control" group of non-lupus membranous glomerulonephritis patients had 4 positives for cryoglobulins and 1 patient positive in each of the Raji and Clq binding assays. These positive specimens in the latter group were obtained from patients with membranous glomerulonephritis associated with neoplasia or hepatitis. The idiopathic membranous patients had negative immune complex assays. Correlations among these assays revealed that the best correlation occurred between the cryoglobulin and Raji cell assay ($r = 0.793$; $p < 0.001$), however a significant correlation was also seen between the cryoglobulin and Clq binding assay and the Clq binding assay and Raji cell assay. It should be noted that 8 of 20 sera which were positive in either the Raji cell assay or Clq binding assay were not reactive in both. These discrepancies reflect the fact that the two assays measure different properties of immune complexes.

The amount of immune complexes varied considerably within each group, however patients with proliferative glomerulonephritis had significantly higher immune complex levels in each of the assays. Within the proliferative group the mean level of Clq binding activity was 156 ± 74 µG/ml (SD); Raji assay revealed 198 ± 216 µG/ml and cryoglobulins revealed 207 ± 194 µG/ml. In membranous lupus Clq binding assay revealed a mean of 73.5 ± 50 µG/ml, while the Raji cell assay revealed a mean of 47.8 ± 38.3 µG/ml and cryoglobulins 61.5 ± 45 µG/ml. These results reveal that proliferative lupus glomerulonephritis is associated with greater levels of circulating immune complexes than membranous lupus. In addition the results suggest that a single immune complex assay may not be adequate for a complete characterization of the circulating immune complexes in a given patient or disease state.

Investigation of the Components of Cryoprecipitable Immuno-globulins

Several investigators have provided evidence that cryopre-cipitable immunoglobulins (cryoglobulins) represent immune complexes (7,8). DNA and antiDNA complexes have been detected in the cryoglobulins from patients with systemic lupus erythematosus. Cryoglobulins from patients with systemic lupus contain antibodies directed against native DNA antigens (8,9). These antibodies may not be readily demonstrable, as they behave as if they are bound to antigen. Pretreatment of the cryoglobulin with acid, in order to dissociate immune complexes, or DNAase II, in order to destroy bound DNA, allows the demonstration of antinative DNA antibody activity using the Farr assay for DNA binding, immunofluorescence technique or counterimmunoelectrophoresis (CIE). DNA can also be demonstrated in cryoprecipitates utilizing either CIE or the ethidium bromide assay for double stranded polynucleotides. However, again, it is difficult to detect DNA unless the samples are pre-digested utilizing protease in order to destroy cryoprecipi-table proteins. Protease digestion of cryoglobulins leaves the DNA component intact and readily detectable. That these two components of cryoprecipitates can behave as antigen and antibody can be shown using CIE. If an aliquot of a cryoglobulin is pre-digested with DNAase and a second aliquot predigested by protease, the DNA and antiDNA components left by these digestions can then be shown to interact and form an immunoprecipitin band utilizing CIE.

In addition to the identification of the components of DNA-antiDNA immune complexes in cryoglobulins, the reactivity of cryoglobulins was tested in other immune complex tests. We have been able to show that serum depleted of cryoglobulin has decreased measurable immune complexes according to either the Clq binding or Raji cell assays. In addition, isolated cryoglobulins added to normal serum can be shown to react as do immune complexes utilizing these latter assays.

Characterization of Cryoprecipitable Immune Complexes

We have studied cryoglobulins from four patients with lupus using sucrose density gradient ultracentrifugation in order to determine the molecular weight of this fraction of immune complexes (10). The highest level of IgG, immune complex reactivity and immune-bound IgG antinative DNA antibody were demonstrated in 6.5 to 10 S fractions in all samples. Immune-bound IgG and IgM antinative DNA antibodies were identified in lower quantity in higher (17-30 S) molecular weight fractions. Protease digestion of the gradient fractions and subsequent testing with ethidium bromide for double stranded DNA revealed reactive material in the 6.5 to 10 S samples, as well as in heavier fractions, indicating double stranded DNA to be present in the same fractions as antiDNA antibody of the IgG class. It therefore appears that a fraction of the circulating immune complexes in lupus are of low molecular weight and contain antinative DNA and double stranded polynucleotides. These low molecular weight cryoprecipitable circulating immune complexes may constitute the major proportion of DNA-antinative DNA immune complexes in lupus patients with glomerulonephritis.

DISCUSSION

The presence of immune aggregates in damaged organs in lupus undoubtedly reflects the immunopathogenesis of that disease. However, the relationship between circulating immune complexes and organ damage remains obscure. Circulating immune complexes are readily demonstrable in the serum of patients with lupus and our studies indicate that these may be of low molecular weight. In view of the decreased affinity of cells of the macrophage-phagocytic system for soluble, low molecular weight immune complexes (11), it is possible that DNA-antiDNA may have a prolonged serum half-life which predisposes to the formation of immune deposits. A second point of view is represented by the possibility that immune aggregates found in damaged organs occur as the result of in situ formation of the aggregates, rather than the deposition of preformed immune complexes. This mechanism, represented experimentally by the Arthus phenomenon, has been suggested by Couser et al (12) and Hoedemaeker et al (13). Indeed, some

of the immunopathologic variation seen in the kidney in lupus
may be due to varying degrees of activity of these two mechanisms.
It is critical that we understand the latter issue, insofar as
we must know whether the diminution of serum immune complex
levels or of free antibody production is central to the management of patients with lupus.

REFERENCES

1. Dixon FJ, Feldman JD, Vazquez JJ: Experimental glomerulo-
    nephritis. The pathogenesis of laboratory model resembling
    the spectrum of human glomerulonephritis. J. Exp. Med. 113:
    899, 1961.
2. Eagen JW, Memoli VA, Roberts JL, Matthew GR, Schwartz MM,
    Lewis EJ: Pulmonary hemorrhage in systemic lupus erythema-
    tosus. Medicine 57:545, 1978.
3. Bidani AK, Roberts JL, Schwartz MM, Lewis EJ: Immunopathology
    of cardiac lesions in fatal systemic lupus erythematosus.
    Amer. J. Med., in press.
4. Atkins C, Kondon J,Jr., Quismorio F: The choroid plexus in
    systemic lupus erythematosus. Ann. Intern. Med. 76:65, 1972.
5. Eagen JW, Roberts JL, Schwartz MM, Lewis EJ: The composition
    of pulmonary immune deposits in systemic lupus erythematosus.
    Clin. Immun. Immunopathol. 12:204, 1979.
6. Robinson MF, Roberts JL, Jones JV, Lewis EJ: Circulating
    immune complex assays in patients with lupus and membranous
    glomerulonephritis. Clin. Immun. Immunopathol. 14:348, 1979.
7. Winfield JB, Koffler D, Kunkel HG: Specific concentration of
    polynucleotide immune complexes in the cryoprecipitates of
    patients with systemic lupus erythematosus. J. Clin. Invest.
    56:563, 1975.
8. Roberts JL, Lewis EJ: Immunochemical demonstration of cryo-
    precipitable antinative DNA antibody and DNA in the serum of
    patients with glomerulonephritis. J. Immunol. 124:127, 1980.
9. Roberts JL, Lewis EJ: Identification of anti-native DNA
    antibodies in cryoglobulinemic states. Amer. J. Med. 65:437,
    1978.
10. Roberts JL, Robinson MF, Lewis EJ: Low molecular weight
    plasma cryoprecipitable anti-native DNA:polynucleotide com-
    plexes in lupus glomerulonephritis. Clin. Immunol. Immuno-
    pathol. in press.
11. Mannik M, Arend WP, Hall AP: Studies on atnigen-antibody com-
    plexes. I.Elimination of soluble complexes from rabbit cir-
    culation. J. Exp. Med. 133:713, 1971.
12. Couser WG, Steinmuller DR, Stilmant MM, Salant DJ, Lowenstein
    LM: Experimental glomerulonephritis in the isolated perfused
    rat kidney. J. Clin. Invest. 62:1275, 1978.
13. Fleuren GJ, Lee RVD, Greben HA, VanDamme BJC, Hoedemaeker PJ:
    Experimental glomerulonephritis in the rat induced by anti-
    bodies directed against tubular antigens.IV. Investigations
    into the pathogenesis of the model. Lab. Invest. 38:498, 1978.

FOCAL GLOMERULOSCLEROSIS - A REVIEW

D.R. TURNER

The precise definition of a disease entity is often
very difficult, and all we are doing in glomerulonephritis
is dividing it up into a number of what we hope are useful
categories. It seems to me that the criticisms which have
been levelled at the acceptance of focal glomerulosclerosis
as an entity, can equally be used to attack a well-accepted
category such as membranous glomerulonephritis. It is
suggested that focal sclerosing lesions can be produced by
different aetiological factors, but this is also true of
membranous glomerulonephritis. It has been pointed out that
patients with segmental sclerosing lesions do not always have
a uniform prognosis and yet we know that 25% of membranous
cases may recover spontaneously. It has also been pointed
out that focal sclerosing lesions may complicate other
patterns of disease. This also applies to the membranous
pattern which can be seen in lupus nephritis and superimposed
on mesangio-capillary glomerulonephritis. Finally we now
have quite good evidence of recurrence of focal glomerulosclerosis in renal transplants, yet this is rare in
membranous glomerulonephritis. On this evidence it would
seem that focal glomerulosclerosis is at least as reliable an
entity as membranous glomerulonephritis. For the purpose of
this account I intend to ignore focal global glomerulosclerosis which several workers have shown to have the same
prognosis as minimal change disease.

Focal segmental glomerulosclerosis can be summarised as
a condition occurring in children or adults with a heavy,
non-selective proteinuria, often of nephrotic proportions,
and often associated with microscopic haematuria. A renal
biopsy shows focal segmental sclerosing lesions early in the
course of the disease, although these may be missed in a
superficial biopsy since they are maximal in the deep
cortex. The segmental lesions may contain cells with
"foamy" cytoplasm or hyaline eosinophilic accumulations of
protein seen by light microscopy, and may be situated
either in the para-hilar position or peripherally. There
may be some proliferation of the overlying epithelial
cells but this is insufficient to warrant the term
"cellular crescent". Associated with the glomerular lesions
which gradually extend to involve a large portion of the
glomerulus and to involve more glomeruli, is an increasing

degree of focal tubular atrophy.

The immuno-peroxidase technique shows that there is intense staining of lgM and C3 in the segmental glomerular lesions but this is normally restricted to these sites, in contrast to the diffuse lgG and lgA staining of mesangical regions seen in proliferative glomerulonephritis with focal scarring. The former pattern of staining for lgM and C3 we find to be a reliable and consistent indicator of focal segmental glomerulosclerosis.

Electron microscopy in most cases of focal glomerulo-sclerosis shows that the "normal" glomeruli by light microscopy have foot-process fusion which indicates that there is a diffuse leakage of protein through all glomeruli. The segmental lesions in some cases show degenerative changes in the overlying epithelial cells, but this change can also be seen in many other forms of severe glomerular damage (Cohen et al., 1977) and I do not regard the electron microscopy as contributing significantly to the diagnosis.

Patients with the condition of F.G.S. as I have defined, differ radically from those with minimal change disease in that they normally are resistant to treatment with cortico-steroids and alkylating agents, have a marked tendency to become hypertensive and the majority progress slowly towards end-stage renal failure.

It is however important to appreciate that some 12% of patients with F.G.S. persue a particularly rapid downhill course to chronic renal failure (Brown et al., 1978) and it has been suggested by some workers that the presence of a hyper-cellular mesangium in F.G.S. indicates a worse prognosis (Schoeneman et al., 1978). However in our experience this was not a reliable indicator, and confirmation has been obtained by White et al., (1980) in a free communication given at this meeting.

The fact that F.G.S. tends to recur in renal transplants is well known. In our series of 25 patients whose original diagnosis was F.G.S. and who have been transplanted, 5 have developed a nephrotic syndrome at an early stage and have also been shown to have the classical histology on renal biopsy of the transplant kidney. It is worth noting that four of the five recurrences were under the age of 15 years and had had a rapid progression to renal failure. The recurrence of F.G.S. in a renal transplant may lead to loss of the graft, but some patients with recurrent disease remain with good function for many years despite profuse proteinuria or the nephrotic syndrome.

It is important to appreciate that focal segmental sclerosing lesions with hyalinosis may occur as a complication of many other conditions including:-

a)   membranous glomerulonephritis

b)   malarial nephropathy

c)   scarred focal proliferative glomerulonephritis.

d)   Alport's syndrome

e)   renal transplants (? recurrent F.G.S.)

f)   diabetic glomerulopathy

g)   heroin addiction

h)   ischaemia/hypertension

i)   reflux nephropathy

Presumably one is looking at a particular pattern of scarring which can occur in glomeruli as a result of a wide range of different aetiological factors. It is clearly important to identify the underlying pathology if one exists.

Aetiology:-

a) Is F.G.S. a complication of relapsing minimal change? Not if one restricts the definition as I have done to cases in which segmental lesions are present early in the course of the disease. One has to admit that in chronically relapsing minimal change disease, the classical histology may be seen in a biopsy taken some 5 years or more after onset of disease. However in this setting the prognosis is not significantly different from relapsing minimal change without segmental lesions, and does not carry the poor prognosis of F.G.S.

b)   Despite the presence of lgM and C3 in the segmental lesions there seems to be little support for the idea that F.G.S. has an immune pathogeneis, and·I intend therefore to reject that hypothesis.

c)   The idea that a chronic intravascular coagulation might be involved is suggested by a number of factors. George et al. in 1974 showed that there was an abnormal consumption of platelets and fibrinogen in F.G.S. These findings were confirmed in more detailed studies by Futrakul et al (1978).

Further support comes from the observations by Taylor and Novak that pregnancy has an adverse effect on patients with F.G.S. We know that pregnancy sensitises the female to intravascular coagulation and it is presumably this process which exacerbates F.G.S. in pregnancy. Certainly the morphology of the segmental sclerosing lesions and their position would be consistent with a low grade chronic intravascular coagulation.

d) The suggestion that F.G.S. may be the result of heavy proteinuria does not really help us to understand what is occurring, even if it were true. It seems more likely that some noxious influence causes both the proteinuria, the damage to epithelial cells and the segmental sclerosing lesions. Indeed, the experimental evidence (Glasser et al. 1977), that repeated doses of aminonucleoside result in lesions identical with focal glomerulosclerosis suggests that in man we should be looking for some form of circulating toxic substance which perhaps acts as a trigger for a chronic form of intravascular coagulation involving preferentially the juxta-medullary glomeruli.

In summary it seems that focal segmental glomerulosclerosis should be regarded as a clinically useful category provided the patient develops the classical histology early in the course of his or her disease and that it should not include examples of focal global sclerosis. Its significance relates to its failure to respond to treatment with steroids and alkylating agents, its poor prognosis and the 1 in 5 chance of recurring following renal transplantation.

REFERENCES

1. Brown CB. Cameron JS. Turner DR. Chantler C. Ogg CS. Williams DG. and Béwick M. (1978). Focal segmental glomerulosclerosis with rapid decline in renal function ("malignant FSGS"). Clinical Nephrology Vol. 10 p51-61.
2. Cohen AH. Mampaso F. and Zamboni L. (1977) Glomerular Podocyte Degeneration in Human Renal Disease. Lab. Invest. Vol. 37 p30-42.
3. Futrakul P. Poshyachinda M. and Mitrakul C. (1978). Focal sclerosing glomerulonephritis. A kinetic evaluation of hemostasis and effect of anti-coagulant therapy. Clinical Nephrology. Vol. 10, 180-186.
4. George CRP. Slichter SJM Quadracci LJ. Striker GE. and Harker LA. (1974). Kinetic evaluation of hemostasis in renal disease. N. Eng. J. Med. 291, 1111-1115.
5. Glasser RJ. Velosa JA. and Michael AF. (1977). Experimental Model of Focal Sclerosis. 1) Relationship to Protein excretion in aminonucleoside nephrosis. Lab. Invest. Vol. 36 p519-526.
6. Schoeneman MJ. Bennett B. and Greifer I (1978). The natural history of focal segmental glomerulosclerosis with and without mesangial hypercellularity in children. Clinical Nephrology Vol. 9 p45-54.
7. Taylor J. Novak R. Christiansen R. and Sorensen ET. (1978) Focal sclerosing glomerulopathy with adverse effects during pregnancy. Arch. Int. Med. Vol. 138 p1695-1696.
8. White RHR. Yoshikawa N. and Cameron AH. (1980) Prognostic factors in segmental glomerulosclerosis (Abstract) Pediatric Research Vol. 14 p997.

ULTRASOUND EVALUATION OF THE CHILD'S URINARY TRACT

G.C. ARNEIL AND E.M. SWEET

Pulsed ultrasound has been used in this hospital since 1972 for investigation of urinary tract disorders in the newborn and older children. As techniques have improved and experience has been gained it has become possible to expand and to evaluate the place of this technique more fully.

Sonar is particularly useful because it demonstrates renal tract anatomy and is not dependant on function. Amongst its good qualities are: -

(1) It is non-invasive and painless.

(2) It is non-ionizing.

(3) Reasonable repetition is believed to be safe.

(4) In acute or chronic renal failure or in renal shut-down accurate data on kidney shape, size and structure are readily obtained.

(5) Differentiation of solid structures from fluids and semi-solids is practicable.

Ultrasound is used for the following purposes:-

(1) Location and definition of the normal renal tract.

(2) Anatomical demonstration of congenital or acquired abnormalities in the site, size and structure of the kidney.

(3) Detection and differentiation of cysts and solid tumours within or outwith organs and of tumour spread.

(4) Demonstration of pyonephrosis.

(5) Demonstration of calculus.

(6) Monitoring of kidney transplant.

(7) Locating site for renal biopsy or cyst puncture.

(8) Demonstrating site and degree of urinary tract obstruction.

(9) Demonstration of bladder abnormalities and tumours.

Conventional radiology, C.A.T. scanning, sonar and nuclear medicine techniques all have their place in renal tract investigation and should be seen as complementing one another. The broad distinctions, between sonar and C.A.T. scanning as the anatomical investigations, as opposed to nuclear medicine providing the physiological facts in a particular situation, with conventional radiography contrast studies in between, are no longer valid. With continually improving techniques the method employed will inevitably vary with local expertise and comparative examination costs as well as with radiation hazards. The non-ionizing radiation employed is still one of the greatest advantages of sonar examination. Despite recent work indicating that sonar may not be completely hazard free it is still believed to be significantly safer than ionizing radiations.

Technical advances in ultrasound equipment introduced grey-scaling enabling enhanced differentiation of echo levels and therefore increased information on internal organ structure permitting differentiation of renal pyramids and medulla from cortex. Recent trends are towards the use of real time contact scanning units which allow immediate recognition of vascular structures by their pulsations, thereby speeding up examinations by allowing more rapid identification of scanning planes. Suitable transducers which adapt readily to paediatric use are now available - those introduced initially were too bulky.

RADIONUCLIDE IMAGING IN PEDIATRIC NEPHROLOGY: AN UPDATE

H.T. HARCKE, M.D.

During the past decade the use of radionuclide imaging in the evaluation of children with disorders of the urinary tract has gained wide acceptance. The development of low radiation dose agents coupled with improvements in imaging systems has made the radionuclide study suitable for use in pediatrics.

Radionuclide, radiographic and ultrasound studies should be viewed as complementary not competing examinations. The principal advantage of radionuclide studies is that images which provide dynamic and functional information are obtained. Radionuclide images, however, lack the precise anatomic and structural detail found in images obtained with x-ray and ultrasound. By the selection of the appropriate radionuclide and imaging sequence it is possible to analyze renal blood flow, filtration function, tubular function, cortical mass or the serial passage of urine through the kidney, collecting system and bladder. In some instances, a single tracer will assess several of these aspects of function.

Radionuclide studies can provide adequate images of the urinary tract in situations where the use of contrast urography is not feasible. The ability to detect the presence of functioning renal tissue, when it cannot be successfully imaged radiographically or sonographically has prompted the use of radionuclide imaging in the search for ectopic and hypoplastic kidneys. Radionuclide imaging of the kidney is successful even when renal function is severely impaired. As a result, radionuclide studies are widely used in evaluating renal transplants.

The ability to quantitate radionuclides has led to the marriage of the scintilation camera or detector and the digital computer. Much of the information we now obtain from radionuclide studies of the urinary tract is derived from individual and serial images which were stored and subsequently processed in dedicated nuclear medicine computer systems. As an illustration of how advantages offered by radionuclide imaging are being applied to work in pediatric nephrology three types of studies are reviewed: 1) Assessment of Relative Renal Function, 2) Radionuclide Cystography and 3) Diuretic Renography.

(1) <u>Assessment of Relative Renal Function</u>

When discrepancies in renal size or function are established it is useful to numerically relate the size or relative function of the two kidneys. In the case of a duplex system the upper and lower poles of the same kidney can be assessed for relative function. Such quantification provides a more objective means for comparing serial studies. Most of the available radionuclides are suitable for relative function studies. After a study has been acquired by a digital computer, selected images from the renal study are displayed and the kidneys are designated as separate regions of interest using the computer. Adjacent areas of the abdomen are also designated and used to measure background activity. Following correction of the radionuclide activity from each kidney for background, the activity in that kidney can be expressed as a percent of the combined renal activity. This provides a relative approximation of each kidney's contribution to the patient's overall renal function. (1)

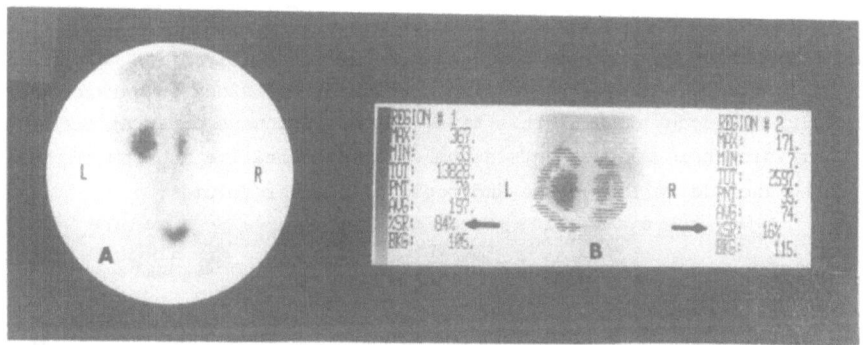

FIGURE I. REFER TO TEXT

The study illustrated in Fig. 1A, was performed with technetium-99m diethylenetrianine pentacetic acid (Tc-99m DTPA). It shows a small right kidney. The image was obtained at 1.5 minutes post injection and represents the nephrogram phase. At this time the radionuclide is in the renal cortex and will be subsequently filtered and fill the collecting system. In the nephrogram phase kidney activity is proportional to the amount of functioning cortex. Fig. 1B shows the computer generated approximation of relative function. Regions of interest have been placed over each kidney and background; averaged background activity has been calculated and used to correct the renal counts. The computer generated approximation indicates that the small right kidney contributes 16% of the child's relative renal function. This calculation can be repeated on successive studies and enables the clinician to follow the patient's course more objectively.

(2) Radionuclide Cystography

Radionuclide cystography is not a new study in pediatric nuclear medicine, but it is still grossly under utilized. Radionuclide images are used to detect vesicoureteral reflux and quantitate some aspects of bladder function. Cystography images detect ureteral reflux with a high degree of sensitivity

360

except when there is minimal reflux entering only the distal ureter since this can be masked by the bladder. The study has the advantage of providing information at a radiation dose 50-100 times less than that received in conventional radiographic cystography. (2,3)

Following catheterization of the urinary bladder, the bladder is filled with saline to which 1.0 millicurie of a Tc-99m labelled agent has been added (Tc-99m pertechnetate alone is suitable). During bladder filling the patient is monitored by a technologist or physician who observes the scintillation camera display oscilliscope (film imaging and/or computer acquisition are customarily obtained as well). Vesicoureteral reflux is seen on the oscilliscope and images as tracer activity above the dome of the bladder. Following complete bladder filling, the catheter is removed and the patient voids into a urinal or bedpan while under observation. We find this can be conveniently done by sitting the patient up with his back against the vertically oriented camera head. It is important that the voiding portion of the study is carried out since reflux may occur only at this time. With continuous observation and recording of volumetric measurements a number of quantitative assessments can be made, these include reflux volume and residual bladder volumes.

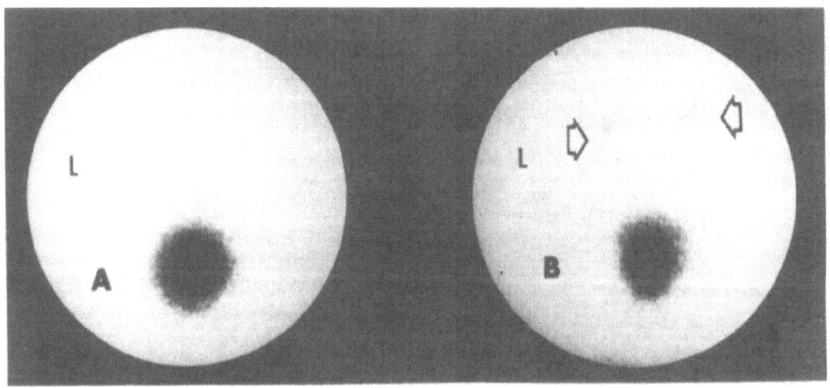

FIGURE 2. REFER TO TEXT

The radionuclide cystogram in Figure 2 illustrates the findings seen with bilateral reflux that occurred during the act of voiding. With passive filling of the bladder (Fig. 2A) activity was seen only in the bladder. During voiding (Fig. 2B) the bladder contracted and reflux to the level of the kidneys occurred.

(3) Diuretic Renography

Hydronephrosis and/or hydroureter secondary to mechanical obstruction can be difficult to differentiate from the same changes secondary to atony or dysmorphism. Diuretic radionuclide renography has provided a non-invasive method which appears to be successful in distinguishing these two entities. This procedure uses diuretic stimulation in conjunction with the conventional radionuclide study performed with Tc-99m DTPA. (1,4) It illustrates several of the advantages of nuclear studies noted above, most notably the ability to quantify function through the use of a scintillation camera/digital computer system.

The patient is injected with the appropriate dose of Tc-99m DTPA and several renal images are obtained. Images can be simultaneously acquired in the computer. When the collecting system and/or ureter of the abnormal system has filled with radionuclide (usually 20-30 minutes post injection) the diuretic phase of the study can be initiated. We use furosemide, 0.5 mg/kg which is administered intravenously. It is our practice to have the patient void prior to receiving the diuretic. Before injection we position the patient prone or erect and begin computer acquisition of serial images to establish the baseline level of activity in the kidneys and/or ureters. After 3-5 minutes the diuretic is injected; sequential imaging is continued for an additional 15-20 minutes without the patient changing position.

Following collection of this series of images the computer is used to designate regions of interest which correspond to the location of the kidneys and/or ureters. The kidney regions should include the collecting system and renal pelvis; ureters should be designated as separate regions if they show retention of the tracer. Time/activity curves can then be generated for each region and recorded. We have not found it necessary to apply background correction.

A dilated collecting system which is unobstructed will show a change in the configuration of its time/activity curve. Approximately 5 minutes after receiving the diuretic there will be a decrease in activity in the system as the increased flow of urine flushes out the tracer. A distinctive change in the slope of the curve is noted. If static images are acquired during this study they may show this change visually; however, in severely dilated systems the count density may be such that the change in activity is difficult to appreciate and curves should always be obtained. The curve generated from a dilated, obstructed collecting system shows no abrupt change in slope in response to the diuretic. A plateau configuration may continue or the curve may rise slightly if the activity in the system countinues to increase. There are occasions where the curve configuration will show a response that must be considered indeterminate. In this instance, the activity in the system shows a slight, gradual decrease, but without a distinct change in slope. Some people utilize slope measurements to more objectively define criteria for classifying the response. It should be noted that a curve obtained from a normal kidney may show little or no response to diuretic stimulation since it will have drained well by the time the diuretic is given and therefore has no significant activity to wash out.

There are pitfalls to be aware of in performing diuretic renography. Experience with this new procedure indicates that many factors influence the study and create the potential for misinterpretation of the results. A crucial consideration in detecting if a dilated system is mechanically obstructed is whether there is a sufficient kidney function to sustain diuresis. The state

362

of hydration, position of the patient, presence of vesicoureteral reflux, and
the amount of urine in the bladder also appears to have the potential for affecting the study. Careful attention must be paid to these factors and presently there is variation in the techniques used in this examination.

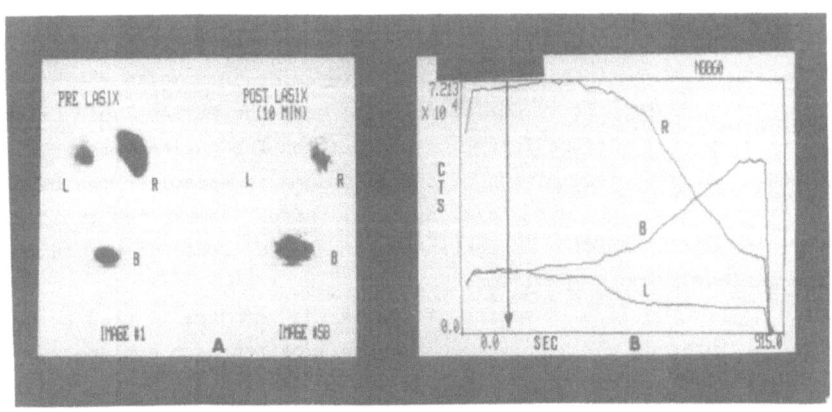

FIGURE 3. REFER TO TEXT

The illustrative case presented in Figure 3 is that of a child who had a
pyelostomy performed to relieve a uretero-pelvic junction obstruction. The
excretory urogram showed a right hydronephrosis which was unchanged in appearance when compared with a pre-operative study. Thirty minutes after the
administration of Tc-99m DTPA the dilatation and stasis in the collecting system of the kidney is evident on the posterior image (Fig. 3A-left). A posterior image (Fig. 3A-right) obtained 10 minutes after diuretic administration
shows that prompt washout occurred. The time/activity curve for the right kidney (Fig. 3B) shows an abrupt change in slope indicating decreasing activity
as the tracer is flushed out. This is the pattern seen in a hydronephrotic
kidney without obstruction. If the hydronephrosis was secondary to an obstruction at the uretero-pelvic junction the curve would have retained a horizontal
configuration. The diuretic was administered at the time indicated by the
vertical arrow. The time/activity curve for the left kidney shows a minimal
slope change reflecting the washout from the renal pelvis. The curve for a
normal kidney has little or no slope change since there was no appreciable retention of radionuclide. The rising bladder curve reflects the increasing
bladder accumulation as the right kidney empties.

The radionuclide studies discussed above touch on three aspects of radionuclide imaging in pediatric nephrology. They illustrate advantages that radionuclide imaging offers over the images obtained with other modalities; (a)
evaluation of function, (b) sensitivity, (c) and the ability to be quantified.
It should be emphasized that radionuclide imaging is often used in conjunction
with other imaging modalities that provide better morphologic or structural

detail. (5) Our objective should be to select the best combination of studies in the proper sequence so that optimal patient care results and unnecessary examinations are eliminated.

REFERENCES

1. Ash, J.M. and Gilday, D.L.: Renal nuclear imaging and analysis in pediatric patients. Urologic Clinics of North America 7:201-214, 1980.
2. Conway, J.J., King, L.R. and Belman, A.B. et al: Detection of vesico-ureteral reflux with radionuclide cystography. Am.J.Roent. 115:720-727,1972
3. Nasrallah, P.F., Conway, J.J., King, L.R., et al: Quantitative nuclear cystogram: Aid in determining spontaneous resolution of vesicoureteral reflux. Urology 6:654-658, 1978.
4. Koff, S.A., Thrall, J.H., Keyes, J.W.: Assessment of hydroureteronephrosis in children using diuretic radionuclide urography. J. of Urology 123:531-534, 1980.
5. Harcke, H.T., Williams, J.L.: Evaluation of neonatal renal disorders: a comparison of excretory urography with scintography and ultrasonography. Ann. Radiol. 23:109-113, 1980.

IMMUNOLOGIC CONSIDERATIONS IN RENAL TRANSPLANTATION

R.B. ETTENGER, S. JORDAN, M. MALEKZADEH, A. PENNISI,
C. UITTENBOGAART, and R.N. FINE

From the Division of Pediatric Nephrology and the Department
of Pediatrics, University of California Los Angeles School of
Medicine.

Dr. Ettenger is the recipient of Clinical Investigator Award
AM 00597-02.

Renal transplantation has been shown to be an effective
form of therapy for end-stage renal disease in children (1).
The major cause of renal allograft loss in children, as in
adults, is immmologic rejection. In an effort to decrease
irreversible renal allograft rejection, a large number of inno-
vative tests, procedures and new drugs have been utilized. It
is impossible to detail here all of the immunologic research
presently being conducted in clinical renal transplantation.
However, research areas receiving a great deal of interest
include: 1) matching for the Major Histocompatibility Complex
(MHC) antigens including a) HLA A and B and b) HLA DR; 2) the
significance of antibodies directed against B lymphocyte
antigens; and 3) the effect of blood transfusions.

1. HISTOCOMPATIBILITY

1.1 HLA A and B matching

Initial optimism over the utility of HLA A and B matching
in clinical renal trasnplantation has become somewhat tempered
over time. The value of HLA A and B matching in intrafamilial
kidney transplantation is unquestioned. Allografts from HLA
identical siblings have a four year cumulative graft survival
of more than 90% (2), and in our experience kidneys from one-
haplotype mismatched donors have a 75% five year cumulative
allograft survival (1). The value of HLA A and B matching in
cadaver renal transplantation is more controversial. Some
studies have shown a marked improvement in cadaver renal trans-

plant outcome with improved HLA A and B matching (2,3), while others have shown a more modest improvement (4). When we examined HLA A and B matching in 84 first cadaver renal allografts, we found no correlation between HLA matching and graft survival (1). The data have now been analyzed for 178 first and 91 second, third and fourth cadaver renal allografts (Table 1). In addition, we have examined the influence of HLA A and B matching in relationship to the degree of recipient presensitization against HLA antigens (Table 1). We examined this since highly presensitized patients (patients with cytotoxic antibodies to greater than 50% of a donor lymphocyte panel) have poorer graft survival than in those with less than 50% cytotoxic antibodies (4).

Table 1. HLA A and B matching in cadaver renal transplantation (Cumulative graft survival (%) ± S.E.)

HLA Matches	First Transplant		Multiple Transplant		Cytotoxic Ab > 50%		Cytotoxic Ab < 50%	
	1 yr	4 yr	1 yr	4 yr	1 yr	4 yr	1 yr	4 yr
0	63±7	42±8	67±9	32±10	43±15	29±15	68±6	41±7
1	64±6	45±7	40±9	37±9	24±11	24±11	62±5	47±6
2	61±7	38±8	53±11	38±11	41±13	29±14	63±7	40±7
3 & 4	80±18	20±18	69±13	69±13	71±17	54±20	73±13	49±16

When considering first cadaver renal transplants, no significant difference between match grades is apparent. However, when considering multiple renal transplants, a trend towards improved graft survival with three or four shared antigens is apparent (P < 0.05 at four years). When patients are not highly presensitized (i.e., cytotoxic antibodies < 50%), there is no significant difference between HLA match grades and cadaver renal allograft outcome. However, in highly presensitized patients (i.e., cytotoxic antibodies > 50%) there is a trend towards improved graft survival when three or four antigens are shared, and this trend is statistically significant (P < 0.05) at two years. Thus, HLA A and B matching appears to be of importance in patients who are highly presensitized to HLA antigens. This is further emphasized by the finding that highly presensitized (> 50% cytotoxic antibodies) recipients who receive a cadaver transplant matched for only 0, 1 or 2 antigens have a significantly poorer graft outcome than those who have less than 50% cytotoxic antibodies ($P < 0.001$ at 1 year, $P < 0.01$ at 2 years, $P < 0.05$ at 3 and 4 years).

1.2. HLA DR matching

In addition to the HLA A and B antigens, a new serologically-defined HLA antigen system, the HLA-DR system, has recently been described. HLA DR antigens are present only on B lymphocytes and monocytes. The HLA DR antigens are the serologic correlates of HLA-D, which is the antigen system responsible for stimulation in the Mixed Lymphocyte Culture (MLC) Test. (The term DR stands for D "Related"). MLC stimulation has been found to be closely associated with renal transplant outcome (5). Since five days are required to perform the MLC, this test is impractical for selection of cadaver renal transplants. However, HLA DR typing is now possible in a matter of hours, making HLA DR matching clinically practical in cadaver renal transplantation. In a recent study, Ting and Morris showed that HLA DR matching had a powerful influence on cadaveric renal transplant outcome (6). They showed that patients receiving kidneys well-matched for HLA DR (no incompatibilities) had a significantly better survival rate (85% at one year) than patients with one or two incompatibilities (64% and 56% respectively at one year). We have obtained similar results. Children receiving allografts with no HLA DR imcompatibility had a 64% one and two year allograft survival rate, compared to 45% and 32% at one and two years respectively for children receiving kidneys with one or two HLA DR imcompatibilities. Other centers have reported similar findings (2).

2. B LYMPHOCYTE CROSSMATCHING

A negative serological crossmatch between recipient serum and donor lymphocytes is a standard requirement for clinical renal transplantation. The crossmatch utilizes the complement-dependent cytotoxicity (CDC) technique to detect preformed

anti HLA A and B antibodies directed against donor lymphocytes
(7). It has been shown that the presence of such preformed
antibodies, as detected by the crossmatch, almost invariably
leads to early irreversible rejection (8).

The policy of excluding transplantation in the presence
of a positive CDC lymphocyte crossmatch has undergone some
revision. B lymphocytes have surface antigens not present on
T lymphocytes (9), as well as HLA A and B antigens which are
present on T lymphocytes. We demonstrated that a positive
crossmatch against donor B, but not T lymphocytes, did not
result in immediate irreversible rejection (10). An examination
of B lymphocyte crossmatching in cadaver renal transplantation
shows no adverse effects of a positive B lymphocyte crossmatch
on long-term graft outcome (Figure 1). This data extends our
previous finding that a positive B lymphocyte crossmatch is
compatible with good long-term cadaveric renal allograft survival
(11). Thus, a weakly positive CDC crossmatch between recipient
serum and unfractioned donor lymphocytes is not a contraindication
to transplantation when the positive crossmatch is attributable
entirely to anti-B lymphocyte antibodies. It has become a
standard practice in many histocompatibility laboratories to
perform fractionated as well as unfractionated CDC lymphocyte
crossmatches pre-transplantation, and to transplant on the basis
of a negative T lymphocyte crossmatch only (12). Such a procedure enlarges the number of potential cadaveric kidneys for
a given recipient, since it eliminates one cause of a "false
positive" CDC crossmatch.

Recently, Iwaki and his colleagues observed improved
cadaver renal allograft survival in patients whose sera contained
B lymphocytotoxins reacting against a B lymphocyte panel at
a $5^{o}C$ incubation temperature (13). They also found decreased
actuarial graft survival in recipients whose sera contained
B lymphocytotoxins reacting at $37^{o}C$ against a similar cell panel.
They have speculated that in direct B lymphocyte crossmatch
testing, a positive "cold" ($5^{o}C$) B lymphocyte crossmatch may
enhance renal allograft outcome, while a positive "warm" ($37^{o}C$)
B lymphocyte crossmatch may be deleterious. We have now examined

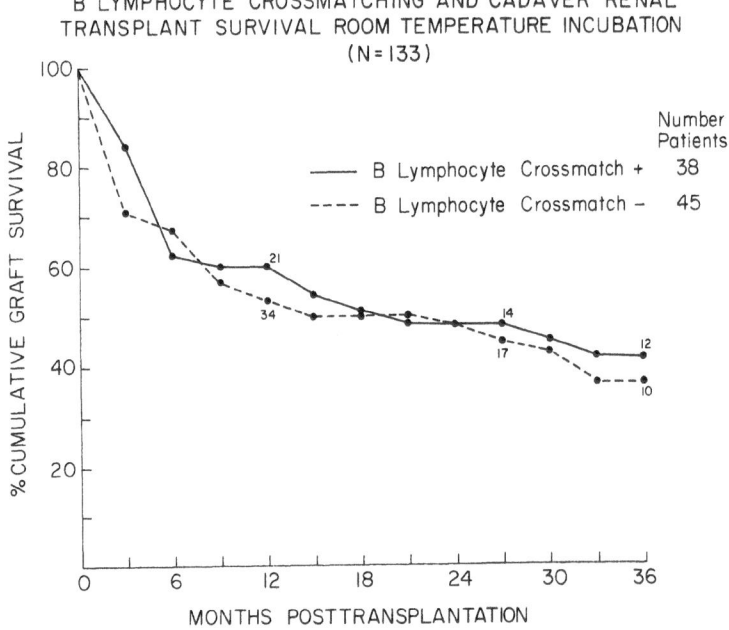

B LYMPHOCYTE CROSSMATCHING AND CADAVER RENAL
TRANSPLANT SURVIVAL ROOM TEMPERATURE INCUBATION
(N=133)

the effect of the incubation temperature of B lymphocyte crossmatching on the outcome of 35 renal allografts (Figure 2).
There is no significant difference between allografts transplanted in the presence of a "cold" vs. a "warm" positive B
lymphocyte crossmatch. In addition, neither of these curves
differs significantly from the curve describing the outcome of
transplants performed with a negative B lymphocyte crossmatch
at all temperatures (curve not shown). One and two year graft
survivals: B+ "warm" 47 ± 11%, 37 ± 11%; B+ "cold" 53 ± 13%,
53 ± 13%; B- 52 ± 9%, 48 ± 7%. While not statistically significant, the trend towards a poorer graft outcome in recipients
with positive B lymphocyte "warm" crossmatches marks this as
an area for further study.

3. EFFECT OF PRE-TRANSPLANT BLOOD TRANSFUSIONS
     In the early and mid 1970's, it was thought prudent to
avoid blood transfusions during maintenance dialysis. It was

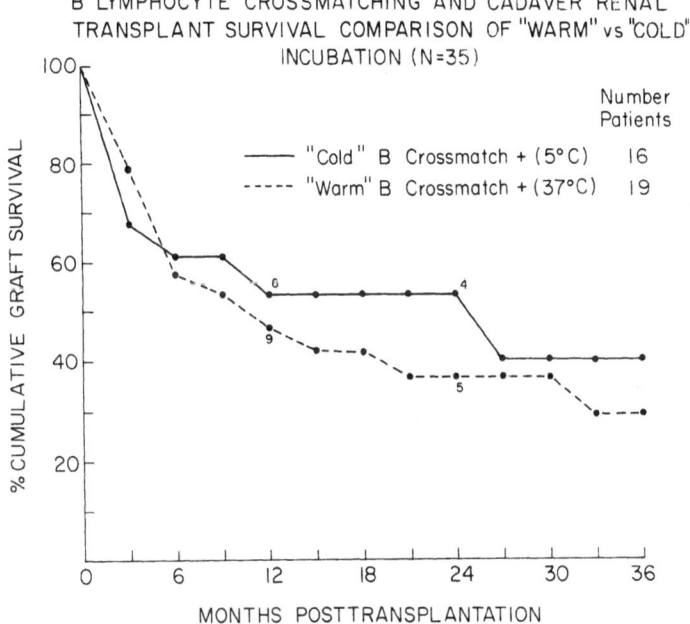

B LYMPHOCYTE CROSSMATCHING AND CADAVER RENAL
TRANSPLANT SURVIVAL COMPARISON OF "WARM" vs "COLD"
INCUBATION (N=35)

felt that transfusions would lead to sensitization which would
adversely affect the outcome of kidney transplantation. It has
now been demonstrated that pre-transplant blood transfusions
have a salutory, and not an adverse effect on renal transplantation (14). The mechanism of this effect is unknown. Opelz
and coworkers have demonstrated that the beneficial effect of
transfusions is "dose-related"--i.e. graft survival is poorest
in those recipients who have never been transfused and improves
as more transfusions are given (14). In contrast, Persijn et
al. found that only one transfusion yields maximal benefits
(15). Both packed red blood cells and whole blood are effective
(14), but it has been found that "leukocyte-free" transfusions
are not beneficial, while "leukocyte-poor" transfusions are
beneficial (16). The beneficial effect of frozen blood is
controversial. In Opelz' study, frozen blood has a significant,
less marked effect than packed red blood cells or whole blood
(14); Fuller et al. on the other hand have found that frozen
blood prepared by the aglomeration technique has a salutory

effect on transplantation without adverse presensitization (17). The beneficial effect of transfusion given during the transplant surgery (i.e. peroperative transfusion) is controversial as well. Stiller et al. (18), and more recently Williams et al. (19) have found that previously untransfused transplant recipients had significantly improved graft survival if they received peroperative blood transfusion. Since this approach avoids problems with presensitization, it has obvious clinical relevance. However, Opelz has been unable to confirm these findings in a large multi-center study (14). The optimal timing of transfusions is also unclear; no association has been found between the interval between last transfusion and transplant and outcome of the graft (14).

The beneficial effect of random blood transfusions has been found in both first and second cadaver renal transplants, as well as in HLA identical and one-haplotype matched related transplants (14). However, Salvatierra et al. have utilized donor-specific transfusions to improve the results of one-haplotype matched related transplants, where the MLC between potential donor and recipient shows marked stimulation (20). They had previously noted that a high MLC stimulation index was associated with poor transplant outcome. Thirty-seven HLA non-identical potential related recipients with high MLC stimulation indices were given three transfusions from prospective donors. Recipient sera were screened weekly for antibodies against donor HLA antigens. Ten of 37 developed antibodies and the related transplants were not performed. Twenty-three of the remaining 27 received the related transplants and all but one (who discontinued immunosuppressives) have excellent graft function at least one year posttransplant.

In summary, developments in histocompatibility, cross-matching, and the effect of blood transfusions are three areas where new developments promise significant improvements in renal transplantation.

References

1. Fine, R.N., Edelbrock, H. et al.: 1977 Urology (Supp)9:61.

2. Solheim, B.G., Flatmark, A. et al.: 1979 Transpl. Proc. 11:748.

3. Festenstein, H., Pachoula-Papasteriadis, C.: 1979 Transpl. Proc. 11:752.

4. Opelz, G., Mickey, R., Terasaki, P.I.: 1977 Transplantation 23:490.

5. Sengar, D.P.S., Opelz, G., Terasaki, P.I.: 1973 Transpl. Proc. 5:641.

6. Ting, A., Morris, P.: 1980 Lancet 2:282.

7. Terasaki, P.I., McClelland, J.D.: 1964 Nature 204:998.

8. Patel, R., Terasaki, P.I.: 1969 N. Engl. J. Med. 280:735.

9. Winchester, R., Fu, S. et al.: 1975 J. Exp. Med. 141:924.

10. Ettenger, R.B., Terasaki, P.I. et al.: 1976 Lancet 2:56.

11. Ettenger, R.B., Uittenbogaart, C. et al.: 1978 Transplantation 27:315.

12. Lowry, R.P., Myrberg, S. er al.: 1980 Proc. Clin. Dial. Transpl. Forum 9:201.

13. Iwaki, Y., Terasaki, P.I. et al.: 1978 Lancet 1:1228.

14. Opelz, G., Terasaki, P.I.: Transpl. Proc. (in press).

15. Persijn, G.G., van Hooff, J.P. et al.: 1977 Transpl. Proc. 9:503.

16. Persijn, G.G.: Transpl. Proc. (in press).

17. Fuller, T.C., Delmonico, F.L. et al.: 1977 Transpl. Proc. 9:117.

18. Stiller, C.R., Lockwood, B.L. et al.: 1978 Lancet 1:169.

19. Williams, K.A., Ting, A. et al.: 1980 Lancet 1:1104.

20. Salvatierra, O., Amend, W. et al.: Transpl. Proc. (in press).

RECURRENCE OF THE ORIGINAL DISEASE IN THE TRANSPLANTED KIDNEY

E.P. LEUMANN, J. BRINER, F. LARGIADÈR
Departments of Pediatrics, Pathology and Surgery A, University of Zürich, Switzerland

Recurrence of the original disease in the transpanted kidney is a relatively rare event and is often of little clinical relevance. According to the EDTA registry (1), recurrence was diagnosed in only 3.2 % of the patients in whom this question (recurrence present or absent) was answered. Recurrence was confirmed histologically in 10 of 177 (= 5.6 %) mainly adult patients who had undergone transplant biopsy in Zurich within a four year period. Recurrence is, nevertheless, of great interest because it provides an opportunity to study pathogenetic mechanisms of the underlying disease and allows to observe the development of renal lesions from the very beginning.

The diagnosis of recurrence is based on clinical findings and histologic examination of both the native and transplanted kidney. The histologic lesions in the grafted kidney should be identical or at least compatible with the original lesions. The interpretation of the transplant biopsy may, however, be difficult, since glomerular lesions which resemble those seen in recurrence are observed in a number of conditions (2, 3), i.e. in transplant glomerulopathy which is part of the host's reaction to the graft (observed in 31 % of the 177 patients mentioned above), in rejection glomerulonephritis (GN) with subendothelial electron-dense deposits (observed in 22 %), in de novo GN (11.3 %), donor GN (1.1 %) and other forms (6.2 %).

Tables 1 and 2 provide some information concerning the rate of recurrence and the clinical implications of recurrence. Since no valid data concerning the overall frequency of recurrence are available, the approximate number of published cases is given instead. It is noteworthy that recurrence is rarely observed in a number of systemic diseases, e.g. in SLE, amyloidosis, Wegener's granulomatosis and anti-GBM-antibody-GN. This may partly be due to the effect of immunosuppressive therapy. However, it casts some doubt on the concept that circulating immune complexes explain most cases of GN. Primary hyperoxaluria type I (= "oxalosis", excluding the pyridoxine-sensitive variant) is in fact the only systemic and metabolic disease where recurrence universally occurs and often, but not invariably, leads to rapid deterioration of renal function.

The different types of GN (Table 2) are classified according to the microscopic appearance. Extracapillary proliferative GN is not listed since crescents are a superimposed feature seen in different types of basic glomerular lesions. Similarly, mesangial proliferative GN is omitted because it forms a heterogenous group. Two types of GN, dense deposit disease (DDD) and focal segmental glomerulosclerosis (FSG), are of special importance because both conditions are predominantly seen in young patients and because recurrence may become clinically relevant. DDD has been shown to recur in nearly all patients in whom electronmicroscopic examination of the allograft has been performed. On the other hand, less than one third of the patients has clinical signs of recurrence, and only a few grafts have been lost due to recurrence so far. However, recurrence might well become a significant factor in determining the ultimate prognosis when more patients are followed over longer periods of time. Two of our patients lost their grafts after 2 years and 5 years, respectively, although urinary abnormalities had been minimal during the first years.

In contrast to DDD, FSG does only recur in a minority of patients. A survey (4) and search of the literature has demonstrated that the risk of recurrence can best be predicted by the duration of the original disease. Patients with a rapid, malignant course (where renal biopsy sometimes shows some mesangial proliferation) are especially prone to develop recurrence, whereas in most other patients, this risk is relatively minor (Figure 1). In fact, 16 of 31 patients (= 52 %) in whom duration of the original disease was less than 3 years, showed recurrence. In contrast, FSG recurred in only 7 of 48 patients (= 15 %) in whom duration of the disease had exceeded 3 years. However, a recent report on a survey in 48 mainly adult patients (5) denies such a correlation, but claims a distressingly high recurrence rate (9 of 11) for 4-antigen matched transplants from sibling donors. - Recurrent FSG usually manifests itself within the first hours or days of transplantation with heavy proteinuria which frequently, but not necessarily, leads to the nephrotic syndrome and early graft failure. Recurrence affects second grafts, too, and is not prevented by bilateral nephrectomy.

374

Recurrence of FSG

Data from survey (n=30) and from literature (n=49)

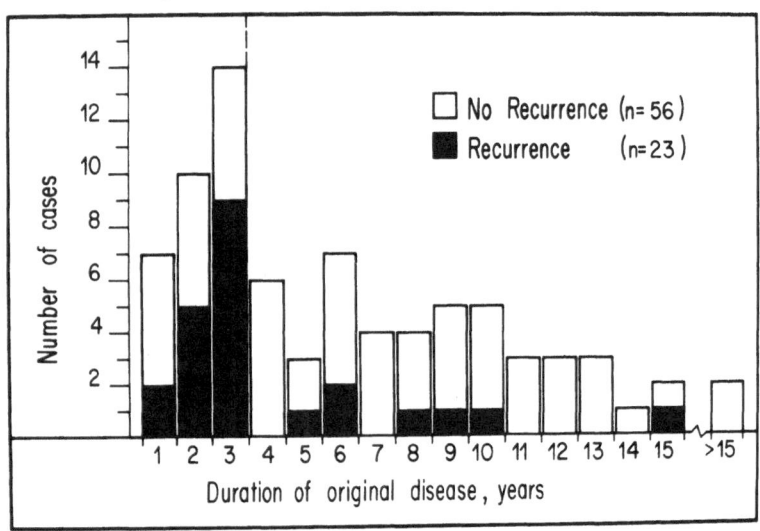

The study of recurrence clearly demonstrates that FSG is not a single entity. Investigations in order to define a postulated circulating humoral substance have failed to date.

It is hoped that a better understanding of the pathogenetic mechanisms of recurrence will ensue in better prediction or even prevention of recurrence. Meanwhile, we do not think any patients should be deterred from transplantation for fear of recurrence.

REFERENCES

1. Wing AJ, Brunner FP, Brynger H, Chantler C, Donckerwolcke RA, Gurland HJ, Hathway RA, Jacobs C, Selwood NH. Combined report on regular dialysis and transplantation in Europe, VIII, 1977. Proc Eur Dial Transplant Assoc 15, 3, 1978.
2. Cameron JS, Turner DR: Recurrent glomerulonephritis in allografted kidneys. Clin Nephrol 7, 47, 1977.
3. Hamburger J, Crosnier J, Noël LH: Recurrent glomerulonephritis after renal transplantation. Ann Rev Med 29, 67, 1978.
4. Leumann EP, Briner J, Donckerwolcke RA, Kuijten R, Largiadèr F: Recurrence of focal segmental glomerulosclerosis in the transplanted kidney. Nephron 25, 65, 1980.
5. Zimmerman CE: Renal transplantation for focal segmental glomerulosclerosis. Transplantation 29, 172, 1980.

Table 1: Recurrence in Systemic Diseases

Disease	Number of published cases with recurrence	Rate of recurrence	Clinical implications of recurrence
Oxalosis	16	100 %	+++
Diabetes mellitus	(12)	(100 %)	—
Amyloidosis	6	infrequent	(+)
Anaphylactoid purpura	7	rare	+
IgA nephropathy	12	~50 %	(+)
SLE	?	very rare	?
Wegener's granulomatosis	1	rare	(+)
Anti-GBM-antibody GN (including Goodpasture)	27	infrequent	?
Hemolytic uremic syndrome	1	rare	+

Table 2: Recurrence in Primary Glomerulonephritis

Type of Glomerulo-nephritis	Number of published cases with recurrence	Rate of recurrence	Clinical implications of recurrence
Membranoproliferative GN			
- type I	32	~ 30 %	in 50 % severe
- type II (= DDD)	50	close to 100 %	often minor
Membranous GN	7	rare (?)	nephrotic syndrome
Focal Segmental Glomerulosclerosis (FSG)	36	~ 50 % if rapid evolution (<3 yrs) ~ 15 % if slow evolution (>3 yrs)	often nephrotic syndrome

HYPERTENSION IN CHILDREN WITH KIDNEY TRANSPLANTS

JULIE R. INGELFINGER, M. D.

In 137 renal transplants performed over a 9½ year period at Children's Hospital Medical Center, hypertension has been seen in over 98% of patients in the immediate post-transplant period, and in 93% of those same patients after the initial post-transplant weeks. Thus post-transplant hypertension, in our experience, is expected.

For diagnosing hypertension, we have used the blood pressure norms published by the American Academy of Pediatrics Task Force for Blood Pressure Control in Childhood (1). Normal blood pressure was defined as within 2 standard deviations for age, mild hypertension as blood pressure over 2 to 3 standard deviations above the mean for age, moderate hypertension as 3 to 4 standard deviations above the mean for age, and severe hypertension as 3 to 4 standard deviations above the mean for age plus evidence of encephalopathy or other acute target organ damage. This paper focuses on the multiple factors involved in post-transplant hypertension as seen in pediatric renal transplant recipients at Children's Hospital Medical Center.

In the immediate post-operative period, acute hypertension is reported to occur with fluids causing volume expansion (2,3), with residual pressor factors (4), with relative hypoperfusion of the allograft (5), with acute thrombosis or stenosis of the allograft artery (6), with acute rejection (7,8), with high-dose steroids (9), or because of decreased perfusion of native kidneys or a previously-failed allograft (10).

Almost all hypertension in the immediate post-operative period in our experience seems related to large intravenous fluid volumes. After fluid status and volume expansion are controlled, blood pressure returns to normal for age.

Immediate post-transplant hypertension occurs in most pediatric transplant recipients, yet in few adults. One clear difference between adult and childhood recipients is the relative mass of the kidney transplant itself.

It has been suggested that the lower cardiac output and arterial pressure in children might stimulate large kidneys to produce extra renin (5) or that conversely, the large kidney could alter cardiac output and/or extracellular volume (5). In order to focus on the relative renal mass and its effect on cardiovascular and renal function, we have measured cardiac output before and after transplant in 7 patients and found no change. However, there are confounding factors such as the use of high-dose steroids, the presence of multiple kidneys, the possible presence of rejection, mechanical difficulties, or recurrent disease. To circumvent these variables insofar as possible, we examined the effect of increasing relative renal mass on cardiovascular and renal function in a group of inbred DLA-matched beagles, and acutely in mongrel pups (11). Blood pressure fell after implanting a large kidney and remained lower than pre-transplant. Cardiac output did not change significantly in these animals, nor did plasma volume. These experiments suggest that renal mass per se does not seem to explain the high frequency of post-transplant hypertension in children.

After the immediate post-operative period, hypertension may occur because of steroids (9,12,13) rejection (acute or chronic) (7,8,14) renal artery disease (6), multiple kidneys (10), recurrent nephritis (14) hydronephrosis (14), or hypercalcemia (15). Some of these factors will be considered in turn:

There is a correlation between prednisone dose and blood pressure. Jacquot et al (12) showed that blood pressure directly varies with prednisone dose. Sampson et al (13) showed a decrease in blood pressure on conversion to alternate-day steroids. We have observed a fall in diastolic blood pressure when steroid dose is converted from daily to alternate day in nearly all patients in whom it is possible (Fig. 1). Furthermore, exogenous steroids may modify the normal pattern of diurnal blood pressure variation, in which blood pressure is lowest during the late evening and early morning hours. Monitoring the blood pressure courses of all patients receiving renal transplants, 66% were found to have reversal of the normal variation.

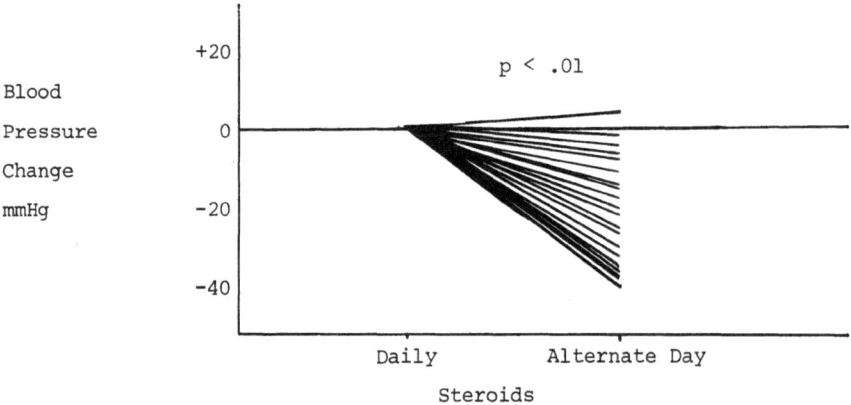

Figure 1

Renal function and blood pressure vary directly. In our patients where blood pressure is rigorously controlled, creatinine level correlates with the number of antihypertensive drugs required (Table 1). Most patients with normal creatinine are on zero or 1 antihypertensive medication, whereas those on multiple antihypertensive medications almost always have some decrease in renal function. An indirect corollary is that blood pressure is higher in recipients of cadaveric transplants than in those with living related donor transplants, possibly due to the better renal function seen in the latter group.

Table 1. Creatinine level and Antihypertensive Agents Needed

Number of Antihypertensives

Creatinine	0	1	2	3	4	Hypertensive on Medication
< 1	18	2		1		
1-2	13	7	10	2		
2-3	3	1	6	5		
3-4			2	8	1	
> 4					1	2

Renal artery stenosis has been a reason for post-transplant hypertension in 3.6% of the transplants in our series. Contributory factors in transplant renal artery stenosis include the technique of nephrectomy prior to implantation, perfusion injury, and technique of implantation (6). Using an interrupted as compared to a continuous suture line cuts down the percentage of allografts developing this complication. External adhesions may still cause stenosis. Rejection, with deposition of fibrin, immunoglobulins, and complement may be associated with transplant renal artery stenosis (16). In some patients with stenosis, even young ones, atheromatous disease may contribute to this problem (6). The approach to diagnosing renal artery stenosis should be aggressive and complete studies including angiography should be done in any child with a renal transplant who has moderate or severe sustained hypertension. The approach to therapy may be resection of the affected area (6), revascularization with a graft (6), and may be correction of the stenosis using the technique of percutaneous angioplasty (17). The most recent patient in our series to suffer the complication of renal artery stenosis had transluminal angioplasty, and the pressure gradient across the stenotic area dropped from 100 mmHg pre-dilatation to 10-20 mmHg. This patient has thus far been followed for 6 months with markedly improved blood pressure.

When multiple kidneys are present, selective renal vein renin determinations and ratios may be helpful in determining whether the transplanted kidney or native kidneys are all contributing to hypertension (10). In addition, as Linas et al (10) have shown, saralasin infusion may also be helpful in this circumstance. In 13 patients with multiple kidneys undergoing arteriography, we found selective renal vein renin determinations lateralizing in 4 (all to native kidneys), but no lateralization in 9. An additional 7 patients with a single transplanted kidney also underwent arteriography. Of all 20 patients, 5 had renal artery stenosis, associated with rejection in 3 of the 5.

Certain groups of patients may be more prone than others to develop post-transplant hypertension. In 137 consecutive renal transplants, we have found that patients with previous glomerulonephritis are especially likely to develop post-transplant hypertension, possibly because they have a high frequency of pre-transplant hypertension (18). When compared to children entering end-stage renal disease due to renal dysplasia, chronic obstructive disease, or other structural lesions, those with glomerulo-nephritis are 2 to 3 times more likely to have moderate or severe post-transplant hypertension. Among individuals who have not had any episode of post-transplant rejection and no recurrent disease, all those with previous nephritis had some post-transplant hypertension, whereas only

17% of those with a previous structural lesion had any blood pressure elevation (19). (Fig. 2).

HTN - 6 MONTHS POST-TX

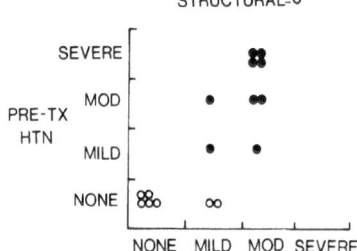

The post-transplant hypertension seen in our 137 transplants is best categorized as shown in Table 2. Most of the patients had rejection-associated hypertension. The next largest category was hypertension associated with steroids which abated upon conversion to alternate day steroids. A minority had recurrent disease, renovascular problems, or peripheral vascular disease. No definite cause could be found in one patient who was fully studied. Only 7% of patients have not experienced hypertension following the initial post-transplant period.

Post-transplant hypertension may be very difficult to control and may be associated with severe morbidity. Of hypertensive patients, up to one-third develop hypertensive encephalopathy, and we have observed 2 intracerebral bleeds and two deaths associated with severe hypertension. Although more patients with nephritis develop hypertension, once an individual becomes hypertensive, the chance of developing a hypertension-related complication is equal no matter what the antecedent history.

Table 2. Etiology of Post-Transplant Hypertension

Rejection	
Acute	15% ⎫ 54%
Chronic	39% ⎭
Steroid-Related	26%
Recurrent Glomerulonephritis	6%
Renal Artery Stenosis	4%
Peripheral Vascular Disease	2%
Unknown	1%
No Hypertension	7%

As shown in Table 3, initial control of post-transplant hypertension may require multiple drugs. Of those who are hypertensive, about 1/3 can

be controlled on a diuretic alone or a diuretic plus 1 antihypertensive
agent. Another 1/3 require diuretic plus 2 antihypertensive drugs, and
the remainder require a diuretic plus 3 or more drugs for blood pressure
control.

Table 3. Drugs Required for Initial Blood Pressure Control

Diuretic Alone	8%	} 29%
Diuretic + 1 Drug	21%	
Diuretic + 2 Drugs	33%	
Diuretic + 3 Drugs (or more)	38%	

After post-transplant hypertension has been controlled, many patients are
able to be managed on decreased amounts of medication over time. The
current blood pressure management is shown in Table 4. Though most
patients are normotensive, many haven't been able to come off antihypertensive medication. A few require multiple antihypertensive agents yet
remain hypertensive, even on agents such as minoxidil.

Table 4. Blood pressure Control 1- 9.5 Years Post-Transplant

Normotensive

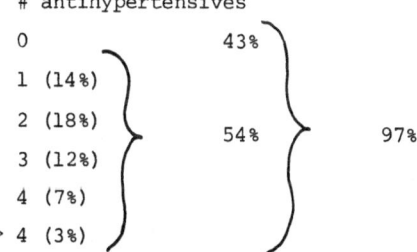

antihypertensives

0	43%	
1 (14%)		
2 (18%)	54%	97%
3 (12%)		
4 (7%)		
> 4 (3%)		

Hypertensive on Medication

3%

Since hypertension is a nearly universal complication of renal
transplantation in children, anticipation of the types of hypertension
which may arise is imperative. Most hypertension in the immediate post-
operative period is volume-mediated and responds to diuresis and vasodilator
therapy. Steroid-induced hypertension also responds well to diuretic and
vasodilator therapy in our experience. On the other hand, much chronic
hypertension, such as that related to rejection, may be renin mediated and
responds to renin-reducing agents such as propranolol (20). Aggressive use
of antihypertensive therapy may prevent continued hypertension and its

382

attendant morbidity.

REFERENCES

1. Report of the Task Force on Blood Pressure Control in Children. 1977. Pediatrics 58 (Suppl): No. 5, Part 2.
2. Gonzales, LL, Martin, L, West, CD, et al: Renal homotransplantation in children. 1970. Arch. Surg. 101:232.
3. Najarian, J.S., Simmons, R.L., Tallent, M.B., et al. Renal transplantation in infants and children. 1971. Ann Surg. 174:583.
4. McDonald, F.D.: Severe hypertension and elevated plasma renin activity following transplantation of "hepatorenal donor" kidneys into anephric recipients. 1973. Am J Med. 54:39.
5. Hume, D.M, unpublished observations.
6. Lacombe, M.: Arterial Stenosis complicating renal allotransplantation in Man: A study of 38 cases. 1975. Ann Surg. 181:283.
7. Smelli, W.A.B., Vinik, M, and Hume, D.M.: Angiographic investigation of hypertension complicating human renal transplantation. 1969, Surg Gynecol. Obstet. 128:963.
8. Gunnells, J.G., Stickel, D.L., and Robinson, R.R.: Episodic hypertension associated with positive renin assays after renal transplantation. 1966. N Engl J Med. 274:543.
9. Sampson, P, Kirdani, R.Y, and Sandberg, A.A. The aetiology of hypertension after renal transplantation in man. 1973. Br J Surg. 61:819.
10. Linas, S.L., Miller, P.D., McDonald, K.M., et al.: Role of the renin-angiotensin system in post-transplantation hypertension in patients with multiple kidneys. 1978. N Engl J Med. 298:1440.
11. Caldicott, W.J.H. and Ingelfinger, J.R.: The effect of increasing renal mass on cardiovascular function in immature dogs. 1981, Ped Res. In Press.
12. Jacquot, C, Idatte, J.M., Bedrossian, J, et al.: Long-term blood pressure changes in renal homotransplantation. 1978. Arch Intern Med. 138:233.
13. Sampson, D., and Albert, D.J.: Alternate day therapy with methylprednisolone after renal transplantation. 1973. J Urol. 109:345.
14. Rao, T.K.S, Gupta, S.K, Butt, K.M.H., et al: Relationship of renal transplantation to hypertension in end-stage renal failure. Arch Intern Med. 138:1236.
15. Weidmann, P, Massry, S.G., Coburn, J.W., et al.: Blood pressure effects of acute hypercalcemia. Studies in patients with chronic renal failure. 1972. Ann Intern Med. 76:741.
16. Collins, G.M, Johansen, K, Bookstein, J. et al: Transplant renal artery stenosis occurring in both recipients from a single donor. 1978. Arch Surg 113:767.
17. Diamond, N.G., Casarella, W.J., Hardy, M., et al: Dilatation of critical transplant renal artery stenosis by percutaneous transluminal angioplasty. 1979. Amer J Roentgen. 133:1167.
18. Ingelfinger, J.R., Lazarus, J.M., Levey, R.H. et al: Hypertension in pediatric renal transplant patients. 1975. Pediatr Res. 9:376.
19. Ingelfinger, J.R., Grupe, W.E, and Levey, R.H.: Post-transplant hypertension in the absence of rejection or recurrent disease. 1978. Ped Res. 12:1074.
20. Potter, E.E., Schambelan, M, Salvatierra, O., et al. Treatment of high-renin hypertension with propranolol in children after renal transplantation. 1977. J Pediat. 90:307.

THE NATURE OF AMINO ACID TRANSPORT DISORDERS

STANTON SEGAL, M.D.

The concept that defective membrane transport function results in clinical disorders is well-recognized and established. Every textbook of pediatrics or books on metabolic disorders has a section concerned with transport disorders. These disorders may involve ions, amino acids, sugars, phosphates, urate and even water. If all the disorders of transport are considered together, their incidence would be about one in 1,000 which makes such abnormalities a common inherited disorder of man. The most common of these is cystinuria with an incidence of 1 in 7000 and iminoglycinuria with 1 in 14,000 births (1).

I would like to present some concepts about transport disorders based on my experience with renal tubule cell handling of amino acids. Aminoacidurias have to be explained with the recognition of the transcellular fluxes that occur through a renal tubule cell in which the membrane is differentiated into a luminal brush border and an antiluminal smooth infolded membrane. The tendency is to focus on the brush border but we have to remember that an amino acid and other substrates in reclamation from tubule urine have to move transcellularly across the cell and enter into the capillary. As a result the molecule has to go through the basolateral membrane as well as through the basement membrane. Although the directional fluxes are for movement through the brush border, across the cell and into the capillary, there is a possibility for outward fluxes through the brush border and, of course, entry from the basolateral side. There is much recent information on the nature of these two membranes since they can be separated. We know from work with membrane vesicles that the brush border contains sodium-dependent transport systems for amino acids and sugars (2,3) and that the basolateral membrane has a facilitated diffusion transport system without sodium dependence for most substances (4). These membranes do have a diversity and the characteristic of each of them with regard to flux of amino acid should determine the various abnormalities that are possible in terms of transport disorders.

Table 1.

Mechanisms of Aminoaciduria

1. Brush border membrane defects - reabsorptive
2. Basolateral membrane defects - cellular efflux
3. Luminal secretion
4. Luminal leakage
5. Tubule basement membrane abnormality

Table 1 summarizes some of the possible abnormalities that could be responsible for aminoaciduria. First, a brush border membrane reabsorptive defect may be present. Second, there could be a defect in the basolateral membrane, so that the downhill movement of amino acids out of the cell into the capillary is prevented. A third defect that could be etiologically related to hyperexcretion of amino acids is an abnormal secretion at the luminal membrane, a process normally associated with organic acid excretion. An analogous abnormality could be a passive backflux or leakage of amino acids anywhere along the tubule. Lastly, penetration of amino acids through the tubular basement membrane which is juxtaposed between the basal membrane and tl capillary might be impeded. The amplification of these concepts is the purpose of this paper.

BRUSH BORDER MEMBRANE DEFECTS

Increasing knowledge of membrane structure and function have provided new insights for understanding transport abnormalities of the luminal brush border which could result in defective reclamation from tubule urine. First, the fluid mosaic model of the membrane presented the concept of glycoproteins embedded in membranes which act as a channel for hydrophilic substances to cross the lipid barrier (5). Second, the properties of active transport of amino acids have been delineated (6). These indicated that 1) a carrier or recognition site exists in the membrane which has an affinity for an amino acid or a group of similar acids; 2) there is a stereospecific preference for the L configuration; 3) sodium ion is usually required; 4) energy input is a necessity and 5) the sites are limited and therefore the transport process is saturable. Another tenet is that the process is asymmetrical and enables a higher concentration of the amino acid to exist in the cell than in the sur- rounding fluid, the hallmark of active transport. Kinetic studies have indicated that there may be several transport processes for an amino acid with varying degrees of specificity.

Figure 1 shows a schematic representation of protein embedded in a lipid matrix and depicts defects that could explain abnormal brush border reabsorptive function responsible for aminoacidurias. The first diagram in Figure 1 represents a normal protein carrier with a binding site, one part of which is drawn as a wider line to represent an area of sodium binding. The second diagram shows an altered binding site which would reveal itself as a change in Km or affinity. This can be due to a primary alteration affecting the attachment of the amino acid or a secondary one affecting sodium binding. The carrier protein could be abnormally placed (Fig. 1-3) or indeed be absent from the membrane (Fig. 1-4). Another possibility is a defect in energy trans-duction resulting in altered configuration of the binding site. This kind of defect might exist for example in a Fanconi syndrome. The last diagram of Fig. 1 shows that the binding site may be normal but that a conformational change in the carrier protein exists. These theoretical possibilities await correlation with known clinical abnormalities. This will, however, depend on further methodologic advances and the ability to isolate renal membranes from affected patients. At present research in this area still involves kinetic measurements of carrier function.

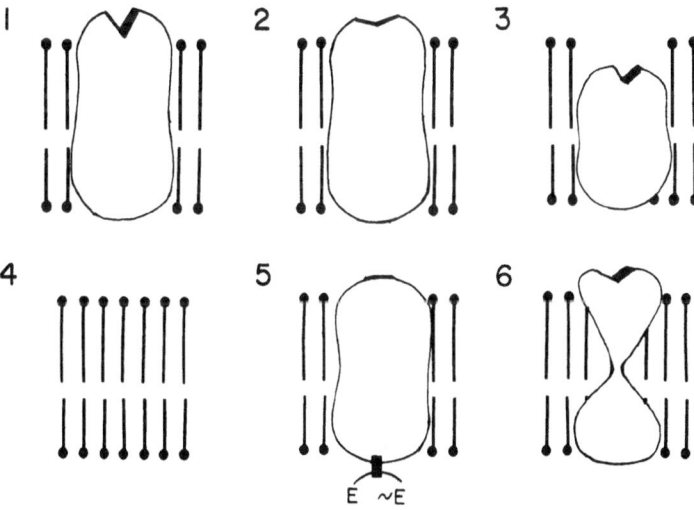

FIGURE 1. Schematic diagram of the fluid mosaic model of the cell membrane depicting possible alterations in a carrier protein that could result in defective transport.

The study of amino acid transport by in vitro techniques has progressed from work with renal cortical slices (7) to tubule fragments (8) and isolated membranes (3). In my laboratory, all of these methods have been used to study cystine metabolism because of an interest in human cystinuria. I will

386

try to give an update on our thinking about cystinuria and the defect as it might be related to the concepts just presented. The postulate first presented by Dent and Rose (9) that there was a common renal tubule transport defect for cystine and dibasic amino acids to account for the clinical manifestations was questioned when patients with only hyperexcretion of cystine (10) and others with only dibasic aminoaciduria (11) were described. In addition, studies in renal cortical slices from cystinuric patients showed a defect in lysine and arginine transport but not that of cystine, (12) and, in rat cortical slices, no interrelationship between cystine and dibasic amino acid transport could be demonstrated (13). Experiments, however, with cortical tubule fragments (14) and isolated brush border membranes (15,16) give a new picture of cystine transport characteristics. Fig. 2 is a Hofstee plot showing the relationship of velocity of cystine uptake from bicarbonate buffer to the concentration of cystine.

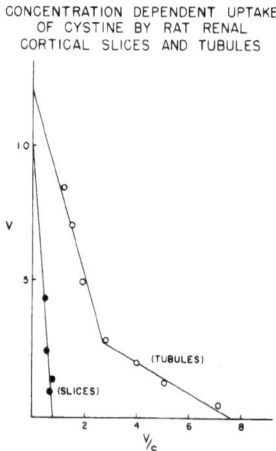

FIGURE 2.   Hofstee plot of the dependence of the velocity of cystine uptake on concentration (7,14)

When rat cortical slices are used there is a single line which designates a single transport system with a Km of 0.8 mM. When tubule fragments are used, a two-limbed curve is obtained. One line is similar to that in slices, the other indicates the presence of a second system with a high affinity (14). These same two systems are observed in isolated brush border membrane vesicles (15,16). The addition of lysine can obliterate the activity of the low Km system (15,16) but does not interact with the high Km system seen in the slice. It seems apparent now that Dent and coworkers were correct in postulating a common carrier for cystine and lysine. Figure 3 shows schematically a possible carrier explanation for the clinical entities involving these amino acids. In cystinuria without dibasic aminoacidurias the cystine specific carrier could be affected. In classical cystinuria a defect could be present in the renal brush border membrane of the shared cystine, lysine, arginine, ornithine carrier with residual normal specific carriers. In hyperdibasic aminoaciduria there could be a defect only in the lysine, arginine and ornithine binding sites of the carrier shared with cystine. These possibilities should be considered as sheer speculation, however.

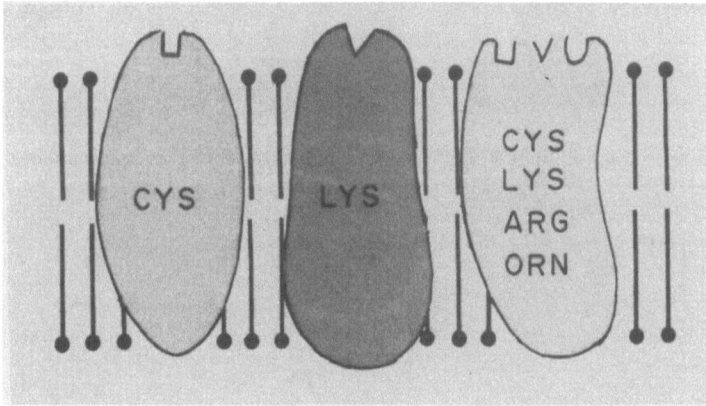

FIGURE 3. Schematic diagram of a membrane showing the possible diversity of carrier proteins for cystine (cys), lysine (lys), arginine (arg), and ornithine (orn)

The Fanconi syndrome with its many etiologies has fascinated those interested in transport disorders. A group of us in Philadelphia have been studying the spontaneous Fanconi syndrome that has a high prevalence in the Basenji

dog (17) (Fig. 4). This animal model has permitted transport experiments with
amino acids and sugars in kidney cortex slices and isolated brush border are
incubated in bicarbonate buffer with labeled substrates, there is defective
uptake of lysine and glycine as well as for a model sugar similar to glucose
(17). We have found defective uptake of amino acids and glucose by brush border
vesicles from affected animals but have no idea yet which of the brush border
abnormalities shown in Fig. 1 is present in Basenji membranes. The multiple
carrier systems involved suggest that the carriers may be abnormally placed in
the membrane or that there is defective energy transduction. Another possibility is that the lipid skeleton of the membrane is abnormal, making it
impossible for normal carrier mediated transport.

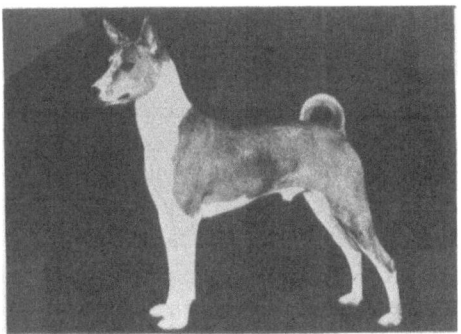

FIGURE 4.   Basenji dog, a breed with a high prevalence of a spontaneous Fanconi
             syndrome.

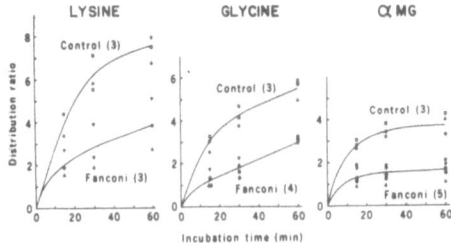

FIGURE 5.   Uptake of amino acids and alpha methyl-D-glucoside (αMG) from
             bicarbonate buffer by renal cortical slices of normal and affected
             Basenji dogs. Distribution ratio is the ratio of radioactive sub-
             strate in intracellular fluid to that in extracellular fluid (17).

LUMINAL EFFLUX AND SECRETION OF AMINO ACIDS

Until the discovery of a spontaneous Fanconi syndrome in the dog, the experimental focus has been on the chemically induced syndrome produced by administration of maleic acid to animals (18) or the incubation of various preparations of proximal tubule cells with the chemical (19,20). Studies of amino acid and sugar uptake by maleic acid treated cortical slices or tubule fragments indicate that there is a disorder involving maintenance of tissue amino acid pools with the primary difference from normal tissue being an accelerated efflux of amino acids from the cells (19). There appears to be no effect of maleic acid on the uptake of amino acids by isolated brush border membranes (21). Bergeron's group in Montreal, as a result of micropuncture and clearance studies, has postulated there is no defect in reabsorption of amino acids at the luminal membrane resulting from maleic acid treatment but that there is an abnormal efflux or leakage at the luminal surface from tubule cells either in the proximal tubule or further along in the nephron (22). Silbernagl's group, however, disagrees with this interpretation (23). There, thus, appears to be multiple explanations for the underlying cellular abnormality in the Fanconi syndrome, especially emphasized by the recent finding that an acetoacetate infusion can protect the animal from the maleic acid induced syndrome (24).

I have tried to discuss brush border membrane defects and have mentioned luminal efflux. I would like to also raise the problem of luminal secretion and whether amino acids can be secreted and whether there can be inherited aminoacidurias resulting from abnormal secretion. In many of the patients that have been studied by clearance techniques for cystine and dibasic amino acids, the clearance of cystine can be found to be higher than the glomerular filtration rate (25,26). We have a young patient about twelve years old who has a clearance of cystine that is four times the glomerular infiltration rate and excretes enormous amounts of cystine daily in the urine. This has given rise to the problem of explaining cystinuria merely on the basis of a reabsorptive defect. We have to think about how and where in the nephron secretion could occur. At this time, I don't think there is an answer to that. We can't do very many studies in human subjects and we are always looking for animal models. In this regard, some cystinuric dogs have been found who "secrete" cystine (27) and recently a South American maned wolf has been described with cystinuria who, in clearance studies, has been shown to secrete not only cystine but also lysine, arginine and ornithine (28). Cystine clearances in dogs have been reported to be increased by lysine infusion (29). If the old data of Weber, Brown and Pitts (29) is carefully examined, there is evidence that lysine infusion in dogs causes cystine clearance to be greater than the glomerular filtration rate. Recent studies in my unit have shown that in some dogs not only can lysine infusion cause cystine secretion but also the secretion of other dibasic amino acids. It appears that under some circumstances secretory processes may play an important role in the excessive urinary excretion of amino acids. Little is known of the mechanisms involved.

BASOLATERAL AND BASEMENT MEMBRANE ABNORMALITIES

So far, my remarks have focused on events at the luminal side of the tubule cell that could cause hyperexcretion of amino acids. I would like to conclude with comments about events at the basal side of the cell as outlined in Table 1. The basal lateral membrane is an additional lipid barrier for reclamation of amino acids and has an important position in handling amino acids. One can imagine a defect in the facilitated diffusion mechanisms of the basolateral membrane such that movement of substrate out of the cell into the capillary would be impeded. At present, there is one instance where this seems to be the case, in the physiological aminoaciduria of the newborn. Studies of amino acid transport and handling by newborn rat kidney indicate that at the same time that there is excessive urinary amino acid excretion, the tubule intracellular pool of an amino acid may be larger than that in adult tissue(30) In vitro experiments with rat renal cortex slices and tubules have indicated that a hallmark of newborn tissue is the continuous high uptake of amino acids (31). The level of accumulation of amino acids is several-fold higher than that of adult tissue during 90 min. incubation periods. During maturation, the ability of cortical cells to accumulate amino acids diminishes.

The continuous high uptake of amino acids is characteristic of a relatively slow efflux rate. If, indeed, the tubule cells are preloaded with amino acids and the efflux rate measured, the efflux is found to be much slower in newborn than adult kidney (32). The exact location of the efflux from tubule cells in vitro is not known but it is thought that this occurs at the basolateral membrane. A maturational event in newborn tubules is the increase in infoldings of the basolateral membrane (33). Both increasing surface area and maturation of transport mechanisms in this membrane may underly the disappearance of hyperaminoaciduria present in the newborn.

In the structure of the tubule, the basement membrane is interposed between the basolateral membrane and the capillary, adding another barrier

to amino acid entry into the capillary. One disorder where there is a characteristic widening of these basement membranes is Lowe's syndrome (34). The
syndrome is associated with a generalized aminoaciduria. Little, however, is
known about how amino acids normally penetrate the basement membrane.

I have tried to present an overall picture of the five physiologic
mechanisms that I think would explain aminoacidurias. There is a great deal of
work ahead of us; we are in our infancy in really studying the gene product
responsible for abnormal amino acid transport. We started looking at whole
kidney with clearances. We looked at transport in slices and we have examined
uptake by tubules. We have studied isolated membranes. I want to emphasize
that if we are really going to get the full picture of mechanisms of abnormal
amino acid excretion, we are going to have to utilize a lot of information
gathered by all these different techniques and not rely on anyone to give the
final answer. There remain many questions relating to membrane structure and
composition, how membranes are synthesized and carrier proteins inserted.
There is much to learn about the nature of transport proteins, the genetic
regulation of their synthesis and the true nature of the abnormality in
inherited transport disorders.

REFERENCES

1. Lery HL. Genetic Screening, in Herns and Herschorn, Progress in Human
    Genetics, Vol. 4, pp. 1-104, Plenum Press, New York, 1973
2. Kinne R. Properties of the Glucose Transport System in the Renal Brush
    Border Membrane, in Current Topics in Membranes and Transport, Bronner
    F and Kleinzeller A, ed. Academic Press, New York, 1976, pp. 209-267
3. McNamara PD, Ozegovic B, Pepe LM, and Segal, S. Proline and glycine
    uptake by rat kidney cortex brushborder membrane vesicles. Proc Natl
    Acad Sci 73: 4521-4525, 1976
4. Reynolds RA, Wald H, McNamara PD, and Segal S. An improved method for
    isolation of basal-lateral membranes from rat kidney. Biochim Biophys
    Acta 601: 92-100, 1980
5. Singer SJ and Nicolson GL. The fluid mosaic model of the structure of
    all membranes. Science 175: 720-721, 1972
6. Segal S. Disorders of amino acid transport. New Engl J Med 294:
    1044-1051, 1976
7. Segal S and Crawhall JC. Characteristics of cystine and cysteine
    transport in rat kidney cortex slices. Proc Natl Acad Sci 59: 231-237,
    1968
8. Roth KS, Hwang SM, London JW and Segal S. Ontogeny of glycine transport
    in isolated rat renal tubules. Am J Physiol 233: F241-F246, 1977
9. Dent CE and Rose GA. Amino acid metabolism in cystinuria. Q J Med
    200: 205-218, 1951
10. Brodehl J, Gellhissen K and Kowelewski S. Isobeile Cystinuric (ohne
    lysin⁻, ornithin and argin-uric) in liver Familie met hypocalcamisher
    Tetanie. Montasschr. Kinderheil. 115: 317-320, 1967

11. Whelan DT and Scriver CR. Hyperdibasic aminoaciduria, an inherited disorder of amino acid transport. Pediatr Res 2: 525-534, 1968

12. Fox M, Thier S, Rosenberg LE, Kiser W, and Segal S. Evidence against a single renal transport defect in cystinuria. New Engl J Med 270: 556-561, 1964

13. Rosenberg L, Downing S and Segal S. Competitive inhibition of dibasic amino acid transport in rat kidney. J Biol Chem 237: 2265-2270, 1962

14. Foreman JW, Hwang SM, and Segal S. Transport interactions of cystine and dibasic amino acids in isolated rat renal tubules. Metabolism 29: 53-61, 1980

15. Segal S, McNamara PD and Pepe LM. Transport interactions of cystine and dibasic amino acids in renal brush border vesicles. Science 197: 169-171, 1977

16. McNamara PD, Pepe LM and Segal S. Cystine uptake by rat renal brush border vesicles. Biochem J 194: 443-449, 1981

17. Bovee KD, Joyce T, Reynolds R, and Segal S. The Fanconi syndrome in Basenji dogs - a new model for renal transport defects. Science 201: 1129-1130, 1978

18. Harrison HE and Harrison HC. Experimental production of renal glycosuria, phosphaturia and aminoaciduria by injection of maleic acid. Science 120: 606-608, 1954

19. Rosenberg LE and Segal S. Maleic acid-induced inhibition of amino acid transport in rat kidney. Biochem J 92: 345-352, 1964

20. Roth KS, Goldmann DR and Segal S. Developmental aspects of maleic acid-induced inhibition of sugar and amino acid transport in the rat renal tubule. Pediatr Res 12: 1121-1126, 1978

21. Reynolds R, McNamara PD, and Segal S. On the maleic acid induced Fanconi syndrome: Effects on transport by isolated rat kidney brush border membrane vesicles. Life Sciences 22: 39-44, 1978

22. Bergeron M, Dubord L, and Haussner C. Membrane permeability as a cause of transport defects in experimental Fanconi syndrome, a new hypothesis. J Clin Invest 57: 1181-1189, 1976

23. Gunther R, Silbernagl S and Dietzen P. Maleic acid induced aminoaciduria, studied by free flow micropuncture and continuous perfusion. Pflugers Arch 382: 109-114, 1979

24. Szczepanoka M and Angielski S. Prevention of maleate induced-tubular dysfunction by acetoacetate. Am J Physiol 239: F50-56, 1980

25. Crawhall JC, Scowen EF, Thompson CJ and Watts RWE. The renal clearance of amino acids in cystinuria. J Clin Invest 46: 1162-1171, 1967

26. Morin CL, Thompson MW, Jackson SH and Sass-Korsak A. Biochemical and genetic studies in cystinuria: observations on double heterozygotes of genotype I/II. J Clin Invest 50: 1961-1976, 1971

27. Bovee K, Thier S, Rea C, and Segal S. The renal clearance of amino acids in canine cystinuria. Metabolism 23: 51-58, 1974

28. Bovee KC, Bush M, Dietz J, Jezyk P and Segal S. Cystinuria in the maned wolf of South America. Science, in press, 1981

29. Weber WA, Brown JL, and Pitts RF. Interaction of amino acids in renal tubular transport. Am J Physiol 200: 380-386, 1961

30. Blazer-Yost B, Reynolds R, and Segal S. Amino acid content of rat renal cortex and the response to in vitro incubation. Am J Physiol 236: F398-404, 1979

31. Reynolds R, Roth KS, Hwang SM and Segal, S. The Fanconi syndrome in Basenji dogs - a new model for renal transport defects. Science 201: 1129-1130, 1978

32. Segal S, Rea C and Smith I. Separate transport systems for sugar and amino acids in developing rat kidney cortex. Proc Natl Acad Sci 68: 372-376, 1971

33. Hay PA and Evan AP. Maturation of the proximal tubule in the puppy kidney: A comparison to the adult. Anat Rec 195: 273-300, 1979

34. Witzleben CL, Schoen EJ, Tu WH and McDonald LW. Progressive morphologic renal changes in the oculo-cerebral renal syndrome of Lowe. Am J Med 44: 319-324, 1968

AMINO ACID TRANSPORT

J. BRODEHL

After the development of chromatographic methods for
quantitation of free amino acids (a.a.) in biological fluids
and their clinical applications by Dent in the late 1940s,
the first two decades in the investigation of tubular a.a.
transport were primarily concerned with clinical studies.
The clinician has available three methods by which he can
investigate the renal handling of a.a.: 1. quantitative
measurement of a.a. in blood and urine of normals and
patients with hyperaminoacidurias due to inborn or acquired
defects of tubular transport; 2. endogenous or exogenous
loading with a.a.; 3. studies of postnatal development of
tubular a.a. reabsorption. With these methods most of the
human hyperaminoacidurias known today were investigated in
the period 1950 to 1970. In the last 10 years only two new
types of renal hyperaminoacidurias have been detected (Table 1).

In the following, a short review of our present knowledge
of tubular a.a. transport is given, as it emerged from such
investigations during the last decade. Clinically hyper-

Table 1. Human renal hyperaminoacidurias

Classical cystinuria	1951	Dent and Rose
Hartnup syndrome	1956	Baron et al.
Hyperglycinuria	1957	DeVries et al.
Iminoglycinuria	1958	Joseph et al.
Hypercystinuria	1966	Brodehl et al.
Hyperdibasic aminoaciduria	1968	Whelan and Scriver
Hyperdicarboxylic aminoaciduria	1974	Teijema et al.
Histidinuria	1976	Sabater et al.

aminoacidurias can be classified into 2 categories, the renal
hyperaminoaciduria and the pre-renal hyperaminoaciduria. Renal types of hyperaminoaciduria can be caused either by defects in specific tubular transport systems or by a generalized cellular dysfunction. The pre-renal hyperaminoacidurias just reflect the renal response to increased loads
of free a.a. derived from disturbances in their metabolism,
and are usually not related to tubular defects. Tubular transport systems are genetically determined carrier proteins which
are either specific for individual a.a. or for groups of related a.a. Group specific transport systems have been postulated for cystine and dibasic a.a., glycine and imino acids,
neutral a.a., dicarboxylic a.a., and beta a.a.

Cystine and dibasic amino acids

The tubular reabsorption of cystine and dibasic a.a. has
been investigated intensively. There are three clinical entities characterized by tubular defects for cystine and/or
dibasic a.a.: 1. Classical cystinuria, in which homozygous
patients excrete large amounts of cystine and dibasic a.a.
and acquire urinary cystine stones; 2. Isolated hypercystin-
uria, which is a very rare tubular abnormality and characterized by excessive excretion of cystine, while dibasic a.a.
exhibit normal reabsorption rates, and absence of urinary
stones so far; 3. Hyperdibasic aminoaciduria, which shows
greatly increased excretion rates for lysine, ornithine and
arginine, while the excretion of cystine remains completely
normal. Many patients with hyperdibasic aminoaciduria have in
addition intestinal resorption defects and experience lysine
or protein intolerance. From these clinical observations at
least two different tubular transport systems for cystine
and dibasic a.a. can be postulated: one, which is shared by
all four a.a., and the other, which is specific for cystine
or the 3 dibasic a.a., respectively.

Loading tests with lysine or arginine have been performed
in patients with all three disturbances. Lysine loading in

classical cystinuria provokes a strong increase in the clearance rates not only of lysine, ornithine and arginine, but
also of cystine (4,11,13). The latter finding is intrigueing,
since the clearance of cystine exceedes already that of inulin before lysine loading. The further increase of cystine
clearance by lysine suggests, that mechanisms other than
tubular reabsorption are involved in this effect. Similar
findings could be obtained in a child with isolated hyper-
cystinuria (4). After elevation of plasma lysine the clearance rates of dibasic a.a. and of cystine increase strongly.
In this case the effect can be explained by a competetive
inhibition of the common transport system for dibasic a.a.
and cystine which should not be disturbed in isolated hyper-
cystinuria.

The postnatal development of tubular reabsorption has also
been studied for cystine and the dibasic a.a. The underlying
hypothesis for such studies is, that differences in the postnatal development, especially in the rate for approaching the
mature level of reabsorption, might be an indication for the
individuality of tubular carrier systems. The individual values for lysine collected in 49 infants and children are shown
in Fig.1 ; each dot represents a single patient. In the same
way data for cystine, ornithine, and arginine were collected
(3). From those individual values growth curves for the tubular
reabsorption were calculated by a computer program using the
one compartment equation $y = a_1 + a_2 \cdot e^{-a_3 x}$. The term a_1
is the asymptotic maximal value which is approached in adulthood, and a_3 is the kinetic constant which denotes the rate,
at which the maximal values of the function is approached.
The computed curves for the percentage tubular reabsorption
of cystine and the dibasic a.a. are shown in Fig.2. As can
be seen, each a.a. seems to exhibit an individual slope on
the approach to the mature level, and the adult mature levels
are reached at different rates. The half time of growth rate
$(T_{1/2})$ can be calculated from the kinetic constant a_3. The

FIGURE 1.
Individual data of
urinary excretion
rates, clearance rates
and percentage
tubular reabsorption
of lysine in 49 infants
and children (3)

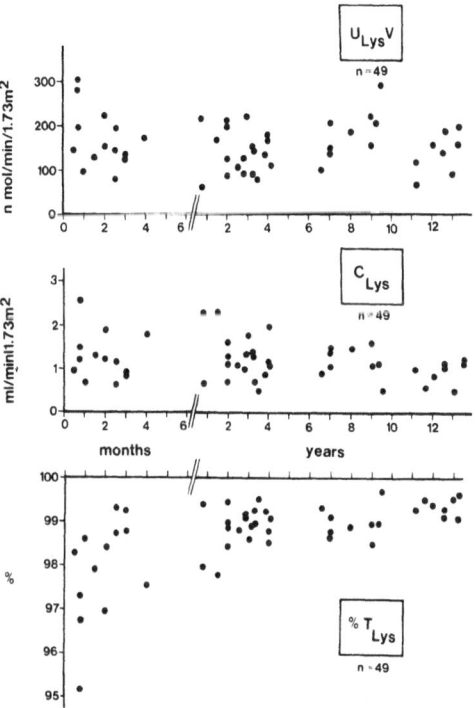

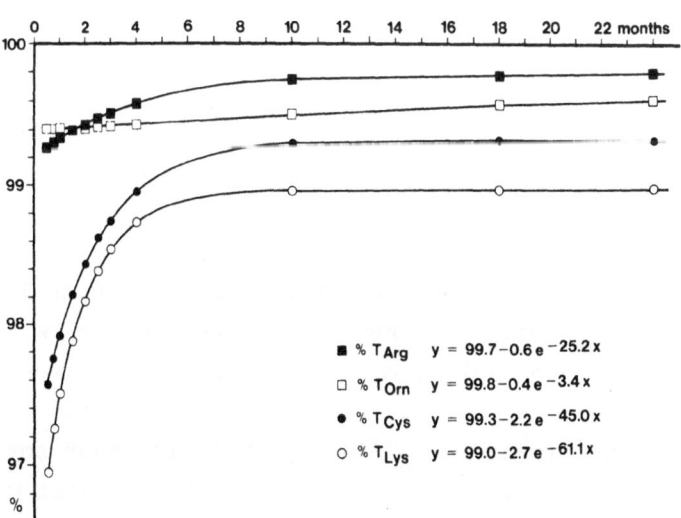

FIGURE 2. Computed curves for percentage tubular
reabsorption of cystine and dibasic a.a. (3)

values of a_3 and $T_{1/2}$ are significantly different for each a.a. The shortest $T_{1/2}$ is for lysine with 1.13 months, followed by cystine (1.54), arginine (2.75) and ornithine (2o.3). These findings support the postulate, that each of the 3 dibasic a.a. might also have its own specific tubular transport system, in addition to the two common transport systems.

Glycine and imino acids

There are two clinical entities in which the tubular reabsorption of these a.a. are specifically disturbed: 1. renal imino-glycinuria, which is characterized by a defect in the tubular reabsorption of both glycine and the imino acids, transmitted as an autosomal recessive trait and sometimes associated with cerebral and neurological disturbances (1o, 15). 2. Isolated glycinuria which demonstrates an isolated defect in the reabsorption of glycine, with completely normal excretion of prolineand hydroxyproline (8.9). It is associated with nephrolithiasis, the pathomechanism of this, however, is not well understood. From these clinical oberservations it was claimed that glycine and imino acids are reabsorbed at least by two tubular transport systems: one is shared by all three a.a., while the other is specific for glycine or the imino acids.

These conclusions are confirmed by developmental studies, which could be performed in the same fashion as described above for cystine and the dibasic a.a. (3). The percentage tubular reabsorption of proline starts at birth from 95 percent of filtered load, and that of glycine from below 8o percent. The calculated half-time for proline is 1.o4 months, while that of glycine is 1.32 months, the difference is statistically significant. This finding indicates that for both a.a. a separate specific transport system might exist which mature at a different rate.

Neutral amino acids

The reabsorption of neutral and cyclic a.a. is disturbed
in a syndrome, which was first described by Baron et al.
in the Hartnup family. The renal defect in the Hartnup syndrome
is characterized by a massive excretion of all neutral and
cyclic a.a. as shown in Fig.3. Clearance rates of affected
a.a. may approach those of glomerular filtration; tubular net
secretion, however, has never been observed. In contrast to
generalized hyperaminoaciduria of the Fanconi syndrome, the
tubular reabsorption of imino acids, glycine, dibasic and
dicarboxylic a.a. are usually not changed in the Hartnup syndrome. In the group of neutral and cyclic a.a. there is only
one, histidin, for which an isolated defect has been described
(14). In isolated histidinuria clearance rates of histidine
are in the range of 25-49 ml/min, while all other a.a. are
reabsorbed completely normal.

Generalized hyperaminoaciduria

Disturbances of tubular cell metabolism lead to generalized
hyperaminoaciduria, as in the Fanconi syndrome. This hyperaminoaciduria follows a very distinct pattern regardless of the
severity of the syndrome. In Fig.4 the clearance rates of free
a.a. from 8 children with the Fanconi syndrome of various
etiologies are depicted. As can be seen all patients seem to
adhere to a general rule; certain a.a. have the highest values
in all cases, for instance glycine and histidine, others are
always in the very low range, as valine or arginine. If one
calculates the mean values for each a.a. and compares these
values with the values of normal controls, one can see, that
a certain rule governs the excretion pattern in generalized
hyperaminoaciduria (4): those a.a. which exhibit the highest
excretion rates in the normal state, show the highest rates in
the Fanconi syndromes also, and vice versa. Thus, the patterns
of the hyperaminoaciduria of Fanconi syndrome seems to be just
an exaggeration of the normal pattern, regardless of the
severity of the tubular disturbance.

The mechanism of increased excretion of a.a. in the Fanconi syndrome is still debated. The original concept was that the urinary a.a. pattern reflects the inability of the proximal tubules to maintain a normal reabsorption rate of filtered a.a. There are, however, some experiments (2), which question this concept, and put forward the postulate that the urinary a.a. profil rather reflect the membrane permeability of the distal tubules. Disturbances of the cellular energy supply could lead to an alteration of the functional integrity of the tubular cell membrane. As a consequence the membrane becomes leaky, and since the pool of intracellular free a.a. is much higher than the extracellular content, this could lead to an increased efflux into the tubular fluid.

Thus although the quantitative aspects of the generalized types of hyperaminoaciduria have been well described in the last decades, the pathomechanism which leads to the disturbances still are not well understood. It is unknown whether the molecular basis of the defect is located in the brush border membranes or is more related to alterations in the energy producing or transferring mechanisms of the cell or both. A further question is, whether all generalized hyperamino-acidurias follow the same pattern which means that this repre-sents a uniform answer of the tubular cell to various toxic agents, or whether there are different types of hyperamino-acidurias which could be related to different etiologies and would let assume that there are different intracellular patho-mechanisms leading to the Fanconi syndrome.

Further studies, both clinically and experimentally, are therefore needed to clarify the mechanisms of the deranged tubular transport in specific and generalized tubulopathies. By understanding the pathological condition a deeper insight in the physiology of these processes is gained.

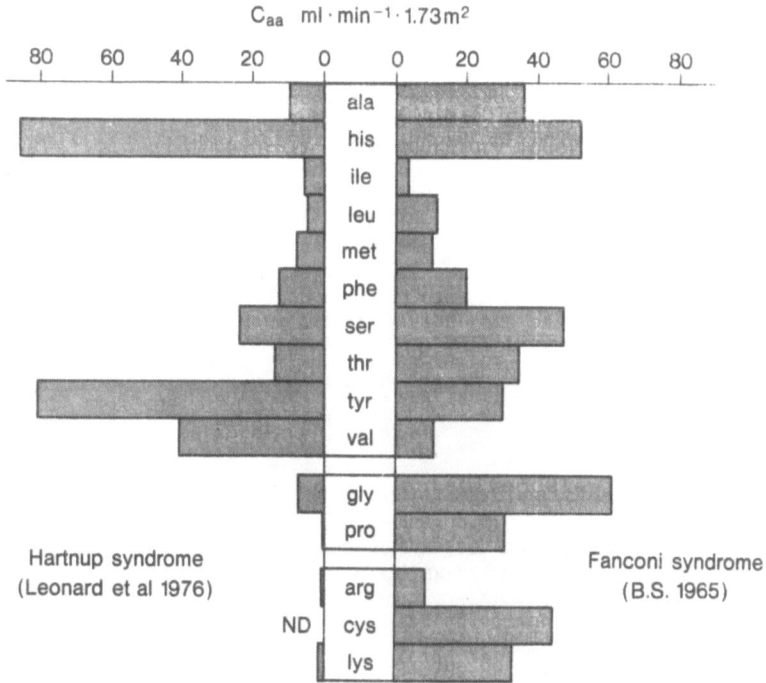

FIGURE 3. Hyperaminoaciduria of Hartnup syndrome as compared with generalized hyperaminoaciduria of Fanconi syndrome.

REFERENCES

1. Baron,D.M., Dent,C.E., Harris,H., Hart,E.W., Jepson,J.B. 1956. Lancet II,421.
2. Bergeron,M., Dubord,L., Hausser,C. 1976. J.clin.Invest.57, 1181.
3. Brodehl,J. 1976. In: "Amino acid transport and uric acid transport". Silbernagel,S., Lang,F., Greger,R. (eds) Thieme Publ. Stuttgart, p.128.
4. Brodehl,J., Bickel,H. 1973. Clin.Nephrol. 1,149.
5. Brodehl,J., Gellissen,K., Kowalewski,S. 1966. III International Congress of Nephrology. Washington. Abstract p.165.
6. Dent,C.E. 1946. Lancet II,637.
7. Dent,C.E., Rose,G.A. 1951. Quart.J.Med. 2o,2o5.
8. DeVries,A., Kochwa,S., Lazebnik,J., Frank,M., Djaldett,M. 1957. Amer.J.Med. 23,4o8.
9. Greene,M.L., Lietman,P.S., Rosenberg,L.E., Seegmiller,J.E. 1973. Amer.J.Med. 54,265.

402

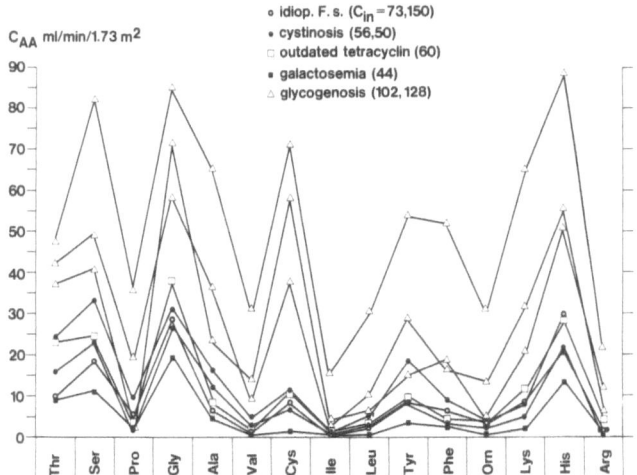

FIGURE 4. Pattern of hyperaminoaciduria in 8 children with Fanconi syndrome due to various etiologies.

REFERENCES (cont.)

1o. Joseph,R., Ribierre,M., Job,J.-C., Girault,M. 1958.
    Arch.Franz.Pédiat. 15,374.
11. Kato,T. 1977. Clin.Scie.Molec.Med. 53,9.
12. Leonard,J.V., Marrs,T.C., Addison,J.M., Burston,D.
    Clegg,K.M., Lloyd,J.K., Matthews,D.M., Seakins,J.W.
    1976. Pediatr.Res. 1o,246.
13. Lester,F.T., Cusworth,D.C. 1973. Clin.Sci. 44,99.
14. Sabater,J., Ferré,C., Puliol,M., Maya,A. 1976. Clin.
    Genet. 9,117.
15. Scriver,C.R. 1968. J.clin.Invest. 47,823.
16. Teijema,H.L., VanGelderen,H.H., Giesberts,M.A.H.,
    Laurent DeAngulo,M.S.L. 1974. Metabolism. 23,115.
17. Whelan,D.T., Scriver,C.R.1968. Pediatr.Res. 2,525.

CURRENT ISSUES IN HYDROGEN ION TRANSPORT

ELISABETH McSHERRY, UNIVERSITY OF CALIFORNIA SAN FRANCISCO

OVERVIEW

The advances in our understanding of clinical hydrogen
ion transport defects presented at this Congress are
summarized in two parts. Elsewhere in this volume Soriano
has considered recent findings in a variant of type 2 Renal
Tubular Acidosis, (RTA), "Pure Proximal" RTA-2. In this
paper, we will specifically address the new findings in the
pathophysiology of the two newest forms of non-azotemic RTA-4
and then consider the secondary effects of chronic hyperchloremic
acidosis in children relating to: (1) growth (2) nephrocalcinosis
and (3) the metabolism of a common pediatric drug,
pseudoephedrine.

RTA is defined as the biochemical syndrome of hyperchloremic acidosis, absence of marked azotemia and an
inappropriate urine pH during mild degrees of acidosis (but
not necessarily during severe acidosis). In each of the 3
prototypic types of RTA, the H+ transport defect is presumed
to occur at a different specific site along the renal tubule.
(See Figure 1.) In RTA-2, the disorder of tubular H+ transport
occurs in the proximal convoluted tubule, usually in
association with the Fanconi syndrome, a complex disorder of
proximal tubular transport of amino acids, phosphate, and
glucose. RTA-4, "mineralo-corticoid deficient (or resistant)
RTA", is a syndrome associated with a H+ transport defect at
the renal tubular transport sites influenced by aldosterone:
the distal convoluted tubule and early collecting duct. RTA-1,
or "classic distal RTA", occurs in the distalmost nephron,
in the distal collecting duct, as is demonstrated by an

inability to generate an H+ gradient and lower urine pH to
normal minima even during severe acidosis. Soriano has
considered RTA-2 elsewhere; we will move further down the
tubule and consider first the new pathophysiologic findings
in RTA-4.

Figure #1

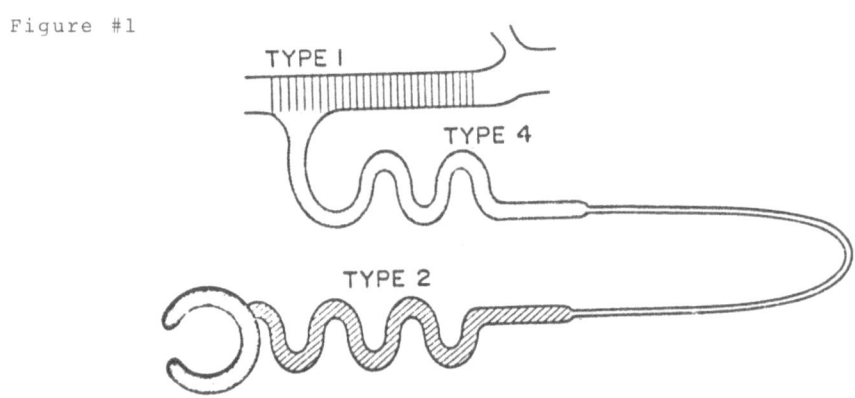

(Reprinted with permission Rudolph and Barnett (3).)

5 NEW SUBTYPES IN RTA-4

RTA-4, a syndrome of hyperkalemic, hyperchloremic
acidosis with acid urine pH during severe acidosis, is
probably the most common of the non-uremic renal tubular
acidification defects in both children and adults. Described
originally in association with Addison's disease, RTA-4 is
now known to occur in 5 etiologically and pathophysiologically
distinct subtypes with different therapeutic requirements
(1-3). (See Table 1.) Subtype 1 RTA-4 is observed in
association with primary mineralocorticoid deficiency
disorders: congenital adrenogenital syndrome, Addison's
disease and isolated hypoaldosteronism (1-3). Subtype 1 and
subtype 4 RTA-4 known as "pseudohypoaldosteronism of infants"
(described by Cheek and Perry in 1958 (4)), are the only two
RTA-4 subtypes characterized by clinical salt-wasting;
thus in addition to the two defining defects of tubular
transport, that of H+ and K+ secretion, these two subtypes

demonstrate a third defect of aldosterone-sensitive transport, that of NaCl. "Pseudohypoaldosteronism" occurs only in infancy and disappears by age 4 years, if the infant receives therapy and survives. Values for 24-hour urinary aldosterone and plasma renin are very high, which suggest a renal tubular unresponsivity to aldosterone. The "pseudohypoaldosteronism" subtype 4 RTA-4 is still seen in Belgium but rarely in the USA. Subtype 2 RTA-4 "hyporeninemic hypoaldosteronism is characteristically non-salt wasting and is found in azotemic patients with a variety of chronic interstitial renal diseases, as described by Schambelan et al in 1973 (5).

TABLE 1 - CLINICAL SPECTRUM OF RTA-4 (HYPERKALEMIC ACIDURIA), SUBTYPED PATHOPHYSIOLOGICALLY

SUBTYPE	CLINICAL FINDING				
Number Designation	Plasma Renin Activity	Urinary Aldosterone	Blood/ Plasma bp	Volume	Salt-Wasting
Aldosterone deficiency without intrinsic renal disease					
1. 1° Mineralocorticoid Deficiency (Addison's; Congenital adrenal hyperplasia; isolated hypoaldosteronism)	↑	↓	↓→	↓→	+
Aldosterone deficiency with chronic Hyporeninemia					
2. 1° Hyporeninemic 2° Hypoaldosteronism of Azotemic Adults (diabetes, gout, pyelnephritis interstitial nephritis, nephrosclerosis)(Sebastian, Schambelan)	↓	↓	↑→	↑→	
3. Adolescent Hyperkalemic Syndrome (?Cl-shunt)(Rector; Gordon-Healy; (Spitzer; Weinstein)	↓	↓	↑	↑	-
Reduced tubular responsiveness to aldosterone					
4. Pseudohypoaldosteronism (Cheek and Perry)	↑↑	↑↑	↓	↓	+
5. "Early Childhood" Type 4 RTA (McSherry)	Not↑	Not↓	Nl	Lo	Nl -

Abbreviations: bp, blood pressure; 1°, primary; 2°, secondary; Nl, normal.

The two subtypes we will consider in depth here, are not associated with azotemia or clinical salt-wasting; both occur mainly in children. Subtype 3 RTA-4 "adolescent type 4 RTA", reported in only 13 young persons, is characterized clinically by frank hypertension (for age); high normal or increased blood volume; and in several patients, by the

finding of hyporeninemic hypoaldosteronism. Findings in
these few reported patients, 6 prepubertals and 7 adolescents,
suggest that NaCl hyperreabsorption occurs apparently, as
proposed orininally by Rector (6), to account for the
clinical findings of increased ECF volume, hypertension, and
reduced values of plasma renin and 24 hour urinary aldosterone.
In the 7 reported patients with this apparent renal
hyperreabsorption of Cl- syndrome who received chlorothiazide
diuretic therapy alone, hyperkalemia and acidosis were
completely corrected (1-3); this was also true in two patients,
a girl and man, who were treated with severe dietary-NaCl
restriction alone (1-3). (See Table 2.)

Table #2

ADOLESCENT TYPE 4 RTA ·SUBTYPE 3
(Renal Cl⁻ Shunt of RECTOR)

PATIENT		BLOOD PRESSURE	PLASMA RENIN ACTIVITY	URINE ALDO	EFFECTIVE Rx?	
REF.#	AGE/SEX				CTZ	LOW Na⁺ DIET
CHILDREN						
1	4 F	↦	↓			
2	9 M	↑	↓	↓	+	+
3	10 F	↑				
1	10 M	↦				
4	11 M	↦	↓	↦	+	
5	15 M	↑	↓	↦		
YOUNG ADULTS						
6	17 M	↑	↓	↦	+	
1	21 M	↑	↓	↦	+	
1	22 M	↦			+	
7	22 M	↑	↓	↓	+	+
8	23 M	↑	↓	↓		
9	23 F	↑			+	
9	28 F	↑				

References

1 Farfel '78
2 Weinstein '74
3 Gordon· '70
4 Spitzer '73
5 Paver/Arnold '64 - 69

6 Grekin '79
7 Langford '81
8 Schambelan '78
9 Bravtbar '78

(Reprinted with permission, Pediatrics Update (2).)

Subtype 5 RTA-4, "early childhood type 4 RTA", the most common type of childhood RTA, is found with equal frequency in males and females and occasionally several siblings of one family are affected (1-3;7). This subtype is unique because with the characteristic RTA-4 hyperchloremic acidosis, hyperkalemia, and aciduria, there is no azotemia, evidence of clinical salt-wasting or hypertension. Physiologic studies reveal a $\leq$ 7% defect in renal tubular reabsorption of bicarbonate at low normal plasma bicarbonate concentrations and a fixed low fractional urinary excretion of potassium (7). The findings in subtype 5 RTA-4 of impaired renal tubular transport of H+ and K+ together with normal or elevated values of aldosterone, are consistent with the formulation that the defect in subtype 5 RTA-4 is a maturational failure of aldosterone-sensitive response by the distal nephron, isolated to H+ and K+ secretion, but not involving mass transfer of Na+ (1-3). The finding that the values of urinary aldosterone excretion and plasma renin activity are increased in these children, but not as greatly as in children with "pseudohypoaldosteronism" (subtype 4 RTA-4), suggests that a tubular transport defect which includes a failure in renal NaCl reabsorption may provide more potent stimulation to aldosterone secretion than an dysfunction of the distal tubule isolated to H+ and K+ secretion alone.

This patient group with subtype 5 RTA-4 provides the unique opportunity to study the pathophysiologic characteristics of the RTA-4 H+ transport defect in a relatively pristine state, free from the secondary effects of azotemia, clinical salt-wasting, or major hormonal imbalance (7). During sustained correction of acidosis with high-dose alkali alone, despite consistently normal or high values of plasma renin activity and 24 hr urinary aldosterone, in each of 13 children renal bicarbonate wasting occurred: (the urinary excretion of net base in amounts $\geq$ 3 meq/kg/d at low or low normal $\underline{/}\,HCO_3^-\,\underline{/}$ p (7). Acute bicarbonate titration studies revealed a 4% fractional urinary excretion of HCO_3^- during mild acidosis, that rose to 7.6% (range 5-15%) at low

normal $\underline{/}^-HCO_3^-\underline{/}$ p. Despite this massive urinary bicarbonate
excretion at low normal $\underline{/}^-HCO_3^-\underline{/}$ p, fractional potassium
excretion remained fixed and low; the mean was 16% for studies
both before and after alkali infusion (7). Such data provide
further support for the hypothesis that distal tubular K+
secretion is defective in children with "early childhood"
subtype 5 RTA-4.

As a metabolic consequence of intracellular K+ depletion,
in adult patients Podolsky demonstrated human growth hormone
(hGH) release is reversibly blunted (8). No studies of
intracellular $\underline{/}^-K+\underline{/}$ have been reported in children with
"early childhood" subtype 5 RTA-4. As we will see later in
this paper, hGH release has been shown to be blunted during
acidosis in children with RTA-1 and RTA-4. There is no
reason to assume that pathophysiologic factors participating
in the metabolic consequences of acidosis in "early childhood"
subtype 5 RTA-4 are obliged to be similar to those for any
other subtypes of RTA-4.

SECONDARY EFFECTS OF HYPERCHLOREMIC ACIDOSIS:(1)NEPHROCALCINOSIS

Nephrocalcinosis (NC has occurred invariably by age 4
years in all children with RTA-1 treated since infancy with
low-dose alkali ($\leq$ 3 meq/kg/d) (1-3;9-11). It was previously
though that the renal tubular defect of RTA-1, not acidosis,
caused this invariable NC. Two years ago, however, we
demonstrated that low-dose alkali (1-3 kg/d) was insufficient
to sustain correction of acidosis in children with RTA-1;
5 - 14 meq/kg was required, as these children underwent both
growth spurts and renal bicarbonate wasting (12-13). In the
7 of 10 children with RTA-1 given such "high-dose" alkali to
sustain correction of acidosis from less than 4 years of age,
radiologically demonstrable NC did not occur over periods
ranging from 10-20 years (9-11). Six of the 7 children were
members of 3 unrelated kindred that include 8 other affected
members. In each of these 8, NC had occured despite low- dose
alkali therapy, instituted as early as 2 years of age. In
all 10 patients of our study, hypocitraturia was invariable
with low-dose alkali therapy; with high-dose alkali therapy,

hypocitraturia and hypercalciuria were invariably corrected.
These results indicate that the renal disorder expressed in
early childhood as RTA-1, does not itself cause or give rise
to NC or cause hypocitraturia. Rather the results support
the hypothesis that in children with RTA-1, metabolic acidosis
(with its attendant metabolic consequences) is a critical
pathogenetic determinant not only of short stature, but also
of NC and hypocitraturia. The results are consistent with
the formulation that in patients with RTA-1, acidosis gives rise
to NC by causing hypercalciuria and hypocitraturia.

A CALCIUM TRANSPORT DEFECT IN SUBTYPE 5 RTA-4

    Infants and children with non-azotemic, "early childhood"
subtype 5 RTA-4 were then investigated, after acidosis had
prevailed of sufficient severity to cause height stunting,
to evaluate the occurrence of NC. Radiologically demonstrable
NC did not occur over 2-10 years observation in 14 children
with non-azotemic RTA-4 all of whom had short stature at time
of diagnosis including 5 patients in whom untreated chronic
acidosis had been documented for 2-4 years duration (14).
These findings are in direct contrast to those in short statured
children with RTA-1 on low-dose alkali ($\leq$ 3 meq/kg/d) since
infancy, in whom NC is invariable (9-11). In children with
RTA-4, possibly of benefit in the prevention of NC, was the
predictable finding that the urinary excretion of calcium
did not increase with acidosis, but persisted significantly
lower than that seen in acidotic normal children or in
acidotic children with RTA-1. Also of possible benefit in
the prevention of NC in patients with RTA-4 was the finding
that during acidosis urinary citrate (a chelator and complexer
of calcium) was higher than the lower normal limits for non-
acidotic children; in normal children given NH_4Cl to induce
acidosis or in acidotic children with RTA-1, urinary citrate
is characteristically low or unmeasurable. During acidosis in
normal adults, citrate is completely reabsorbed by the proximal
and distal convoluted tubules and none appears in the urine;
normal amounts of citrate are excreted in the urine only after
acidosis is corrected fully. In reported cases of proximal

RTA-2 with the Fanconi syndrome, urinary citrate excretion
is very high despite acidosis, and in these patients, despite
massive hypercalciuria, NC and nephrolithiasis do not occur.
We postulated that the children with non-azotemic RTA-4, as
well as the ones reported with RTA-2, may be protected from
the occurrence of NC despite chronic hyperchloremic acidosis
sufficient to cause height stunting, in part because the
abnormally high urinary citrate excretion,which occurs
during acidosis as a characteristic part of their respective
multiple renal tubular transport defects, protects against
calcium precipitation (14).Our study provided the first
evidence in patients with non-azotemic RTA-4, that renal
tubular transport defects for both calcium and citrate are
characteristically found in association with the transport
defect of RTA-4: during acidosis, renal tubular reabsorption of
citrate is significantly reduced and that of calcium, significantly increased in patients with subtype 5 RTA-4 (14, 15).

RTA RADIOLOGIC FINDINGS: A 10-YEAR STUDY

In the recent report of a decade of radiographic findings
in 92 patients, (56 children and 36 adults), with the three
prototypic types of RTA, (1969-1979), bone disease was rarely
observed in non-azotemic RTA, and then only in patients with
RTA-2 (11). Radiologically demonstrable nephrocalcinosis was
seen only in patients with RTA-1, but was not observed in
children with RTA-1 who received high-dose alkali (5-14 meq/kg/d)
since infancy (11).

2^{O} EFFECTS OF ACIDOSIS: (2)GROWTH AND HUMAN GROWTH HORMONE (hGH)

As the next issue related to H+ transport, we will
consider our recent findings on the effect of hyperchloremic
acidosis on hormonal and metabolic factors related to growth.
In children with non-azotemic RTA-1 (12, 13) and RTA-4 (10),
acidosis caused short stature which was reversed if high-dose
alkali therapy (5-14 meq/kg/d) was sustained. In a recent
report in the 13 patients with early childhood subtype 5
RTA-4, mean height was low (- 2.4 SD) before alkali therapy;
6 patients were frankly stunted. With 5-15 meq/kg/d alkali
therapy, in 6 months normal height was attained by each

child (17). The effect of acidosis, and its correction by
alkali therapy alone, on the release of human growth hormone
(hGH), was investigated in 11 children with RTA-1 and 4 children
with RTA-4 by measuring peak hGH concentration during standard
arginine and L-dopa stimulation tests. During chronic acidosis
($\geq$ 6 months), in each of 7 prepubertals, peak hGH concentration
was blunted (< 8ng/ml) (mean 5.2). The absolute value of blunted
hGH varies with age in children and is higher in pubertals
(<12ng/ml); therefore when values of hGH were expressed as %
non-acidotic values, in 15 children, ages 2 - 19 years, mean
peak hGH release during acidosis was found to be 57.9% of
non-acidotic values; in 12 of the 15 children, peak hGH was
absolutely blunted for age (17). The findings of this study
provide no support for the suggestion that serum potassium
concentration correlates positively with peak hGH release
(8): in our study mean serum potassium concentration was
lower during correction of acidosis than during acidosis.
The results of this study demonstrated that acidosis reduces
peak hGH release after standard stimulation tests in non-
azotemic children with RTA-1, RTA-4 and in normal children
(17). The study suggests that plasma $\underline{/}\overline{HCO_3^-}\underline{}\underline{/}$ is a critical
determinant of hGH release for children undergoing standard
hGH stimulation tests (17).

SECONDARY EFFECTS OF ACIDOSIS: (3) COLLAGEN SYNTHESIS

The synthesis of collagen has 7 major enzymatic steps,
the last of which is catalyzed by the extracellular enzyme,
lysyl oxidase (LO), after the partially-completed collagen
molecule is extruded from the cell. In rats with experimental
hepatic fibrosis plasma LO levels are elevated and, the
activity of LO is elevated in both tissue and plasma, in
chicks with vitamin D-deficiency, a syndrome in which, as in
RTA, acidosis and growth retardation are characteristic. In
10 children (6 months to 18 years), 7 with RTA-1 and 3 with
RTA-4, LO activity was measured by the method of Pinnell
and Martin modified by Siegel (18). Mean LO activity was
elevated by 8-10 fold during acidosis, but after sustained
correction of acidosis with alkali therapy alone, fell

immediately to normally low values in each patient (18).
In steady-states each pertaining for at least one week
duration, plasma LO activity inversely correlated with plasma
concentration of $\underline{/}HCO_3^-\underline{}/$ over the range 15-23 meq/L (15
studies of 10 patients) (18). In a 3-year-old child with
RTA-4, during chronic partially-treated acidosis, activity
of LO was measurable and mildly, but not markedly, increased,
but with complete withdrawal of alkali therapy for 4 days,
LO increased by 4 fold to significantly elevated levels; LO
activity then fell to unmeasurable levels within 24 hours of
institution of fully-corrective alkali therapy (18). The
findings of this study provided the first demonstration that
acidosis directly affects collagen metabolism.

PSUEDOEPHEDRINE (SUDAFED) EXCRETION AND RTA

"Sudafed", pseudoephedrine (Ps), is a decongestant used
ubiquitously in the practice of pediatrics. In a child with
RTA-1, severe toxicity was observed after the administration
6 weeks of Ps for chronic otitis: the 6-year-old girl had a
weight loss of 6 pounds, toxic organic-psychosis like that
of "speed" or amphetamine toxicity, and greatly elevated
levels of blood Ps. We presumed the drug accumulated because
her persistently alkaline urine pH favored the renal tubular
reabsorption of the weak base, Pseudoephedrine ($PK_a = 9.4$).
The renal determinants of the urinary elimination of Ps were
assessed in 15 studies in 8 subjects: 3 normal adults, 3
normal children and one adult and one child each with RTA-1.
Ps (5 mg/kg) was administered orally; blood and urine levels
were serially measured by liquid chromatography. Urine pH
was controlled at various levels by the administration of
$NaHCO_3$ or NH_4Cl. In all studies the administered Ps dose was
excreted 45% as Ps, and 6% $\pm$ 1.0% as norpseudofed. Elimination
half-life, significantly and directly, correlated with the
urine pH; mean, for the 15 studies, was 7.0 $\pm$ 1.2 hours,
range 1.0 to 21 hours over the observed physiologic range of
urine pH values (19). At alkaline urine pH, in each subject
the renal excretion of Ps and its metabolite, norpseudoephedrine,
was also directly and significantly correlated to urine flow

rate. These findings suggest that, as with amphetamine and ephedrine, the elimination of Ps and its metabolite are importantly determined by both urine pH and urine flow rate in man (19).

CONCLUSION

In the review of the most recent findings in clinical defects of hydrogen ion transport, we see that RTA-4 is presently considered the most common of the 3 prototypic RTA types and is now separable into 5 subtypes with distinct diagnostic, therapeutic and prognostic implications. In considering the new pathophysiologic findings in the two most recently described non-azotemic subtypes of RTA-4, we see that the renal tubular defect of hyporeabsorption of citrate and a relative hyperreabsorption of Ca^{++} during acidosis, now further characterizes the renal tubular defect of at least one non-azotemic form of RTA-4, "early childhood" subtype 5. Chronic hyperchloremic acidosis has now been shown to be causal of both nephrocalcinosis and its associated hypocitraturia in RTA-1. In RTA-1, RTA-4 and in normal children hyperchloremic acidosis has shown to affect reversibly at least two human growth factors, human growth hormone and the collagen synthetic enzyme, LO. Finally the high urine pH, characteristic of patients with RTA $\lceil$ at all levels of plasma bicarbonate concentrations (RTA-1) or during alkali therapy only (RTA-2 and RTA-4) $\rfloor$, severely reduces the normal urinary excretion of a weak-base, pseudoephedrine. Sudafed administered to a patient with consistently high urine pH will rapidly induce a severe and debilitating intoxication like the organic toxic-psychosis of amphetamine or "speed". A critical implication of this last Sudafed study was, that in children with RTA on alkali therapy, doses of Pseudoephedrine, a component of nearly all cold remedies and decongestants, must be reduced to at least one-third or entirely withdrawn.

REFERENCES

1. McSherry, E. 1981, Renal Tubular Acidosis - Nephrology Forum: Kidney International (presented July 14, 1980)

REFERENCES (Continued)

2. McSherry, E. 1981, "Current Issues in Renal Tubular Acidosis" in Pediatrics Update, Editors, Smith, F.G., Jr., and Moss, A., Volume 4, Elsevier Publishers

3. McSherry, E. 1981, "Renal Tubular Disorders of Childhood" in Rudolph and Barnett's Textbook of Pediatrics, 17th Edition

4. Cheek, D.B., and Perry, J.W., 1958, A salt-wasting syndrome in infancy Arch. Dis. Child 33:252

5. Sebastian, A., McSherry, E., Schambelan, M., Connor, D., Biglieri, E., and Morris, R.C., Jr. 1973, Renal Tubular Acidosis (RTA) in patients with hypoaldosteronism caused by renin deficiency, Clin. Res. 21:706

6. Shambelan, M., Sebastian, A., Rector, R.C., Jr., 1978, 81, Mineralo-corticoid (MC) resistant renal K+ secretory defect: Proposed distal tubule chloride shunt. Clin. Res.26:54A, and 1978, and Kidney International, 1981 (In press)

7. McSherry, E., Portale, A., Gates, J., 1978, Non-areninemic Type 4 renal tubular acidosis (RTA) of infancy. American Society of Nephrology, 11th annual meeting ((Presented November 21, 1978), 135.

8. Podolsky, S., Zimmerman, H.J., Burrow, B.A., et al 1973, Potassium depletion in liver cirrhosis: A reversible cause of impaired growth hormone and insulin response, New Eng.J. Med.288:644-648.

9. McSherry, E., Pokroy, M., 1978, The absence of nephrocalcinosis in children with Type 1 RTA on high-dose alkali therapy since infancy. Clin. Res. 26:470A, Presented May 1, 1978.

10. Morris, R.C., Jr., Sebastian, A., McSherry, E., 1978, Therapeutic evidence in patients with classic renal tubular acidosis. Proceedings of the IVth International Congress of Nephrology, Montreal, Canada, 345-349.

11. Brenner, R.J., Spring, D., McSherry, E., Sebastian, A., Genant, H., Morris, R.G., Jr., and Palubinskas A.J., 1981, Radiologic findings in 92 patients (56 children - 36 adults) with the 3 major types of RTA Radiology

12. McSherry E., Morris, R.C., Jr., 1978, Attainment of normal stature with alkali therapy in infants and children with classic renal tubular acidosis (RTA): Evidence that acidosis is critical to the pathogenesis of impaired growth. J. Clin. Invest. 61:509-527.

13. McSherry, E., 1978, Acidosis and growth in chronic non-uremic renal disease. Kidney International, 14:349-354.

REFERENCES (Continued)

14. McSherry, E., Gates, J., Pialaet, M., 1981, Nephrocalcinosis and the urinary excretion of citrate and calcium in non-azotemic Type 4 RTA.Proceedings IVth International Workshop in Urolithiasis Research, Williamsburg, VA 6/23/1980, January 81.

15. McSherry, E., Gates, J., Pialaet, M., 1980, Urinary excretion of citrate and calcium and the incidence of nephrocalcinosis in the major types of non-azotemic RTA. American Society of Nephrology, November 1980, 25.

16. McSherry, E., Portale, A.A., Gates, J., 1978, The predictable occurrence of impaired growth in infants with Type 4 RTA. VIIth International Congress of Nephrology, Proceedings, Montreal, Canada. Presented June 21, 1978

17. McSherry, E., Weberman, J., Kaplan, S., Grumbach, M.M., 1980, The effect of acidosis on human growth hormone (hGH) release. (Presented at National Meeting, ASCI) Clin. Res. 28:535

18. Griger, C., Siegel, R., McSherry, E. The modulation of the plasma of lysyl oxidase activity by plasma bicarbonate concentration. American Society of Nephrology, for 11th annual meeting. Presented November 2, 1978, p. 18.

19. Brater, D.C., Kaojarern, S., Benet, L.Z., Lin, E.T., Lockwood, T., McSherry, E., Morris, R.C., Melmon, K.L., 1980, and 1981, Renal excreti of pseudoephedrine by man. Clin. Pharm. and Therapeutics, 1981, Clin. Res. 28:238, 1980 and in press.

THE MANAGEMENT OF RESISTANT HYPERTENSION - THE ROLE OF
MINOXIDIL

PETER R. LEWY, M.D.
CHILDREN'S MEMORIAL HOSPITAL, CHICAGO, IL. USA

Minoxidil is an antihypertensive agent that acts by
direct peripheral vasodilatation.It has recently been made
available for use in the U.S. Between 1973 and 1979 we had
the opportunity to utilize minoxidil on 25 occasions for the
treatment of severe refractory hypertension in 21 children
(11 males, 10 females) between the ages of 6 months to 16
years. All patients were treated according to an investigational emergency protocol approved by the Research and Human
Ethics Committee of the Children's Memorial Hospital, Chicago.
Informed consent for the use of minoxidil was obtained from
parents and all older children.

Of the 21 patients treated with minoxidil, 12 had normal
renal function, (serum creatinine less than 2.0mg/dl), 8 were
given to children with renal insufficiency and 3 were on
recently initiated maintenance hemodialysis. .The 12 patients
with normal renal function included four on high dose of
corticosteroids early in the course of renal transplantation
and five with renal artery stenosis of a single kidney. Those
with stenosis included 4 with renal transplants and one with
a single kidney 4 years after nephrectomy from Wilm's Tumor.
The remaining 3 were a 6 month old with infantile polycystic
diseaseof the kidney and liver, a 9 year old with a stable
liver transplant on prednisone therapy, and a 12 year old with
newly diagnosed focal lupus nephritis on prednisone therapy.
Of patients with renal insufficiency 2 had acute transplant
rejection, 3 had chronic rejection and four had progressive
primary renal disease. Two of the 3 dialysis patients had
recent hemolytic uremic syndrome and the third had severe

glomerulosclerosis of unknown origin. Altogether 15 patients were receiving prednisone and this was considered to be a definite factor in the hypertension of _eight_ patients.

The indications for recommending the use of minoxidil were 1) a blood pressure exceeding 140/100mmHg in children under 6 years of age or exceeding 150/110mmHg in older children, despite the use of limiting oral doses of routinely available antihypertensive agents in combination or 2) the need for continual use of parenterally administered antihypertensive agents to achieve or maintain such levels and/or 3) the occurrence of hypertensive encephalopathy or heart failure despite such treatment. The oral antihypertensive agents in routine use in our clinic were hydralazine,alphamethyl dopa propranolol and furosemide. In hospitalized patients with abrupt elevations of blood pressure in excess of 150/110mmHg intravenous hydralazine was often utilized as initial parenteral therapy. For refractory hypertensive episodes or encephalopathy, diazoxide was given as needed.

In each case minoxidil therapy was initiated in the hospital with a single dose of one milligram. Subsequent doses of 2,3,5,7.5 and 10mg, respectively were then given every 12 hours as needed to achieve a blood pressure of 140/100 to 130/90mmHg. The effective dose was then continued on a 12-hourly basis for several doses. Further increases to a maximum of 40mg/day were made as needed to lower blood pressure into the normal range. In general, all parenteral antihypertensives were withdrawn at the onset of minoxidil therapy while all prior oral antihypertensives were continued until satisfactory blood pressure control had been established. The doses of hydralazine and alphamethyldopa were then reduced as long as satisfactory control was maintained.

The mean blood pressure for the entire group just prior to initiation of minoxidil therapy was 157 ± 12 (S.D.)mmHg systolic and 112 ± 12mmHg diastolic with a range of 190/130-140/100mmHg. All patients were receiving a variety of antihypertensive agents and 9 patients required diazoxide to reverse or prevent serious hypertensive sequelae.

In fact, sixteen children suffered serious hypertensive complications prior to minoxidil therapy, including twelve with hypertensive encephalopathy and/or papilledema, and six with congestive heart failure; two had both complications. All six patients with congestive failure had chronic renal insufficiency, and volume expansion undoubtedly contributed to both the hypertension and the congestive failure. Nineteen patients had electrocardiographic evidence of left ventricular hypertrophy, and cardiomegaly was apparent in thirteen.

RESULTS

Prompt control of unacceptably elevated blood pressure was obtained in all but one patient. The average of the blood pressures achieved when a stable dose of minoxidil had been reached was 118 ± 20 (S.D.)mmHg systolic and 74 ± 16mmHg diastolic with a range of 160 - 92mmHg systolic and 110-50mmHg diastolic. The median time required to reach this response was 10 days with a mean of 17 and a range of 1-105 d. Blood pressure control was accomplished with an average daily dose of minoxidil of 0.48mg/Kg/day with a range of 0.07-1.6mg/kg/day. In absolute terms, doses of minoxidil at or below 2.5mg q 12 hr. was effective in 11 patients. On the other hand, the blood pressure of an adolescent boy with relentless polyarteritis nodosum and intractable edema remained refractory to a dose of 30mg q 12 hours. Interestingly, diazoxide remained effective in this boy. Patients remained on minoxidil for a mean of 124 days over a range of 7-20 days, plus a patient who required treatment for $4\frac{1}{2}$ years (1660 days).

There was a tendency to a gradual increase in blood pressure with time in 8 patients. This was related to fluid retention in 6 patients who had renal insufficiency, and to continued use of high dose prednisone in two patients with episodes of acute reversible transplant rejection.

During minoxidil therapy, the dosage of alphamethyldopa and of hydralazine could be reduced, while the doses of propranolol and furosemide were essentially unchanged. At the time minoxidil could be discontinued the mean dose of hydralazine had been reduced from 6.0mg kg/day in 21 patients to 3.3mg kg/day in the 12 patients who still required it. Similarly, alphamethyldopa was reduced from a mean of 47 mg kg/day in 22 patients to 30 mg kg/day in 16 patients who still required it. In contrast, during minoxidil, propranolol was required at an average daily dose of 3.0 mg kg in 18 children. This dose was comparable to the 3.5mg kg/day used prior to minoxidil treatment. The average daily dose of furosemide was 4.2 mg/kg in 12 of 15 patients who were not in renal failure during minoxidil treatment, compared to 4.7 mg/kg in 13 patients just prior to treatment.

In qualitative terms the overall control of severe hypertension was considered to be good (diastolic pressure - 85mmHg) in 15 cases, fair (diastolic pressure 85-100mmHg) in 3 cases and poor (diastolic pressure $\geq$ 100mmHg) in 4 cases. Five of the 7 cases with less than good control had renal insufficiency and relative fluid overload. The remaining two had multiple arterial stenoses in well functioning renal transplants.

COMPLICATIONS

Hypertrichosis was noted in all patients receiving minoxidil for more than three weeks. Increased hair growth was noted on forehead and face, as well as on the back and limbs. The occurrence of hypertrichosis appeared to be independent of daily dose minoxidil. It was more apparent in children with darker complexions. Upon discontinuing minoxidil excess hair growth ceased and a normal hair pattern returned within 6-8 weeks.

The relationship of minoxidil therapy to tachycardia and to fluid retention was not clear in this group of patients none of whom had uncomplicated stable hypertension. These effects would have been masked by the diuretics and beta blocking agents that most patients were already receiving when minoxidil was initiated.

Two children experienced asthamatic episodes for the first time while on minoxidil and large doses of propranolol (6mgkg/day and 9mg/Kg/day, respectively). Propranolol dosage was reduced and no further episodes were experienced. One of

these patients, a 5 year old boy with transplant artery
stenoses and three courses of minoxidil therapy also
experienced a variety of other complications during minoxidil
therapy. He had split cranial sutures early in the first
course of therapy. There was no papilledema. The skull film
was taken during evaluation for a seizure. Resolution was
spontaneous. A diagnosis of pseudotumor cerebri related to
prednisone therapy was considered most likely. This patient
also had several seizures, always in mid-morning after
missing breakfast due to minor illness. Severe elevations
of blood pressure to 180/130mmHg or higher were common during
and after the seizures despite ongoing minoxidil therapy.
These blood pressure elevations responded to diazoxide 5mg/
Kg IV. Several of these seizures were related to hypoglycemia
(blood glucose < 40mg/dl). This in turn was considered to be
related to the fasting state and the effects of propranolol
on hepatic glycogenolysis. This same child developed a
transient pericarditis on two occasions, neither related to
renal failure or apparent fluid overload. The pericarditis
resolved spontaneously within several days each time.
Finally, this patient had two brief episodes of acute
parotitis while on minoxidil. This was not associatedwith
any of the other complications.

Two important complications of therapy were observed in
other patients. The first was the development of abrupt renal
shutdown in a 16 year old boy with a chronically rejecting
cadaveric transplant. He had an initial blood pressure of
160/120, a serum creatinine of 6mg/dl, and a daily urine
output of 800 ml. He was receiving alphamethyldopa,
metroprolol, and furosemide. The blood pressure fell to
120/75 at 10 mg of minoxidil q 12hr. A decreased urine output (< 200cc/24 hr) was noted on day 7 and the serum
creatinine had risen to 12 mg/dl. Minoxidil was discontinued.
Urinary output and serum creatinine concentration reverted
to their previous levels. Interestingly, the blood pressure
rose to only 140/100mmHg where it remained for several weeks.

The other significant complication related to the abrupt appearance of congestive heart failure in the boy with the stable liver transplant and normal renal function when he abruptly failed to take his minoxidil early in the 4½ year course of his treatment. Blood pressure control was promptly re-established with his usual dose of minoxidil. The congestive failure resolved without further treatment.

Finally, it may be worthy of note that symptomatic hypotension was not a complication noted in this series, even in a patient who inadvertently was given a single dose of minoxidil four times the effective dose.

Only one patient remains on minoxidil at the present time. In 6 patients improved blood pressure was related to decrease in prednisone therapy. In 6 patients with progressive renal failure minoxidil could be discontinued when the initiation of maintenance hemodialysis permitted improved regulation of extracellular fluid volume. In 3 patients already on dialysis, bilateral nephrectomy resulted in improved blood pressure control without minoxidil. In 6 instances in patients with renal arterial stenosis minoxidil was discontinued after surgical repair or bypass. The minoxidil was restarted a few months later following each of two unsuccessful repairs in one transplant recipient. Five patients have died while on minoxidil: four with chronic renal failure (all refused dialysis) and one with sepsis. In a final patient, minoxidil was withdrawn after 7 days because of renal shutdown presumed due to renal hypoperfusion.

In conclusion, minoxidil has proved to be a very useful agent in the management of severe complicated or refractory hypertension in children. Patients can be titrated rapidly to an effective dose without evident risk of hypotension. The case of minoxidil has permitted hospital discharge of patients otherwise dependent upon parenteral antihypertensive therapy.

Though not free from side effects, the drug is generally safe especially in the context of present or potential hypertensive complications. Notwithstanding its relative

safety, but because of the cosmetic problem of hirsutism and
because of the often perceived need for the concomitant use
of beta-blockers and diuretics, minoxidil should be reserved
for use in severe hypertension where unacceptable side effects
occur with other agents or when parenteral therapy would
otherwise be needed to treat or to avert the serious
complications of hypertension itself.

CHLORAMBUCIL THERAPY IN THE NEPHROTIC SYNDROME

H.J. BALUARTE, M.D., A.B. GRUSKIN, M.D., M.S. POLINSKY, M.D., J.W. PREBIS,M.D., H. ROSENBLUM, M.D.   St. Christopher's Hospital for Children, Phila., PA.

In an attempt to reduce corticosteroid toxicity and to induce long-term remission, immunosuppressive agents such as cyclophosphamide and chlorambucil have been used in combination with corticosteroids to treat the frequently relapsing and steroid resistant nephrotic syndrome.[1-5] The effectiveness of cyclophosphamide has been established and its long-term results have been reviewed by Rance and co-workers.[6] These studies indicate that the duration of remission following a course of cyclophosphamide is approximately proportional to the length of the course. When low doses of the drug were given for sufficiently short periods of time to reduce toxic side effects, relapse subsequently occurred in as many as 48% of the patients during the first 12 to 26 months after therapy. Data from Grupe and co-workers [7] indicate that the combination of prednisone and chlorambucil, produces a longer remission than steroids alone, and that this combination also alters the subsequent course of relapses. In a more recent publication [8] by the same authors, a life table analysis of two dosage schedules of chlorambucil at four years shows that 91% of patients on low doses and 80% of those on high doses are still in remission.

We have carried out a prospective controlled clinical trial whose purpose was to determine if a stable dose regime of chlorambucil was as effective as an increasing dose in inducing immediate response, and to evaluate the immediate toxicity and the long-term effects. Twenty-two children with the idiopathic nephrotic syndrome as defined by the International Study of Kidney Disease in Children were investigated.[9] After inducing a remission the patients were randomly divided into two groups: Group I received chlorambucil 0.2 mg/kg/day for 8 weeks. Group II received chlorambucil 0.2 mg/kg/day initially and increments of approximately 0.1 mg/kg/day every two weeks for 6 to 11 weeks or until leukopenia developed, which marked the end of the therapy. Both groups also received prednisone 60 mg/m^2 as a single dose on alternate days.

Twenty-two patients were studied. Their ages at the onset of the nephrotic syndrome averaged 3.4 and 3.7 years. The mean ages at the onset of chlorambucil therapy were 7.7 and 8.7 years. The mean total dose in relation to body weight were 11.3 mg and 18 mg and the mean total cumulative doses of chlorambucil were 363 and 680 mgs. respectively. The highest daily dose given to children in Group II ranged from 0.25 to 0.63 mg/kg/day.

TABLE I   RESULTS OF CHLORAMBUCIL THERAPY

	GROUP I	GROUP II
Follow up (yr)	5.2 (3.6 - 6.8)	5.28 (4.5 - 6.0)
Onset of Relapse (Mos)	#Patients	#Patients
0 - 12	2	0
12 - 24	0	1
24 - 36	1	2
36 - 48	0	0
48 - 60	0	0

Table I displays the results of chlorambucil therapy. Follow-up averaged 5.2 years in Group I and 5.28 years in Group II. Three patients in each group had relapses. In Group I, patients relapsed 6, 10 and 26 months after completion of therapy. In Group II, patients relapsed at 15, 31 and 32 months. One patient in Group II received a second course of low dose chlorambucil because of her frequently relapsing pattern. She has had only one relapse in the last four years. Preliminary data reported in 1978[10] demonstrated that a stable dose regimen of chlorambucil for 56-60 days was as effective in altering the relapse pattern as in increasing dose, given over 42 to 72 days, even though the stable dose regimen furnished a lower cumulative dose. Evaluation of our data without actuarial analysis showed that 19% of the children had relapses during an observation period that averaged 2.4 and 2.3 years in both groups. Extension of the follow up to cover 5 years continues to indicate the lasting effectiveness of the stable dose regimen of chlorambucil in the treatment of the idiopathic nephrotic syndrome of childhood.

Focal sclerotic lesions of glomeruli are found in about 10% of children with the nephrotic syndrome and account for approximately 40% of steroid resistant.[11] The impression from various clinical surveys of patients with focal segmental glomerulosclerosis is that such a lesion is associated with high risk of progression to renal insufficiency.[12-16]

The response to corticosteroid therapy in patients with focal sclerotic lesions and the nephrotic syndrome has not been encouraging. The International Study of Kidney Disease in Children is currently conducting a controlled therapeutic trial of patients with focal segmental glomerulosclerosis in which patients are randomly assigned to a group treated with prednisone alone or a group receiving cyclophosphamide and prednisone. A preliminary report of the I.S.K.S.C. presented at the Fifth International Pediatric Nephrology Symposium[17] indicated that neither therapeutic regimen is superior to the other. The reported use of other cytotoxic agents in the treatment of focal segmental glomerulosclerosis is limited.[11,18,19,20]

We have now studied 22 children with nephrotic syndrome and focal glomerulo-sclerosis, 12 males and 10 females with their onset of nephrotic syndrome between 0.9 and 14 years (average 4.3 years). Renal biopsies were performed when they became resistant to steroid therapy or after several years of steroid sensitive-frequently relapsing or steroid dependent disease. Nineteen had the lesion of focal segmental glomerulosclerosis and three had focal global sclerosis on initial renal biopsy. All patients presented with the nephrotic syndrome, 54% had hematuria, 27% hypertension and 9% a GFR less than 80 ml/min/ $1.73m^2$.

Before treatment with chlorambucil, all patients were treated with standard prednisone regimen recommended by the International Study of Kidney Disease in Children. The clinical course of these patients associated with their steroid therapy was as follows: two patients were frequent relapsers, three steroid dependent and ten steroid resistant. In the other seven late non-responders, steroid resistance appeared 0.5 to 7 years after the clinical onset of the nephrotic syndrome.

Chlorambucil therapy was undertaken once the diagnosis of focal glomerulo-sclerosis was made. As it is shown in Table II, chlorambucil therapy was given at a starting dose of 0.2 mg/kg and increased every other week by 0.1 mg/kg. Alternate day prednisone, 60 mg/m^2 was also given. The age of the children at the onset of chlorambucil therapy ranged between 1 and 19.5 years. The total cumulative dose of chlorambucil ranged between 7.7 and 39.8 mgs with a mean of 18.2 mg/kg. Their highest daily dose ranged from 0.2 to 0.83 mg with the mean value being 0.43 mg/kg.

TABLE II   SCHEME OF CHLORAMBUCIL THERAPY

Dosage 0.2 mg/kg/day (increments 0.1 mg/kg)
with Prednisone 60   mg/m^2/qod

	6.8
Age at treatment (yr)	(1 - 19.5)
Days of therapy	28 - 72
Total cumulative dose (mg/kg)	18.2 (7.7- 39.8)
Highest daily dose (mg/kg)	0.43 (0.2-0.83)

The results of 26 courses of chlorambucil therapy in 22 patients are sum-marized in Table III. These patients have been followed for 1 to 7 years. Of the 22 patients treated with chlorambucil, 15 patients went into remission within 11 weeks of the onset of therapy. The other 7 failed to respond. Of the 15 patients who responded to chlorambucil, 7 subsequently relapsed. Among the children that failed to respond to chlorambucil therapy, one is on hemo-dialysis, one has mild renal insufficiency and the other underwent a successful cadaveric renal transplant.   All 15 chlorambucil responders continue to have a normal urine sediment and renal function.

TABLE III   RESULTS OF CHLORAMBUCIL THERAPY

Follow up (yr)   Mean 3.95   (1.0 - 7.0)

		FR	SD	LNR	SR
Remission	(15/22)	2(2)	3(3)	6(7)	4(10)
No response	(7/22)	-	-	1	6
Relapse	(7/15)	1	2	3	1
CRF,Dialysis,Tx				1(DX)	1(CRF) 1(TX)
Normal urine-GFR		1	3	6	4

The Table IV describes in more detail the 7 patients that had relapses 0.5 to 7 years after chlorambucil therapy. One patient in the frequent relapser group relapsed after 3 years and at the time of this evaluation he was in relapse. Two patients in the steroid-dependent group relapsed 0.8 to 3 years after chlorambucil, one received a second course of chlorambucil because of the same steroid-dependent pattern, but both are presently in remission. Among the late non-responders 3 patients have relapsed 0.5, 1 and 2.5 years after chlorambucil, one had 3 courses of chlorambucil 2 and 4 years apart, but all are presently in remission. One patient in the steroid resistant group relapsed after 1 year post chlorambucil, was resistant to steroids again but responded to a second dose of chlorambucil and she has remained in remission for the last 5 years.

TABLE IV   RELAPSES POST-CHLORAMBUCIL THERAPY

Category	Number of Patients	Onset of Relapse(YR)	Number Courses	Present Status
FR	1	3	1	Relapse
SD	2	0.8	1	Remission
		3	2	"
LNR	3	0.5	1	Remission
		1	3	"
		2.5	1	"
SR	1	1	2	Remission

To summarize, 15/22 or 68% of the children with nephrotic syndrome and pathology compatible with the diagnosis of focal glomerulosclerosis have responded to chlorambucil therapy. It is apparent that children who are or were steroid responsive respond well to chlorambucil. Chlorambucil as we have used it in our mixed patient population has been effective in the treatment of children with nephrotic syndrome and focal sclerotic lesions. In our opinion further controlled clinical trials would seem to be indicated.

Chlorambucil shares with other cytotoxic drugs the potential for considerable immediate and long-term toxicity. Leukemia has been noted in children given a total dose in excess of 22 mg/kg.[21,22] Focal seizures occurred in 7.5% of patients treated with chlorambucil.[23] Chlorambucil has been implicated in causing gonadal dysfunction when given alone or in combination with other agents.[24] In most cases, the great variability of the administered doses and the fact that the same patient has frequently received two or more drugs, makes it difficult to obtain useful conclusion on the real threshold dose for its gonadal toxicity. When chlorambucil is used as the only cytotoxic agent without steroids, azoospermia has been reported to occur when cumulative doses exceed 7 mg/kg, and at 17 mg/kg if given with steroids.[24] It seems that dosage and length of treatment are both important in determining long-term toxicity. As with cyclophosphamide, the duration of treatment may be more important than dosage as regards the development of azoospermia.[6]

Our experience with complications following 48 courses of chlorambucil therapy is summarized in Table V. Reversible leukopenia was the most consistent side effect. Since leukopenia is dose related, it was more common in those patients given an increasing dose regime. Reversible thrombocytopenia occurred in two patients. Mild gastrointestinal symptoms occurred in two patients shortly after the onset of therapy. Viral and bacterial infections occurred during therapy or developed shortly after it was discontinued in a number of children. Herpetic infections developed in five patients within 2 weeks after completion of therapy. The relationship of these treatment regimens to long term gonadal function in our patients is in the process of evaluation.

TABLE V ACUTE COMPLICATIONS OF CHLORAMBUCIL IN 48 COURSES AMONG 44 PATIENTS

	Group I	Group II	Group III
Leukopenia	3	7	14
Thrombocytopenia	-	2	-
Gastrointestinal	1	1	-
Infections	-	3	4
Seizures	-	-	-
Cystic,Alopecia,Leukemia	-	-	-
Death	-	-	-

In conclusion:

1. Chlorambucil is an effective drug in the treatment of minimal change nephrotic syndrome of childhood. Its use should be limited to the frequently relapsing steroid-dependent or steroid resistant patient.

2. Present evaluation indicates the lasting effectiveness of the stable dose regime in the treatment of the idiopathic nephrotic syndrome. The lowest effective dose of chlorambucil still remains to be established.

3. Chlorambucil appears to be effective as we have used it among children with nephrotic syndrome and focal glomerulosclerosis.

4. There is a need for caution in the management of these patients because of the immediate and long-term side effects of chlorambucil.

REFERENCES

1. Barratt, T.M. and Soothill, J.F.: Controlled trial of cyclophosphamide in steroid-sensitive relapsing nephrotic syndrome of childhood. Lancet 2:479, 1970.
1. Prospective, controlled trial of cyclophosphamide therapy in children with the nephrotic syndrome: Report of the International Study of Kidney Disease in Children, Lancet 2:423, 1974.
3. Moncrieff, M.W., White, R.H.R., Ogg, C.S. and Cameron, T.S.: Cyclophohphamide therapy in the nephrotic syndrome in childhood. Br.Med.J. 1:666, 1969.
4. Grupe, W.E.: Chlorambucil in steroid-dependent nephrotic syndrome. J.Pediatr. 82:598, 1973.
5. Barratt, T.M., Osofsky, F.G., Bercowsky, A., et al: Cyclophosphamide treatment in the steroid-sensitive nephrotic syndrome of childhood. Lancet 1:55, 1975.
6. Rance, C.P., Arbus, G.S. and Balfe, J.W.: Management of the nephrotic syndrome in children. Pediatr.Clin.North Am. 23:735, 1976.
7. Grupe, W.E., Makker, S.P. and Ingelfinger, J.R.: Chlorambucil treatment of frequently relapsing nephrotic syndrome. N.Engl.J.Med. 295:746, 1976.
8. Williams, S.A., Makker, S.P., Ingelfinger, J.R. and Grupe, W.E.: Long-term evaluation of chlorambucil plus prednisone in the idiopathic nephrotic syndrome of childhood. N.Engl.J.Med. 302:929, 1980.
9. Abramowicz, M., Arneil, G.C., Barnett, H.L., Barron, B.A., Edelmann, C.M., Gordillo, G., Greifer, I., Hallman, N., Kobayashi, O. and Tiddens, H.S.: Controlled trial of azathioprine in children with nephrotic syndrome. Lancet 1:959, 1970.
10. Baluarte, H.J., Hiner, L. and Gruskin, A.B.: Chlorambucil dosage in frequently relapsing nephrotic syndrome. A controlled clinical trial. J.Pediatr. 92:295, 1978.
11. Nash, M.A., Greifer, I., Olbing, H., Bernstein, J., et al: The significance of focal sclerotic lesions of glomeruli in children. J.Pediatr.88:806,1976.
12. Cameron, J.R., Ogg, C.S., Turner, D.R. and WEller, R.O.: Focal glomerulosclerosis, in Kincaid-Smith, P., Mathew, T.H., and Becker, E.L., editors: Glomerulonephritis, New York, 1973, John Wiley & Sonc, Inc. p.249.
13. Habib, R.: Focal glomerular sclerosis, Kidney Int. 4:355, 1973.
14. Hyman, L.R. and Burkholder, P.M.: Focal sclerosing glomerulonephropathy with hyalinosis. J. Pediatr. 84:217, 1974.
15. McGovern, V.J. and Lauer, C.S.: Focal sclerosing glomerulonephritis, in Glomerulonephritis, New York, 1973, John Wiley & Sons, Inc.,p.223.
16. White, R.H.R., Glasgow, E.F. and Mills, R.J.: Focal glomerulosclerosis in childhood, in Glomerulonephritis, New York, 1973, John Wiley & Sons, Inc. p.231.
17. A controlled therapeutic trial of cyclophosphamide plus prednisone versus prednisone alone in children with focal segmental glomerulosclerosis: A preliminary report of the International Study of Kidney Disease in Children. Pediatr.Res. 14:1006, 1980.
18. Siegel, N.J., Kashgarian, M., Spargo, B.H. and Hayslett, J.P.: Minimal change and focal sclerotic lesions in lipoid nephrosis. Nephron 13:125,1974.
19. Schoeneman, M.J., Bennett, B. and Greifer, I.: The natural history of focal segmental glomerulosclerosis with and without mesangial hypercellularity in children. Clin. Nephrol. 9:45, 1978.
20. Cameron, J.S., Turner, D.R., Ogg, C.S., Chantler, C. and Williams, C.G.: The long-term prognosis of patients with focal segmental glomerulosclerosis. Clin.Nephrol. 9:213, 1978.

21. Westberg, N.G. and Swolin, B.: Acute myeloid leukemia appearing in two patients after prolonged continuous chlorambucil treatment for Wegener's granulomatosis. Acta. Med. Scand. 199:373, 1976.
22. Cameron, S.: Chlormabucil and leukemia. N.Engl.J.Med. 296:1065, 1977.
23. Williams, S.A., Makker, S.P., Grupe, W.E.: Seizures: A significant side effect of chlorambucil therapy in children. J.Pediatr.93:516, 1978.
24. Guesry, P., Lenoir, G., Broyer, M.: Gonadal effects of chlorambucil given to prepubertal and pubertal boys for nephrotic syndrome. J.Pediatr. 92:299, 1978.
25. Supported in part by NIH General Research Grant RR-75.

ANTICOAGULANT THERAPY

JERRY M. BERGSTEIN, M.D.

Histopathologic and biochemical studies demonstrate that the
coagulation system is activated in certain forms of human and
experimental renal disease. Studies of experimental models of
intravascular coagulation and immune-mediated glomerulonephritis
suggest that anticoagulant or fibrinolytic therapy may significantly
reduce the severity of the glomerular lesions. This review will
summarize the results of anticoagulant therapy in human renal disease.

HEMOLYTIC-UREMIC SYNDROME

Although more than 100 children with Hemolytic-uremic Syndrome have
been treated with heparin,[1-33] the value of such therapy remains
unconfirmed. Comparison between studies is difficult due to
differences in diagnostic criteria, severity of the disease process,
and variation in the natural history in different geographic areas.
The results of heparin therapy are difficult to interpret because of
variations in the dose, time of initiation, duration, and means of
administration of the drug.

In the majority of patients, the renal lesion seems established by
the time the patient is initially seen and evidence for active
coagulation is not detected.[34-36] Heparin therapy seems unlikely to
help this group. However, a small percentage of patients have been
found who show evidence of active coagulation when first seen[1,37] and
these might benefit from anticoagulant therapy.

If the renal lesion is already established at the time of
presentation, then glomerular survival would depend upon the kidneys'
capacity to remove glomerular fibrin deposits. We have previously
shown that the human glomerulus possesses fibrinolytic activity
mediated by the elaboration of plasminogen activator.[38] Stimulation
of fibrinolytic activity might be of value in removing glomerular

fibrin thrombi. Streptokinase, an indirect plasminogen activator, has
been used in the treatment of a few children with the Hemolytic-uremic
Syndrome.[19,30,39-44] Analysis of such therapy is confounded by the
same problems that prevent analysis of heparin therapy. It is clear
that a small percentage of patients with the Hemolytic-uremic Syndrome
fail to recover from the disease process; these might be helped by
fibrinolytic therapy. Unfortunately, we have no method to identify
these patients early in the course of their disease. Since
fibrinolytic therapy is most helpful when given shortly after
thrombosis occurs (when those who will have a poor result are not yet
evident) and has a definite risk of hemorrhage and in view of the high
rate of recovery following conservative management of the renal
failure,[23,31,45] we have abandoned this form of treatment.

THROMBOTIC THROMBOCYTOPENIC PURPURA

Thrombotic thrombocytopenic purpura is uncommon in
childhood.[46,47] As in the Hemolytic-uremic Syndrome,
microangiopathic hemolytic anemia and thrombocytopenia are common;
evidence of disseminated intravascular coagulation is generally
absent.[47-49] Severe neurologic involvement appears more common in
Thrombotic Thrombocytopenic Purpura whereas severe renal disease
appears more common in the Hemolytic-uremic Syndrome.

The pathogenesis of Thrombotic Thrombocytopenic Purpura seems
related to intravascular platelet aggregation.[49] In view of the high
mortality rate in untreated patients, some form of therapy should be
attempted. I agree with the therapeutic recommendations of Amorosi and
Karpatkin[50] who suggest starting treatment with high-dose
corticosteroids and inhibitors of platelet aggregation (e.g.,
dipyridamole) and adding exchange transfusion[51] or plasmapheresis[52]
in the absence of prompt clinical improvement.

GLOMERULONEPHRITIS

Little information is available concerning anticoagulant therapy in
children with glomerulonephritis. Most studies have not been
controlled and also include the use of immunosuppressive and/or
antiplatelet agents. Herdman and associates[53] demonstrated improved

renal function in 5 children treated with heparin alone (two with rapidly progressive glomerulonephritis, and one each with membranoproliferative glomerulonephritis, anaphylactoid purpura, and Wegener's granulomatosis). Robson et al.[54] treated six children having proliferative glomerulonephritis, necrosis and/or crescents, and biochemical evidence of active intravascular coagulation with heparin followed by phenindione, azathioprine, and dipyridamole; all improved. Cunningham et al.[55] found improvement in four of five children having rapidly progressive glomerulonephritis after treatment with heparin, immunosuppressive agents and, in two, dipyridamole. However, post-Streptococcal glomerulonephritis was the etiology in three of the four that recovered and this has been shown to recover spontaneously.[56]

In adults, uncontrolled studies using anticoagulants, immunosuppressive and antiplatelet agents have shown benefit in certain patients with rapidly progressive, chronic proliferative, and membranoproliferative glomerulonephritis.[57-67] However, negative reports also exist.[68-70]

As the natural history of untreated rapidly progressive glomerulonephritis is poor, treatment should be attempted in view of the occasional successes reported in the literature. Treatment should be restricted to patients with some degree of residual renal function as those with oligo-anuria rarely respond. Studies suggest an initial course of high-dose corticosteroids in combination with other immunosuppressive drugs (azathioprine or cyclophosphamide), heparin, and dipyridamole. Plasmapheresis[71,72] should be considered in the absence of a prompt clinical response.

REFERENCES

1. Willoughby MLN, Murphy AV, McMorris S, Jewell FG. Coagulation studies in haemolytic uraemic syndrome. Arch Dis Child 1972;47:766-771.
2. Berman W Jr. The hemolytic-uremic syndrome: initial clinical presentation mimicking ulcerative colitis. J Pediatr 1972;81:275-278.
3. Brain MC, Baker LRI, McBride JA, Rubenberg ML, Dacie JV. Treatment of patients with microangiopathic haemolytic anemia with heparin. Br J Haematol 1968;15:603-621.
4. Chan JCM, Eleff MG, Campbell RA. The hemolytic-uremic syndrome in nonrelated adopted siblings. J Pediatr 1969;75:1050-1053.
5. Clarkson AR, Lawrence JR, Meadows R, Seymour AE. The haemolytic uraemic syndrome in adults. Quart J Med 1970;39:227-244.
6. Egli F, Stalder G, Gloor F, Duckert F, Killer F, Hottinger A. Heparin therapie des haemolytisch-uramischen syndroms. Helv Paediatr Acta 1969;13:24-28.
7. Gervais M, Richardson JB, Chiu J, Drummond KN. Pathology of the hemolytic-uremic syndrome. J Pediatr 1971;47:352-359.
8. Habib R, Courtecuisse V, Leclerc F, Mathieu H, Royer P. Etude anatomo-pathologique de 35 observations de syndrome hemolytique et uremique de l'enfant. Arch Franc Pediatr 1969;26:391-416.
9. Habib R, Leclerc R, Mathieu H, Royer P. Comparison clinique of anatomo-pathologique entre les formes mortelles et curable du syndome hemolytique et uremique. Arch Franc Pediatr 1969;26:417-426.
10. Hitzig WH. Therapie mit antikoagulantien in der padiatrie. Helv Paediatr Acta 1964;19:213-222.
11. Kaplan BS, Katz J, Krawitz S, Lurie A. An analysis of the results of therapy in 67 cases of the hemolytic-uremic syndrome. J Pediatr 1971;78:420-425.
12. Kibel MA, Barnard PJ. Treatment of acute haemolytic-uraemic syndrome with heparin. Lancet 1964;2:259-260.
13. Kunzer W, Aalam F. Treatment of the acute haemolytic-uraemic syndrome with heparin. Lancet 1964;1:1106.
14. Lieberman E. Hemolytic-uremic syndrome. J Pediatr 1972;80:1-16.
15. McCredie DA, Dixon SR. The hemolytic-uremic syndrome. In: Kincaid-Smith P, Mathew TH, Becker EL, eds. Glomerulonephritis. New York: John Wiley and Sons, 1973:1069-1078.
16. Moncrieff MW, Glasgow EF. Haemolytic-uraemic syndrome treated with heparin. Br Med J 1970;3:188-191.
17. Monnens L, Schretlen E. Haemolytic-uraemic syndrome. Lancet 1968;2:735-736.
18. Piel CF, Goodman JR, Beck J. Ultramicroscopic glomerular lesions in hemolytic uremia. Clin Res 1970;18:225.
19. Powell HR, Ekert H. Streptokinase and anti-thrombotic therapy in the hemolytic-uremic syndrome. J Pediatr 1974;84:345-349.
20. Seiler G, Tietze HU. Haemolytisch-uramishes syndrom. Z. Kinderheilkd. 1969;106:249-252.
21. Sharpsone P, Evans RG, O'Shea M, Alexander L, Lee HA. Haemolytic-uraemic syndrome: survival after prolonged oliguria. Arch Dis Child 1968;43:711-716.
22. Troelstra JA, Visser HKA. Haemodialysis in the haemolytic-uraemic syndrome. Lancet 1965;1:770-771.

23. Tune BM, Leavitt TJ, Gribble TJ. The hemolytic-uremic syndrome in California: a review of 28 nonheparinized cases with long-term follow-up. J Pediatr 1973;82:304-310.
24. Vitacco MJ, Avalos S, Gianantonio CA. Heparin therapy in the hemolytic-uremic syndrome. J Pediatr 1973;83:271-275.
25. Westra B. Recurrent haemolytic-uraemic syndrome treatment with and without heparin. N Zeal Med J 1974;80:209-210.
26. Ekberg M, Holmberg L, Denneberg T. Hemolytic uremic syndrome. Results of treatment with hemodialysis. Acta Paediatr Scand 1977;66:693-698.
27. Sorrenti LY, Lewy PR. The hemolytic-uremic syndrome. Experience at a center in the midwest. Am J Dis Child 1978;132:59-62.
28. Shashaty GG, Atamer MA. Hemolytic-uremic syndrome associated with infectious mononucleosis. Am J Dis Child 1974;127:720-722.
29. Ray CG, Portman JN, Stamm SJ, Hickman RO. Hemolytic-uremic syndrome and myocarditis. Am J Dis Child 1971;122:418-420.
30. Monnens L, Van Collenburg J, De Jong M, Zoethout H, Van Wieringen P. Treatment of the hemolytic-uremic syndrome. Helv Paediatr Acta 1978;33:321-328.
31. Riella MC, George CRP, Hickman RO, et al. Renal microangiopathy of the hemolytic-uremic syndrome of childhood. Nephron 1976;17:188-203.
32. Gianantonio CA, Vitacco M, Mendilaharzu F, Gallo GE, Sojo ET. The hemolytic-uremic syndrome. Nephron 1973;11:174-192.
33. Proesmans W, Eeckels R. Has heparin changed the prognosis of the hemolytic-uremic syndrome. Clin Nephrol 1974;2:169-173.
34. Harker LA, Slichter SJ. Platelet and fibrinogen consumption in man. N Engl J Med 1972;287:999-1005.
35. Katz J, Krawitz S, Sacks PV, et al. Platelet, erythrocyte, and fibrinogen kinetics in the hemolytic-uremic syndrome of infancy. J Pediatr 1973;83:739-748.
36. Kisker CT, Rush RA. Absence of intravascular coagulation in the hemolytic-uremic syndrome. Am J Dis Child 1975;129:223-226.
37. Avalos JS, Vitacco M, Molinas F, Penalver J, Gianantonio C. Coagulation studies in the hemolytic-uremic syndrome. J Pediatr 1970;76:538-548.
38. Bergstein JM, Michael AF Jr. Cortical fibrinolytic activity in normal and diseased human kidneys. J Lab Clin Med 1972;79:701-709.
39. Bergstein JM, Edson JR, Michael AF Jr. Fibrinolytic treatment of the haemolytic-uraemic syndrome. Lancet 1972;1:448-449.
40. Guillin MC, Boyer C, Beaufils F, Lejenne C. Utilisation de streptokinase dans deux cas de syndrome hemolytique et uremique. Arch Franc Pediatr 1973;30:401-412.
41. Heimsoth VH, Blumcke S, Bohlmann HG, Haupt H, Kuster F. Erfolgreiche thrombolytische therapie bei bilateralen nierenrindennekrosen. Deut Med Woshenschr 1973;98:1895-1898.
42. Monnens L, Kleynen F, Van Munster P, Schretlen E, Bonnerman A. Coagulation studies and streptokinase therapy in the haemolytic-uraemic syndrome. Helv Paediatr Acta 1972;27:45-54.
43. Stuart J, Winterborn MH, White RHR, Flinn RM. Thrombolytic therapy in haemolytic-uraemic syndrome. Br Med J 1974;2:217-221.
44. Sutor AH, Schindera F, Jacobi H, Kunzer W. Haemolytic-uraemic syndrome; thrombocyturia after treatment with streptokinase and aspirin. Lancet 1972;2:762.

45. Kaplan BS, Thomson PD, de Chadarevian JP. The hemolytic-uremic syndrome. Pediatr Clin North Am 1976;23:761-777.
46. Berman N, Finklestein JZ. Thrombotic thrombocytopenic purpura in childhood. Scand J Haematol 1975;14:286-294.
47. Berberich FR, Cuene SA, Chard RL Jr, Hartmann JR. Thrombotic thrombocytopenic purpura. J Pediatr 1974;84:503-509.
48. Jaffe EA, Nachman RL, Merskey C. Thrombotic thrombocytopenic purpura-coagulation parameters in twelve patients. Blood 1973;42:499-507.
49. Neame PB, Hirsch J, Browman G, et al. Thrombotic thrombocytopenic purpura: a syndrome of intravascular platelet consumption. Can Med Assoc J 1976;114:1108-1112.
50. Amorosi EL, Karpatkin S. Antiplatelet treatment of thrombotic thrombocytopenic purpura. Ann Intern Med 1977;86:102-108.
51. Pisciotta AV, Garthwaite T, Darin J, Aster RH. Treatment of thrombotic thrombocytopenic purpura by exchange transfusion. Am J Hematol 1977;3:73-82.
52. Myers TJ, Wakem CJ, Ball ED, Tremont SJ. Thrombotic thrombocytopenic purpura: combined treatment with plasmapheresis and antiplatelet agents. Ann Intern Med 1980;92:149-155.
53. Herdman RC, Edson JR, Pickering RJ, Fish AJ, Marker S, Good RA. Anticoagulants in renal disease in children. Am J Dis Child 1970;119:27-35.
54. Robson AM, Cole BR, Kienstra RA, Kissane JM, Alkjaersig N, Fletcher AP. Severe glomerulonephritis complicated by coagulopathy: treatment with anticoagulant and immunosuppressive drugs. J Pediatr 1977;90:881-892.
55. Cunningham RJ, Gilfoil M, Cavallo T, et al. Rapidly progressive glomerulonephritis in children: a report of thirteen cases and a review of the literature. Pediatr Res 1980;14:128-132.
56. Leonard CD, Nagle RB, Striker GE, Cultler RE, Scribner BH. Acute glomerulonephritis with prolonged oliguria. Ann Intern Med 1970;73:703-711.
57. Kincaid-Smith P, Saker BM, Fairley KF. Anticoagulants in irreversible acute renal failure. Lancet 1968;2:1360-1363.
58. Kincaid-Smith P, Laver MC, and Fairley KF. Dipyridamole and anticoagulants in renal disease due to glomerular and vascular lesions. Med J Austral 1970;1:145-151.
59. Cade JR, de Quesada AM, Shires DL, et al. The effect of long term high dose heparin treatment on the course of chronic proliferative glomerulonephritis. Nephron 1971;8:67-80.
60. Arieff AI, Pinggera WF. Rapidly progressive glomerulonephritis treated with anticoagulants. Arch Intern Med 1972;129:77-84.
61. Suc JM, Conte J, Conte M. Treatment of glomerulonephritis with indomethacin and heparin. In: Kincaid-Smith P, Mathew TH, Becker EL, eds. Glomerulonephritis. New York: John Wiley and Sons, 1973:927-947.
62. Brown CB, Wilson D, Turner D, et al. Combined immunosuppression and anticoagulation in rapidly progressive glomerulonephritis. Lancet 1974;2:1166-1172.
63. Cameron JS, Gill D, Turner DR, et al. Combined immunosuppression and anticoagulation in rapidly progressive glomerulonephritis. Lancet 1975;2:923-925.

436

64. Fye KH, Hancock D, Moutsopoulos H, Humes HD, Arieff AI. Low-dosage heparin in rapidly progressive glomerulonephritis. Arch Intern Med 1976;136:995-999.

65. Rathaus M, Bernheim JL. Low-dose heparin in rapidly progressive glomerulonephritis. Arch Intern Med 1979;139:251.

66. Kincaid-Smith P. The treatment of chronic mesangiocapillary (membranoproliferative) glomerulonephritis with impaired renal function. Med J Austral 1972;2:587-592.

67. Kincaid-Smith P. The natural history and treatment of mesangiocapillary glomerulonephritis. In: Kincaid-Smith P, Mathew TH, Becker EL, eds. Glomerulonephritis. New York: John Wiley and Sons, 1973:591-609.

68. Freedman P, Meister HP, De La Paz A, Ronaghy H. The clinical, functional, and histologic response to heparin in chronic renal disease. Invest Urol 1970;7:398-409.

69. Wardle EM, Uldall PR. Effect of heparin on renal function in patients with oliguria. Br Med J 1972;3:135-138.

70. Suc JM, Durand D, Conte J, et al. The use of heparin in the treatment of idiopathic rapidly progressive glomerulonephritis. Clin Nephrol 1976;5:9-13.

71. McKenzie PE, Taylor AE, Woodroffe AJ, Seymour AE, Chan YL, Clarkson AR. Plasmapheresis in glomerulonephritis. Clin Nephrol 1979;12:97-108.

72. Lockwood CM, Peters DK. Plasma exchange in glomerulonephritis and related vasculitides. Ann Rev Med 1980;31:167-179.

GROWTH FAILURE, END STAGE RENAL DISEASE AND SOMATOMEDIN

JOHN E. LEWY, M.D.

The growth failure associated with severe renal failure in children
undoubtedly results from the interaction of multiple factors. A
possible role for the somatomedins in this pathophysiologic state has
received considerable attention during the past five years.

The somatomedins are a family of circulating peptides with similar
biologic actions, bound to large carrier proteins which originate
primarily in the liver and appear to be degraded at least in part by
the kidney. Our knowledge regarding the role of somatomedins in
chronic renal failure has been slow in developing, due primarily to
difficulties in measurement. The first assay, which evolved from the
pioneering work of Salmon and Daughaday (1) in 1957, was dependent on
either the incorporation of radioactive chondroitin sulfate into
cartilage or the incorporation of tritiated thymidine into DNA. The
bioassays are generally not specific for the various somatomedins and
are sensitive to inhibitors in human serum. One of these inhibitors,
sulfate, is particularly relevant in children with end stage renal
disease because of its high concentration in the uremic serum. High
doses of glucocorticoids also have an inhibitory effect on the
bioassay.

Radio receptor assays were developed when it was recognized that each of the somatomedins competes with ^{125}I insulin for binding the insulin receptors in a number of cell membranes. In addition, the somatomedins bind to specific somatomedin cell membrane receptors which are distinct from the insulin receptors. Thus, competitive membrane binding assays to measure somatomedin levels in serum have been developed. These assays have the advantage of not being subject to inhibitors such as a variation in sulfate concentration in the serum.

Specific radioimmunoassays have now been developed for somatomedin A and somatomedin C. The assay of somatomedin C described by Furlanetto et al, (2) has the advantages of avoiding interference from carrier proteins and allowing determination in small volumes. These assays are so new, that little work has been done evaluating somatomedin levels by radioimmunoassay in children with growth failure associated with chronic renal failure.

Normal values by each of these assays differs from adult values both early and late in childhood. The numbers are still too small to have clearly defined standards for children. However, the data suggests that in the first two or three years of life, somatomedin levels as measured by bioassay or radioimmunoassay are lower than adult normals and that values in the adolescent age group are higher than adult normals. (3) It has been suggested, that the infants cartilage might be more sensitive to somatomedins and thus able to respond with rapid growth despite lower circulating levels. It is certainly also possible that circulating somatomedin is not the "correct" marker.

Serum levels of somatomedin as measured by bioassay have been either

normal or decreased in children with end stage renal failure associated
with growth failure. Growth hormone levels measured in the same
children have been either normal or increased. (4-6) Saenger and
co-workers (4) measured somatomedin by bioassay in nine growth retarded
male children before and after renal transplantation. Serum somatomedin
levels were corrected for sulfate, a known inhibitor, in this study.
Prior to renal transplantation, somatomedin levels were uniformly low.
Following renal transplantation, there was a significant and linear
correlation between growth velocity expected for bone age and somatomedin
levels. Somatomedin levels also correlated with creatinine clearance
following transplantation. In the figure shown, all somatomedins
increased by at least 60% with a return to the normal range in those
patients with normal renal function. Growth hormone levels were also
normal and the paradoxical rise in growth hormone noted during glucose
tolerance testing no longer occured. Phillips (7-9), et al and Pennisi
(10) found somatomedin levels to be decreased by bioassay in four of
ten children prior to dialysis and normal in the remainder.

Spencer and co-workers (10) have recently reported on the use of the
radio receptor assay in the measurement of somatomedin A in thirty-nine
children aged 2 to 17. The study by Spencer evaluates somatomedin
levels in normal children, children with growth hormone deficiency and
excess and 22 children with chronic renal insufficiency. The children
with chronic renal failure had somatomedins in the acromegalic range.
The same study shows a significant increment in somatomedin measured
prior to hemodialysis (2.95 $\pm$ 0.39 U/ml) to that seen in 17 children
receiving hemodialysis (5.7 $\pm$ 0.3). A single dialysis did not
significantly alter the level but successful renal transplantation led

to a return in somatomedin level to or just above normal.

The radioimmunoassay for somatomedin C as described by Furlanetto et al, is currently being studied in order to develop data concerning normals in children. The mean level in the 0-5 year age group is 0.79, while the range is quite wide. The 8-18 year age group reveal a higher mean and higher upper limits than other normals.

Somatomedins by radioimmunoassay have not yet been reported in young children with end stage renal disease. However, Takano and co-workers (11-12) recently reported that five adolescents between the ages of 11 and 18 years showed increased somatomedin A levels, although not as high as those reported by Spencer. Successful renal transplantation was associated with a fall in somatomedin levels to or toward normal levels when measured by either the radio receptor or radioimmunoassay technique.

What does all of this mean? The decreased somatomedin found in uremic children prior to transplantation may be accounted for by inhibitors. However, correction for sulfate as performed by Saenger, et al still results in decreased somatomedin levels in this population. The normal or increased somatomedin as measured by radio receptor assay could be due to the loss of renal tissue as a principal site for the catabolism of somatomedin. Several of the measurements of somatomedin were in the acromegalic range or higher. Clearly these patients show growth failure and no evidence of growth excess suggesting the possibility that somatomedin like somatotropin may be produced in increased amounts associated with decreased somatomedin activity either related to inhibitory factors or decreased end organ sensitivity.

End organ resistance to somatomedins, the influence of somatomedin inhibitors on target tissues, i.e., end organ suppression, or decreased sensitivity to the action of somatomedin has received too little attention. The relationship of assayable somatomdein to its in vivo effect on cartilage and bone is an area that must be a major investigative focus in the future.

BIBLIOGRAPHY

1. Salmon, W.D., Jr. and Daughaday, W.H., A Hormonally Controlled Serum Factor Which Stimulates Sulfate Incorporation by Cartilage in Vitro. J. Lab. Clin. Med. 49:825-828, 1957.

2. Furlanetto, R.W., Underwood, L.E., VanWyk, J.J. and D'Ercole, A.J., Estimation of Somatomedin-C Levels in Normals and Patients With Pituitary Disease by Radioimmunoassay. J. Clin. Invest. 60:648-657, 1977.

3. VanWyk, J. and Underwood, L., Growth Hormone, Somatomedins, and Growth Failure. Hospital Practice. Vol. 13, No. 8, 57-67, August, 1978.

4. Saenger, P., Wiedemann, E., Schartz, E., Korth-Schutz, S., Lewy, J.E., Riggio, R., Rubin, A., Stenzel, K. and New, M., Somatomedin and Growth After Renal Transplantation. Ped. Res. 8:163-169, 1974.

5. Lewy, J.E. and VanWyk, J., Somatomedin and Growth Retardation in Children With Chronic Renal Insufficiency. Kidney Intern. 14:361-364, 1978.

6. Lewy, J.E. and New, M.I., Growth in Children With Renal Failure. Am. J. Med. 58:1; 65-68, 1975.

7. Phillips, L.S. and Vassilopoulou-Sellin, R., Somatomedins. Medical Progress I.N. E.J., 302:371-380, 1980.

8. Phillips, L.S. and Vassilopoulou-Sellin, R., Somatomedins. Medical Progress II. N.E.J. 302:438-446, 1980.

9. Phillips, L.S., Pennisi, A.J., Belosky, C., Somatomedin Activity and Inorganic Sulfate in Children Undergoing Hemodialysis. J. Clin. Endocrinol. Metab. 46:511-4, 1977.

10. Pennisi, A.J., Phillips, L.S., Uittenbogaard, C., Ettenger, R.V., Malezadeh, M.H. and Fine, R.N., Nutritional Intake, Somatomedin

442

Activity and Linear Growth in Children Undergoing Hemodialysis. Proc. Clin. Dial., Transp. Forum. 6:181, 1976.

11. Takano, K., Hall, K., Kastrupk, Hizuka N., Shizume, K., Kawai, K., Mitsuko, A., Takehide, T. and Sugino, N., Serum Somatomedin A in Chronic Renal Failure. J. Clin. Endoc. and Metab. 48:371-376, 1979.

12. Hall, K., Brandt, J., Enberg, G. and Fryklund, L., Radioimmunoassay of Somatomedin A in Human Serum. J. Clin. Endocrin. and Metab. 48:271-278, 1979.

AN APPROACH TO STUDY THE ROLE OF PROSTAGLANDINS

O. Oetliker, F. Mestel, Prostaglandin laboratory,
Division of pediatric nephrology, University Children's
Hospital Berne, Switzerland

Prostaglandins are accused of many different biological
actions. Everybody is familiar with e.g. the antiaggregatory
effect of certain prostaglandins on platelets, as well as
with the aggregatory effect of others. Prostaglandins are
also involved with vasodilation and with vasoconstriction,
with uterus contraction, with inflammation, etc. It is difficult to get an overview on the real role of prostaglandins.
Are they regulators, modifiers or mediators of a variety of
biological processes ? These questions certainly await clarification.

The evidence for the many different actions comes from experiments performed on a large variety of study models. Prostaglandins are almost ubiquitously detectable and it seems
worth thinking about the investigational technics and models
available for study, since such reflections may lead to weigh
the implications obtained from different approaches,and to
justify the introduction of yet another, hitherto rarely
used approach as we intend to do in this presentation.

Radioimmunoassays, bioassays and chromatographical technics
are clearly defined and their pitfalls are reasonably well
known to all those who use the respective technics. Combina-
tions of these analytical technics should always be used if
feasible.

Animal models, used in prostaglandin research,reach from
physiology to cell- and molecular biology. Each approach
can contribute only partly to the understanding of the

prostaglandin system. Physiological studies, for instance, using radioimmunoassays for PG's in body fluids of whole animals, give a crude general information. The combination with local investigation in animal preparations, isolated organs, cell preparations or subcellular fractions can however yield important information concerning the role of prostaglandins .Thus, none of the possible approaches is meant to be less important than another. In fact they all are complementary.

Animal models are ideal tools for the study of prostaglandin metabolism. But, problems may arise, when species differences are observed, or might be suspected. Therefore our interest must also be directed towards the possibilities of human investigation. Studies of prostaglandin metabolism in man are of special interest to the clinician, who treats his patients with inhibitors of prostaglandin synthesis, who may use prostaglandins as therapeutic measures, who deals with diseases in which he has a suspicion that prostaglandin metabolism might be involved or who wants to learn about prostaglandin metabolism during development.

There is obviously a limited number of possibilities for human investigation, and, in addition, some practicable models are rarely used. Firstly, it is almost impossible to perform systematic studies on many preparations mentioned in animal experimentation. One is left with "whole man" studies and a restricted number of possibilities to study human cells and the corresponding subcellular fractions.

Cell systems like kidney-, or liver-cells, lung endothelia and others, are only occasionally available from surgical-, biopsy- or postmortem specimens. For systematic, prospective investigation one is however dependent on easily accessible cells like lymphocytes, umbilical   endothelia, amniotic cells and skin fibroblasts, which are well accessible from the operating rooms as well as from skin biopsies of patients. This human cell approach has only recently been aborded in a few laboratories and has not yet reached the widespread use it probably deserves.

Skin fibroblasts are culturable cells which grow not only in primary cultures, but in subcultures as well, and therefore are available in an almost unlimited amount of reproduced samples. This fact is possibly of special importance, when primary cultures are compared to quiescent subcultures, since the first might reflect regulated metabolism as opposed to the basal metabolism of subcultures.

Cultured human skin fibroblasts, incubated simultaneously with 14C-labelled, and large amounts of cold arachidonic acid (AA), show a time dependent uptake of this substrate for PG-cyclooxygenase. The uptake reaches an equilibrium value of 80 - 90 % after 12 hours. After a 1-day exposure to AA, one can observe a basal production of prostaglandins, released into the medium. When, after 24 hours, the medium is replaced with a buffer, and the fibroblasts are stimulated with 1 ug/ml bradykinine, one can observe the production of important amounts of prostaglandins within minutes. The different prostaglandins are separated on thin-layer-chromatography. Formation of radio labelled 6-oxo-PGF$_{1\alpha}$, the acid degradation product of prostacyclin, of PGF$_{2\alpha}$, PGE$_2$, PGA$_2$ and unchanged AA is regularly observed. It is possible to produce a dose dependent inhibition of prostaglandins by the well-known cyclooxygenase inhibitors, acetylosalicilic acid and indomethacine. Thus, fibroblasts exhibit an AA metabolism which is qualitatively not different from many other cell systems (1).

The standardized model of cultured human fibroblasts, combined with radioactive labelling and thin-layer-chromatography for detection, offers a detailed look at the cellular AA-metabolism, which yields additional and complementary information to implications derived from observations on other

models. This becomes evident with the following examples:
Tranylcypromine, a mono-amine-oxydase inhibitor, is said to
inhibit prostacyclin synthetase. The implication is derived
from studies on human platelets. It is known that aortic
microsomes produce prostacyclin, which in turn was shown to
inhibit AA-induced platelet aggregation (2).Mechanically stimulated human endothelial cells also produce prostacyclin
(3), which therefore shows an antiaggregatory effect in the
platelet bioassay. Both effects can be reversed,when the
microsomial preparations or human lung endothelial cell cultures had been exposed to tranylcypromine (4, 5). Therefore,
it seems likely that tranylcypromine is inhibitory for prostacyclin synthesis, but this does not necessarily mean that
tranylcypromine inhibits the enzyme prostacyclin synthetase.

In cultured human skin fibroblasts, we have examined prostacyclin synthesis, and, as described before, had simultaneously the opportunity to look at other prostaglandins (6). We
found that increasing doses of tranylcypromine decrease progressively, not only prostacyclin production, but PGE_2 production as well. Simultaneously we found that tranylcypromine
clearly stimulates the production of a PGD_2 like substance,
and, in addition, that the most important changes of PG production were associated with severe morphological changes
of the cultures and even with a slight decrease of creatine-
phosphokinase, a cytosol-enzyme used for monitoring cell
damage. This example should demonstrate the complementary
character of the human skin fibroblast model.

Now let us examine three possible uses of the fibroblast
model. First we want to describe another example of studying
actions of drugs. Secondly, we will demonstrate the possibility to study a genetically determined disease. The third
example will then deal with a developmental aspect of the
PG-production by fibroblasts.

We have performed a study on the effect of furosemide on
prostaglandins formation of cultured human skin fibroblasts
(7). The cells were stimulated with bradykinine after different times of incubation with furosemide. Among other findings we were able to show a maximal stimulation of 6-oxo-
$PGF_{1\alpha}$- and of PGE_2-production, present already after 1 hour
of incubation with furosemide. There is no difference of
the increased prostaglandin-production, whether incubation
with furosemide was extended to 24 or to 48 hours. Apart
from directly showing the effect of furosemide on prostaglandin production by living cells, these data demonstrate the
possibility of such a model to further elucidate the dynamics of the action of a drug. The model can also be used to
characterize in more detail the site of action of a drug,
since not only prostaglandins and unchanged AA, but also parts
of the lipid pools of AA are accessible to study.

Although it is the experience of ourselves and others (8),
that there might be large differences in prostaglandin production between cell lines in culture, we believe that with
better standardization of the model differences between individual cell lines will become smaller, and that one can
start now to think of establishing normal values of prostaglandin patterns in man. This has not been done thus far ,
and yet it is of utmost importance, since it should be possible to use the human skin fibroblast model for the study
of genetic as well as developmental aspects in man.

Since the study of Sir Archibald Garrod (9) it has been
known that some diseases have a genetic determinant on enzymes. This fact is used since years to diagnose certain
inborn errors of metabolism, or to search for new genetic
defects. Fibroblasts are an accepted model for this kind of
studies. It seems logical therefore to use the fibroblasts
model for the study of genetic aspects of prostaglandin-
production as well. Since there are barely such studies
available in man we would like to show part of analogous

studies which we performed on cultured rat lung fibroblasts
(10). We asked the question whether the genetically determined spontaneous hypertension of rats might express itself in
a characteristic prostaglandin pattern of fibroblasts.

If one compares bradykinine stimulated PG-production of lung
fibroblasts from controls and from spontaneously hypertensive rats, one can observe, that the latter produce significantly less 6-oxo-PGF$_{1\alpha}$ and PGE$_2$ than controls. There was no
difference in protein content of the cultures, and during
incubation with arachidonic acid its uptake was the same in
controls and spontaneously hypertensive rats, and all fibroblasts were examined as the third subculture. We believe
that it was possible to detect such differences because
all technical aspects of the cultures, including feeding
media, number of subcultures, environmental conditions were
exactly identical in both groups.

Similarly, significant differences could be observed in
another preliminary study where the bradykinine stimulated
prostaglandin production by rat lung fibroblasts was compared in young and adult normal rats. Adult rats produced more
6-oxo-PGF$_{1\alpha}$ and PGE$_2$ than young. The data were   obtained
under the same strictly standardized conditions.

These last two examples of the use of the fibroblast model
had to be adopted from animal experimentation, since similar
studies are not available in cultured human fibroblasts.
The data, however, from animal experimentation encourage us
to abord this kind of studies in human skin fibroblasts as
well.

Since cultured human fibroblasts show metabolization of
arachidonic acid to prostaglandins, and since their AA-metabolism is well accessible to differential cellbiological
studies, this human model is a useful complementary tool to
examine actionsof drugs, or AA-metabolism of diseases which

might express themselves by a characteristic prostaglandin pattern (including genetic diseases), and to study developmental aspects.

In conclusion : AMONG THE APPROACHES TO STUDY THE ROLE OF PROSTAGLANDINS, CULTURED HUMAN FIBROBLASTS ARE AN OUTSTANDING COMPLEMENTARY MODEL BECAUSE THEY ARE PROSPECTIVELY AVAILABLE AND THEY BRING A LINK BETWEEN CLINICAL MEDICINE, AND CELL-BIOLOGY AND MOLECULAR PHARMACOLOGY.

REFERENCES

1. Baenziger NL, Becherer BR,Majerus PhW.1979 Characterization of prostacyclin synthesis in cultured human arterial smooth muscle cells, venous endothelial cells and skin fibroblasts. Cell 16, 967- 974.
2. Moncada S, Gryglewski R, Bunting S, Vane JR.1976. An enzyme isolated from arteries transformes Prostaglandin Endoperoxide to an unstable substance that inhibits platelet aggregation. Nature 263, 663.
3. Marcus AJ, Weksler BB, Jaffe EA. 1978. Enzymatic conversion of Prostaglandin Endoperoxide H_2 and Arachidonic acid to Prostacyclin by cultured human endothelial cells. J Biol Chem, 7138 - 7141.
4. Gryglewski RI, Bunting S, Moncada S, Flower RI and Vane R. 1976. Arterial walls are protected against deposition of platelet trombi by a substance (Prostaglandin X) which they make from Prostaglandin Endoperoxides. Prostaglandins 12, 685 - 713.
5. Johnson AR. 1980. Human pulmonary endothelial cells in culture. Activities of cells from arteries and cells from veins. J Clin Invest 65, 841 - 850.
6. Mestel F, Brunner R, Oetliker OH. 1980. Abstract: The effect of Acetylosalicycilic acid (ASA) and Tranylcypromine (Tc) on the production of Prostacyclin and PGE in the human fibroblast model. The First World Conference on Clinical Pharmacology, London.Compl. publication in preparation.
7. Mestel F, Oetliker OH. 1980. Abstract: Furosemide potentiates Prostacyclin and PGE release in human fibroblasts in culture. Prostaglandins and the cardiovascular system, a Symposium sponsored by the European Society for Cardiology, Belgium.Compl. publication in preparation.
8. Weksler BB, Ley ChW and Jaffe EA. 1978. Stimulation of endothelial cell Prostacyclin production by Thrombin, Trypsin and the Ionophore A 23187. J Clin Invest 62, 923 - 930.
9. Garrod AE. 1908. Inborn errors of metabolism. Lancet 2, 217.

10. Mestel F, Oetliker O. 1980. Abstract: The fibroblast
    model, a possible way of studying arachidonic acid meta-
    bolism in Hypertension. Kidney International, 17,
    859. Compl. publication in preparation.

POINTS TO REMEMBER IN PHARMACOLOGIC GLUCOCORTICOID
TREATMENT OF NEPHROTIC SYNDROME

O. KOSKIMIES and S. LEISTI

1. THE PHYSIOLOGY OF GLUCOCORTICOID SECRETION

The hypothalamus, anterior pituitary and adrenal cortex from the HPA axis,
which is the mechanism for regulating glucocorticoid production. The secretion of
ACTH from the anterior pituitary is dependent on a releasing factor (CRF) from the
hypothalamus. Cortisol can be regarded as the principal secretory product of the
adrenal cortex. Both hypothalamus and anterior pituitary are under negative feedback
control whereby an increase in circulating cortisol inhibits CRF and ACTH secretion.
Any disturbance in the function of this HPA axis may cause deficient production of
cortisol. The most common cause of HPA axis suppression and adrenal atrophy is, of
course, exogenous administration of glucocorticoids.

Under normal physiologic circumstances the adrenal cortex secretes approximately
6-17 mg of cortisol/24 h/m^2 of body surface area. ACTH and thus also cortisol are
secreted pulsewise, the activity of the HPA axis being maximal during the early
morning hours. Thus the peak of cortisol secretion in the morning suppresses the HPA
axis and the lowest level of plasma cortisol in the evening re-activates it.

2. THE EFFECT OF PHARMACOLOGIC GLUCOCORTICOID THERAPY ON ADRENOCORTICAL FUNCTION

The pharmacologic use of glucocorticoids such as prednisone, prednisolone
and dexamethasone is common for the control of diseases in which an immunologic or
anti-inflammatory effect is required. The relatively large doses and long periods of
treatment often required carry a risk of insufficient HPA axis function and adrenal
cortical atrophy. The primary goal in the clinical use of corticosteroids is, of course,
to balance maximal therapeutic efficacy with a minimum of side effects.

As shown by several workers (1, 2), suppression of ACTH secretion and subsequent atrophy of the adrenal cortex are less marked if short-acting steroid is given as a single dose in the morning at the physiologic peak secretion of cortisol than if the dose is divided throughout the day or given in the afternoon or in the evening. Nichols (1) and coworkers gave 0.5 mg of dexamethasone to healthy human volunteers at various times on 2 consecutive days and compared the effects of these regimens on 17-OH corticosteroid production. When dexamethasone was given at 8 AM on 2 consecutive days only temporary suppression of cortisol secretion was noted, the secretion being normal by the third morning. The same dosage, when given at 4 PM, caused partial suppression and when given at midnight total suppression of cortisol secretion for a full 24-h period. Thus not only the dose and the length of treatment but also the time of glucocorticoid administration should be adjusted to fit the normal physiologic pattern. Of course suppression is even less marked if one morning dose is given every other day or less frequently.

We then come to the obvious question whether a dose of glucocorticoid in the morning every day or every other day can suppress an ongoing immunologic disease such as we see in the field of pediatric nephrology. Our experience in treating the nephrotic syndrome, for example, tells us that it cannot - thus we need a suppressive daily divided dose treatment but, as soon as remission has been induced, the dose should be reduced in the way causing a minimum of side effects. The most serious side effect, of course, is post-prednisone adrenal insufficiency with circulatory collapse, which is usually precipitated by an infection or some other stress. The other risk that has been demonstrated is the reactivation or relapse of the disease, e.g., the increased risk of early relapse of idiopathic nephrotic syndrome (INS) associated with hypocortisolism. (Table). The latter phenomenon, which is less well known, will be briefly described.

Effect of prednisone treatment on HPA axis in nephrotic syndrome - 5 new patients and 22 relapses. (Subnormal/total)

	Before prednisone	After daily prednisone	After 4 weeks intermittent p.
Basal cortisol	8/27	26/27	4/27
ACTH test	13/27	27/27	10/27

3. HYPOCORTISOLISM AND RELAPSE OF INS

We used two parameters to evaluate the function of the HPA axis in nephrotic children, namely the morning basal cortisol level and the level of cortisol 2 hours after i.v. injection of ACTH. The plasma cortisol level was measured by an ultra-micro modification of the fluorometric method (3). In this way the basal and reserve capacities of the adrenal cortex can be measured accurately and the risk of potential adrenal insufficiency estimated.

After treatment of the first episode of INS an ACTH test was performed on 23 children; the length of the first remission was correlated with the response to the postmedication ACTH test. In 11 children this was subnormal; 10 of them had their first relapse within a year. Of the 7 children who stayed in remission for more than a year, 6 had normal responses (4). The results for another group of nephrotic children, who had had one or more relapses of INS, showed a similar trend (5). The results for the latter group were used to calculate the cumulative risk of relapse in 52 children with INS. After 3, 6 and 12 months of steroid treatment the cumulative percentages of children who had relapsed were 75, 84 and 92 % in the group with a subnormal ACTH test response and 26, 41 and 63 % in the group with a normal response.

As the next step it was felt necessary to test whether early relapse of INS was due to the hypocortisolism - whether the relapse could be prevented by giving cortisol substitution to those who had a subnormal response in the ACTH test after prednisone therapy. Thus a double-blind cross-over study was performed on nephrotic children with subnormal ACTH responses at the end of the treatment period. 26 relapses in 13 children were evaluated. At 3 months 8 children receiving cortisol substitution and one receiving placebo were in remission, but at 6 months the difference was less marked (6). Thus, although substitution did not alter the natural long-term course of INS, it seems possible to identify individuals at risk of early relapse due to hypocortisolism, and to prevent relapse in some patients at least, by physiologic cortisol substitution.

Glucocorticoid medication in INS should be adjusted so as to cause minimal adrenocortical suppression. One morning dose causes less suppression than treatment divided throughout the day; this may not be sufficient to control the disease in the early active phase but is enough for control as soon as a state of remission has been achieved. After prednisone treatment the patient should be given a 2-hour ACTH test, and those with a deficient response should be given hydrocortisone substitution at least during stress. If adrenocortical suppression is severe, partial daily substitution is recommended for a period of 2-3 months. In this way the risk of acute adrenal insufficiency can be avoided and the number of early relapses due to a subnormal plasma cortisol level can be reduced.

REFERENCES

1. Nichols T, Nugent CA, Tyler FH. Diurnal variation in suppression of adrenal function by glucocorticoids. J Clin Endocr 25:343, 1965.
2. Grant SD, Forsham PH, DiRaimondo VC. Suppression of 17-hydroxycortico-steroids in plasma and urine by single and divided doses of triamcinolone. N Engl J Med 273:1115, 1965.
3. Leisti S, Perheentupa J. Two-hour adrenocorticotropic hormone test: accuracy in the evaluation of the hypothalamic-pituitary-adrenocortical axis. J Pediat Res 12:272, 1978.
4. Leisti S et al. Association of postmedication hypocortisolism with early first relapse of idiopathic nephrotic syndrome. Lancet 2:795, 1977.
5. Leisti S, Vilska J, Hallman N. Adrenocortical insufficiency and relapsing in the idiopathic nephrotic syndrome of childhood. Pediatrics 60:334, 1977.
6. Leisti S et al. Idiopathic nephrotic syndrome: prevention of early relapse. Br Med J 1:892, 1978.

RENAL METABOLIC ALKALOSIS

PHILIP L. CALCAGNO

In]960 at the First International Congress of Endocrinology held in Copenhagen, Pronove, MacCardle and Bartter presented a new syndrome describing a unique renal lesion associated with aldosterone and hypokalemia in a 5 year old boy.(1) Two years later,the patient was reported as Hyperplasia of the Juxtaglomerular Complex with Hyperaldosteronism and Hypokalemic Alkalosis.(2) The clinical findings have become well known to all, yet during the course of two decades the prevailing physiologic interpretation of certain features have been modified.

Initially, the described syndrome of hyperaldosteronism characterized by juxtaglomerular hyperplasia and hypertrophy was considered to be a primary cause of hyperaldosteronism. The histologic lesion was newly described and the alleged association between hypokalemic alkalosis and hyperaldosteronism was made easily. The onset of clinical problems occurred at 4 months of age with growth failure,polydipsia and salt craving suggesting a congenital defect, an aspect not highlighted in the initial publication. Potassium chloride supplements to the patient's diet showed improvement in the appetite and growth rate.

The second patient described was a 25 year old man whose history demonstrated an early onset in that as a child he was not allowed to enter school until 12 years of age. The previous history revealed enuresis and a slow growth rate with weakness and fatigue. These tow patients certainly pinpointed the disorder early in life and both demonstrated a clinical response to KCl supplements and to the intravenous administration of human serum albumin. Most revealing was the fact that with clinical improvement and replenishment of body potassium, urinary aldosterone levels did not decrease and even rose in one instance. The aldosterone levels could be modified with aldosterone antagonist (SC9420) Another striking feature of these two patients was that human

serum albumin administration was able to lower the urinary losses to zero,suggesting that renal sodium wasting was related to effective circulatory volume. The authors concluded that a renal defect was not present as is seen in RTA involving hydrogen ion excretion. In fact the excessive loss of potassium was explained on the basis of large amounts of aldosterone.

The problem with this explanation, in addition to the faulty in-reasoning regarding aldosterone was that hypertension should have been one of the clinical consequences, as was appropriately noted with adrenal cortical adenoma and aldosteronism; indeed, hypertension is the rule and, moreover, is not prevented by potassium depletion. Yet these patients had normal blood pressure determinations. Renin and pressor agents resembling angiotension were shown to be elevated on bioassay. The attributed hypothesis for the lack of hypertension then required an explanation of the juxtaglomerular apparatus which was unknown; insensitivity of the arterial wall to the pressor effects of angiotension was considered and proved. The kidney then sensed a contracted blood volume and responded by oversecreting renin. Excess renin in turn stimulates aldosterone secretion with potassium loss and metabolic alkalosis. This hypothesis seems to fit all aspects of the disorder. Initially, the authors associated the juxtaglomerular apparatus lesion and aldosteronism to a common cause.

In 1960, the year of the Pronove et al report, an abstract of a similar case was presented at the Society of Pediatric Research by Camacho and Blizzard (3) which was subsequently published.(4) This child was 4 years and 2 months old, dwarfed with hypokalemic alkalosis. The child was given high dosages of sodium chloride with potassium supplements which accentuated the electrolyte disturbance. A low salt diet was beneficial in restoring serum pH and electrolytes to nearly normal levels and the authors concluded that primary potassium loss by the kidney was probably at fault in this child. Following three days of NaCl loading (12gm/dy) which normally suppresses aldosterone production, the urinary aldosterone remained elevated at 7 ug/day (normal 1-2). These authors excluded the adrenal glands as a primary defect. In fact, they argued that a low salt syndrome (Na111;Cl 73) developing without serum K elevation (3.5) secondary to administration of an aldosterone antagonist was confirmatory evidence that this was a secondary hyperaldosteronism. These authors were later proven to be correct.

The following year, a 2 and 1/2 year old child was presented to the Society of Pediatric Research with a similar clinical expression entitled,"Congenital Renal Alkalosis" by Calcagno, Rubin, Esperanca and Mattimore (5) and subsequently published.(6) This patient did not have renal juxtaglomerular hyperplasia and hypertrophy. Unlike patients with primary aldosteronism this patient did not improve on a low sodium diet but did mimic the patients of Camacho and Blizzard. The excretion of chloride was persistently greater than sodium and the aldosterone activity was not excessive and was considered to be a secondary feature augmenting losses of potassium. Renin levels were elevated.

The clinical features common to these patients are; metabolic alkalosis, absence of hypertension, onset early

in life, growth failure during the developmental phase of
life, and aldosterone antagonist have little effect in
raising serum K to normal.

The areas which led to the initial hypotheses involving
the hormonal system were the elegance of the histologic
changes which were noted for the first time. Yet, today,
hyperplasia of the JG cells as distinctive for Bartter"s
Syndrome is no longer tenable and, more plausible is the
concept that it represents a secondary phenomenon as
found in other disorders. (7,8,9)

The normalization of the arterial vascular response to
angiotensin following expansion of the blood volume by
saline infusion remains a clouded issue. Vascular insensitivity to angiotensin II appears to be specific since the
response to norepinephrine is usually normal (10,11)
Moreover, indomethacin can normalize this response.(12)
Indeed, saralasin, a competitive antagonist of angiotensin II
causes a fall in blood pressure, suggesting an interesting
supportive homeostatic role for angiotensin II in this
syndrome.

The concept of a fault in the mechanism of renal sodium
transport stems from studies defining sodium loss on a
restricted sodium intake.(6) Impaired sodium transport
in the ascending limb of Henle's loop was found in some
patients.(13) Furthermore, renal sodium wasting is well
documented in other patients. (4,6,14) Others achieve a
normal sodium balance with salt restriction.(2,11) Indeed,
in others salt restriction caused a shock-like syndrome.(4,6)
These opposed observations require explanation and should be
considered when an hypothesis is presented involving the
handling of sodium by the kidney. It should be clear that
sodium loss unto itself will not give metabolic alkalosis,
nonetheless, excess sodium delivery distally could augment
potassium losses. Sodium does not appear to be the main
actor in this scenario.

Renin and aldosterone secretions seem to be related in
most patients, however there are reports of lowered or
normal aldosterone excretions (3,5) Reports of dissociation
of renal levels and aldosterone have been documented in
dialysis patients when compensatory feedback mechanisms are
not operative.(15) During isokalemic ultrafiltration
hemodialysis increments in both plasma aldosterone and
renin are observed. With ultrafiltration dialysis allowing
for a fall in plasma potassium to 3.4 mEq/L,plasma renin
activity rose but aldosterone fell significantly. Most
investigators acknowledge that primary control of aldosterone
secretion is via renin-angiotensin system which is responsive
to electrolyte balance, pressure changes in afferent arterole
and directly to serum potassium levels (16,17,18,63,64}
yet all aspects of the regulation of aldosterone secretion
cannot be fully explained. It should be suspected that since
there is a dissociation with regard to renin-aldosterone

relationship, it would be difficult to give aldosterone the principal role for renal potassium losses.

Prostaglandins have recently been placed into this mystifying physiologic ploy.(19) Urinary PGE was noted to be elevated in four patients. Moreover,indomethacin,an inhibitor of prostaglandin synthesis, resulted in a reduction of urinary excretion and of renin-aldosterone secretion, a return to a positive sodium balance,however serum hypokalemic metabolic alkalosis was maintained.

Hypokalemia is a hall mark of this disorder. Potassium deficit results from excessive urinary losses. Indeed, in 1961 (5) it was shown that urinary potassium excretion exceeded that quantity filtered. These deficits were noted without excessive aldosterone excretion. Suppressing aldosterone secretion with feedback inhibitors does not allow for a normalization of serum potassium. It is clear that potassium appears to be one of the main actors in this scenario. Although it is generally accepted that severe K deficits per se can cause metabolic alkalosis, there is little evidence to support this view in the uncomplicated state. Potassium losses can be coupled to sodium losses however, as previously noted, sodium losses are not an invariable feature of this syndrome.

It is strange that only until recently, in 1975,have the unenlightened referee journals begun to discuss chloride as playing a possible major role in this syndrome even though it was suggested in 1961 (5) and again in 1965 (6) with clear excretion data. A statement published in the New England Journal of Medicine in 1979 noted," unfortunately, data on urinary excretion of chloride are not available in this syndrome". Such data have been published in the pediatric literature.(4,6,20)

In 1975 chloride transport defect in the ascending limb of Henle's loop was suggested.(21) In 1978 evidence was given for a prostaglandin-independent defect on chloride reabsorption in the loop of Henle.(22) Also, in 1979 (23) an excess cf a chloruretic hormone was put forth as another possible explanation. The renal chloride loss defect requires further study to define its exact role,however it is clear that some patients demonstrate this renal anion leak as noted in those patients who became dehydrated and developed a negative sodium balance and azotemia on a restricted sodium intake.(4,6)

The data todate suggest that a multifactorial nature to causation of this disorder be invoked as etiologic mechansims. It is time we identified the malfunctioning unit,"The Kidney". Many years ago,"renal hypokalemic metabolic alkalosis" was suggested and today appears to be an appropriate category. The data further suggest a basic defect in renal hydrogen conservation and in the young,particularly,a defect in anion handling by the kidney. It may be that the disorder in early life is related to a developmental defect in nephron develop- ment. In necropsy reports (24) descriptions of hypoplastic and immature or fetal glomeruli and associated tubules appear to be non-functioning and inactive. In distribution

90% of these hypoplastic glomeruli were located in the cortex. It was particularly interesting to note that the largest maculae densae were associated with mature glomeruli which were exclusively in the juxtamedullary regions of the deeper cortex. This histologic data supports a developmental process in the last trimester which includes the superficial nephron population.

In Comacho and Blizzard's patients the administration of chlorothiazide for four days produced no resultant changes in serum and urinary electrolytes. More to the point,is the patient of Calcagno et al wherein diuretics were administered to attempt to define the site of renal abnormality. The response of this child to acetazolamide showed a dramatic increase in urine volume, osmolar excretion and an unexpected chloruresis when compared to an alkalotic control. Mercuhydrin administration resulted in a more brisk chloruresis, natriuresis and kaliuresis greater than controls. However,of special note was the chlorthiazide reaponse. The expected chloruresis and natriuresis were blunted suggesting faulty reabsorptive processes in the diluting segment of the nephron in the renal cortex.

In the older age group a 37 year old man with hypokalemic metabolic alkalosis (25) was reported with interstitial fibrosis representing one-half of the renal cortex. This report supports a renal cortex disorder. It is interesting that in 1953 a reversible lesion was described by Fashena and Martin in a 7 month old child with hypospadias, cryptorchism and malnutrition with congenital alkalosis of renal origin.(26)

A unifying concept of Bartter's Syndrome should first exclude the role of the adrenals as maintaining a primary defect. Secondly, the kidney appears far and away to be primarily involved. In addition, the function of the distal segment appears at fault and,in particular, the diluting segment of the distalnephron in the patients described by Calcagno et al. Since identification of this lesion is observed early at birth, a congenital nature is evident and in some pedigrees, a familial aspect has been described. I propose, as has been done in 1960,that these children be labelled "Congenital Renal Metabolic Alkalosis",and in those children without an early onset,or a familial basis,an acquired form of the renal metabolic alkalosis should be entertained. The basic renal defect would need to be differentiated from known renal disorders demonstrating excessive urinary potassium losses such as RTA associated with Fanconi Syndrome or distal RTA. Renin secreting tumors of the kidney are associated with hypertension and should pose no problem. Salt losing nephritis would require histologic proof of interstitial or glomerular-tubular pathology.

The basic mechanism would be an increased excretion of net urinary acid in association with an excessive anion loss such as chloride and a gain in body bicarbonate. Potassium urinary loss is thought to be regulated by the intracellular

potassium content in the distal tubule,however the kidney in
urinary K excretion is also influenced by the nature of the
filtered anion, the degree of urinary acidification, the
level of adrenocortical hormones as well as distal tubular
flow and distal sodium delivery. Most of these factors are
present at one time or another in these patients,promoting
excessive losses of urinary potassium. Moreover,body K
deficits could be replenished in patients without altering
the plasma biochemical changes of metabolic alkalosis. The
role of excessive distal tubular flow has received scant
notice even though it is a constant feature. The renal
hydrogen losses are maintained, either related to or independent of anion excretion,allowing for a failure to normalize
blood pH,plasma K concentration and bicarbonate levels.

Recently (27) loop diuretics have been shown to inhibit
electrogenic chloride reabsorption in the rabbit loop of
Henle and reduce the lumen potential difference.In human
beings, furosemide did lower the transtubular potential
difference in the cortical collecting tubule.(28) These
changes allow for an inhibitory effect on chloride
reabsorption. Similar changes could be operative in the
mechanism for renal alkalosis unassociated with diuretic
administration.

Indeed, the rate of renal acidification and changes in
the potential difference in the toad bladder epithelium has
been demonstrated (29). Should such data be applicable to
human beings, then voltage oriented hydrogen ion secretion
could reflect in disorders such as renal alkalosis associated
with excessive urinary chloride excretion and increased net
acid excretion.

A classification of renal metabolic alkalosis could
include disorders of nephrogenic development particularly
in the distal segments of the nephron,a defect in electrogenic dependent mechanisms as well as transport and
hormonal imbalances.

RENAL METABOLIC ALKALOSIS
(↑ Net Acid Excretion)

- **Inhibition of chloride reabsorption**
- **Increase organic anion excretion**
  Ketoacidosis
  Lactic acidosis
- **Increase in poorly or unabsorbable anion**
  Bicarbonate (distal nephron)
  Sulfate

Fig. 1

1. Pronove P,MacCardle R,Bartter FC: Aldosteronism,hypokal-
    emia and a unique renal lesion in a 5 year old boy. Acta
    Endocr (suppl) 51:167,1960.
2. Bartter FC,Pronove P.,Gill JR,MacCardle RC: Hyperplasia
    of the juxtaglomerular complex with hyperaldosteronism
    and hypokalemic alkalosis.A new syndrome.Am J Med 33:
    811,1962.
3. Camacho AM, Blizzard RM: Congenital hypokalemia of renal
    origin due to an inherited metabolic defect. Am J Dis
    Child 100:173, 1960.
4. Camacho AM, Blizzard RM: Congenital Hypokalemia of prob-
    able renal origin. Am J Dis Child 103:43, 1962.
5. Calcagno PL, Rubin MI, Esperanca MJ, Mattimore JM: Con-
    genital renal tubular alkalosis. Am J Dis Child 102:726,
    1961.
6. D'Albora JB, Calcagno PL: Renal acid-base disorder. Path-
    ogenesis and management. Pediat Clin North Am 11:611, 1964
7. Pasternack A, Perheentupa J., Launiala K, Hallman N: Kid-
    ney biopsy findings in familial chloride diarrhoea. Acta
    Endo 55:1, 1967.
8. Cannon PJ, Leeming JM, Winters RW, Laragh JH: Juxtaglom-
    erular cell hyperplasia and secondary hyperaldosteronism
    (Bartter's Syndrome) A re-evaluation of the pathophysio-
    logy. Medicine 47:107, 1968.
9. Fleischer N, Brown H, Graham DY, Delena S: Chronic Laxa-
    tive-induced hyperaldosteronism and hypokalemia simulat-
    ing Bartter's Syndrome. Ann Int Med 70:791, 1969.
10. White MG: Bartter's Syndrome: A manifestation of renal
    tubular defects. Arch Int Med 129:41, 1972.
11. Goodman AD, Vagnucci HH, Hartroft PM: Pathogenesis of the
    Bartter's Syndrome. N Engl J Med 87:281, 1977.
12. Halushka PV, Wohltmann H, Privitera PJ, Hurwitz G,
    Margolius HS: Bartter's Syndrome: urinary prostaglandin
    E-like material and kallikrein: indomethacin effects.
    Ann Int Med 87:281, 1977.
13. Chaimovits C, Levi J, Better OS, Benderli A: Studies on
    the site of the renal salt loss in a patient with
    Bartter's Syndrome. Pediat Res 7:89, 1973.
14. Schwartz GJ, Cornfeld D: Bartter's Syndrome: clinical
    study of its treatment with salt loading and propanolal.
    Clin Neph 4:45, 1975.
15. Henrich WL, Katz FH, Molinoff PB, Schrier RW: Competitive
    effects of hypokalemia and volume depletion on plasma
    renin activity, aldosterone and catecholamine concentra-
    tions in hemodialysis patients. Kidney Int 12:279, 1977.
16. Laragh JH: Aldosteronism in man; factors controlling se-
    cretion of the hormone. In Christy NP (ed) The Human
    Adrenal Cortex, New York Harper and Row P 483, 1971.
17. Muller J: Regulation of aldosterone biosynthesis. Berlin,
    Springer-Verlag, 1971.
18. Blair-West JR, Cain MD, Catt KJ, Coghlan JP, Scoggins BA,
    Wright RD: The dissociation of aldosterone secretion and
    systemic renin and angiotensin II levels during correc-
    tion of sodium deficiency. Acta Endocrinol (KGH) 66:229,
    1971.

462

19. Gill JR, Frolich JG, Bowden RE, Taylor AA, Kreiser HR,
    Seyberth WN, Oates JA, Bartter FC: Bartter's Syndrome:
    A disorder characterized by high urinary prostaglandins
    and a dependence of hyperreninemia on prostaglandin
    synthesis. Am J Med 61:43, 1976.
20. Arant BS, Brackett JR MD, Young MD, Still WSJ: Case stud-
    ies of siblings with juxtaglomerular hyperplasia and sec-
    ondary aldosteronism associated with severe azotemia and
    renal rickets - Bartter's Syndrome or disease? Pediatrics
    46:34, 1970.
21. Kurtzman NA, Gutierrez LE: The pathophysiology of
    Bartter's Syndrome. JAMA 234:758, 1975.
22. Gill JR, Bartter FC: Evidence for a prostaglandin inde-
    pendent defect in chloride reabsorption in the loop of
    Henle as a proximal cause of Bartter's Syndrome. AM J
    Med 65:766, 1978.
23. Grekin RJ, Nicholls MG, Padfield PL: Disorders of chlor-
    iuretic hormone secretion. Lancet 1116,1979.
24. Sutherland LE, Hartroft P, Balis JV, Bailey JD, Lynch MJ:
    Bartter's Syndrome. A report of four cases including
    three in one sibship with comparative histologic evalua-
    tions of the juxtaglomerular apparatuses and glomeruli.
    Acta Paediat Scand (suppl) 201:1970.
25. Potter WZ, Trygstad CW, Helmer DM, Nance WE, Judson WE:
    Familial hypokalemic associated with renal interstitial
    fibrosis. AM J Med 57:971, 1974.
26. Fashena GJ, Martin RJ: Congenital alkalosis of renal
    origin. Am J Dis Child 79:1127, 1950.
27. Burg M, Green N: Effect of ethacrynic acid on the thick
    ascending limb of Henle's loop. Kidney International
    4:201, 1973.
28. Jacobson HR, Gross JB, Kawamura S, Waters JD, Kokko JP:
    Electrophysiological study of isolated perfused human
    collecting ducts. Ion dependency of the transepithelial
    potential difference. J Clin Invest 58:1233, 1976.
29. Ziegler TW, Fanestil DD, Ludens JH: Influence of trans-
    epithelial potential difference on acidification in the
    toad bladder. Kidney International 10:279, 1976.

PATHOGENESIS OF Neo-Mull-Soy (Syntex) Alkalosis

Harold L. Harrison, M.D., Michael A. Linshaw, M.D. and Alan Gruskin, M.D.

Depts. of Pediatrics Univ. of Louisville, Univ. of Kansas Med. Center and St. Christophers Hospital for Children.

During the last year several reports of metabolic alkalosis associated with soy protein formula have appeared. We were involved in the evaluation of thirteen infants who developed alkalosis while ingesting a formula with a low chloride content. Ten cases are presented below.

Table

Age of onset* (mo)	Height (°)	Weight (°)	Clinical findings	Blood Na	K	Cl	CO_2 (mEq/l)	pH	BUN (mg/dl)	Creatinine (mg/dl)	Renin† (ng/ml/hr)	Aldosterone† ng/dl	Urine Na	K	Cl (mEq/l)	RBC/hp‡
10. F +	25	5	Poor feeding	125	2.9	70	43	7.6	11			122.1	3	15	3	8-10
6. M −	10	<3	Spitting up	137	2.4	59	50		40	0.5			16	5	1	+
6. F +	25	<5	Weight loss	132	2.8	72	31	7.71	13	0.5	266	83	18	15	0	75-80
2. F −	25	25	Spitting. seizure	115	3.2	69	28	7.56	12				7	5	2	+
3½. F +	3	<3	Mild diarrhea—lethargy	131	3.5	61	34	7.63	7							0
6½. M +	2.5	<3	Poor feeding	121	2.4	63	43		5	0.5			7	7	<1	2-5
8. F +	5	<5	Spitting	136	2.8	86	29	7.57	20	0.6	133	62	26	39	0	0
5. M −	25	5	Spitting	133	2.5	67	41	7.55	20	0.6	156	39	19	31	0	15-17
5. M +	25	5	Spitting	131	2.4	66	32	7.6	26	0.8	328	60	8	63	0	10-15
2. M −	5	5	Mild vomiting and diarrhea	143	4.6	92	30	7.49	19							0

*Letter F or M following age in months (first column) indicates female or male respectively. A + under the sex in same column denotes that the infant was taking supplemental baby food; − indicates no supplemental food.

†Mean PRA and plasma aldosterone levels in normal infants 3 months to one year of age are 6.3 ng/ml/hr and 42 ng/dl. respectively.'

‡The + in the last column (RBC) indicates a positive dipstick reaction to blood but no quantitative determination.

We studied one patient extensively in an effort to define the mechanism for generation and maintenance of the observed alkalosis. This work was published in the Journal of Pediatrics and forms the basis of this report.[1]

We believe that the alkalosis in these infants was generated from a potential bicarbonate load in the form of citrate and maintained by the low chloride content of the formula.

This infant was a 6½ month old white male who was admitted to the Kansas University Medical Center for evaluation of severe recurrent metabolic alkalosis. Perinatal and past history were significant in that on two occasions this child at 4½ and 5½ months of age had been hospitalized and treated for severe hypochloremic metabolic alkalosis. There had been no history of excessive sweating or diarrhea and only minimal spitting up. At the time of the evaluation the infant was taking metaproterenol 1 ml tid for ten days as treatment for an upper respiratory infection. His diet consisted entirely of NeoMullsoy formula which he had been receiving since 1 month of age. By history he consumed 40-48 ozs. per day.

PHYSICAL EXAM

HR - 120/min   RR - 50/min   BP - 98/56 mm Hg   Wt - 7.14 k₅

LABORATORY

Serum:				
Na	- 141 mEq/1		BUN	- 20 mg/dl
K	- 3.1 mEq/1		Cr	- 0.6 mg/dl
Cl	- 83 mEq/1		Uric acid	- 9.9 mg/dl
CO_2	- 38 mEq/1		Rennin	- 150 mg/ml/hr
pH	- 7.56		Aldosterone	- 96.4 mg/dl

Urine:	Na	10 mEq/1
	K	16 mEq/1
	Cl	<1 mEq/1

Physical examination was entirely normal with no clinical evidence of dehydration. Laboratory investigations demonstrated a severe hypochloremic metabolic alkalosis with mild azotemia and avid urinary chloride retention.

Initial serum renin and aldosterone determinations were markedly elevated.

Since beta stimulators such as isoproterenol may cause release of renin, the child's hospitalization was initially designed to evaluate the possibility that metaproterenol induced hyperaldosteronism and alkalosis.[2] The child's hospital course is illustrated.

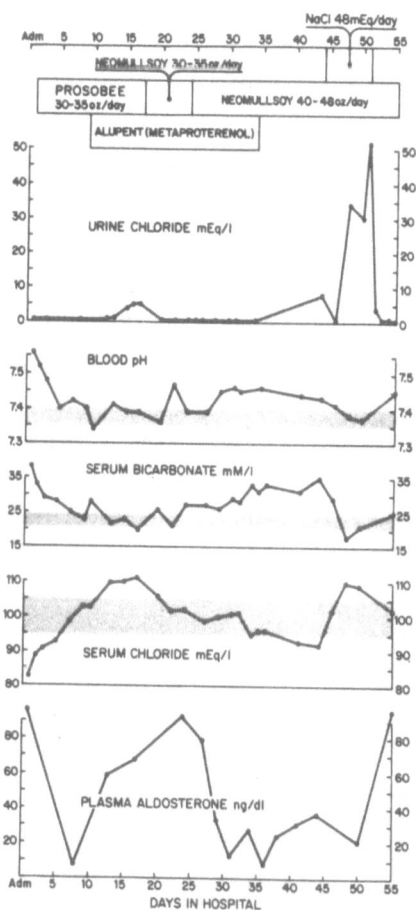

Fig. 1. Hospital course. Blood determinations, including pH, were performed on venous blood. Admission day was 5/23/79.

Within eight days while ingesting 30-35 ozs. of Prosobee,® plasma aldosterone, serum pH and serum electrolyte values returned to normal. We continued the Prosobee and then restarted the metaproterenol to see if the drug might induce the alkalosis. Although plasma aldosterone did dramatically increase, alkalosis was not observed. We then wondered if NeoMullsoy, a formula low in chloride, might be contributing to the alkalosis and, therefore, fed the child this formula. Alkalosis was not observed after seven days while ingesting 30-35 ozs. of formula per day. On this volume the child's weight steadily increased. However, by increasing the volume to 40-48 ozs., the volume provided at home by the mother, the alkalosis reoccurred within one week. Since the alkalosis appeared to relate directly to the NeoMull soy, we discontinued the metaproterenol. The alkalosis persisted for ten days as long as the infant continued to ingest 40-48 ozs. of formula. We then supplemented the formula with 48 mEq of sodium chloride (5-6 mEq per kilo body weight). Within seven days blood pH and electrolyte values returned to normal. When we discontinued the supplemental sodium chloride, urine chloride quickly decreased and within five days, plasma aldosterone and serum pH increased.

The child was moderately hypokalemic on admission with a value of 3.2 mEq/l; however, his serum potassium values were otherwise normal throughout his hospital stay. His BUN and serum creatinine values by day eight of hospitalization were normal and remained constant thereafter. Serum uric acid decreased to 4.9 mg/dl while receiving 30-35 ozs. of formula per day, increased to 7.7 mg/dl when the alkalosis developed, and decreased to 5 mg/dl with addition of dietary sodium chloride.

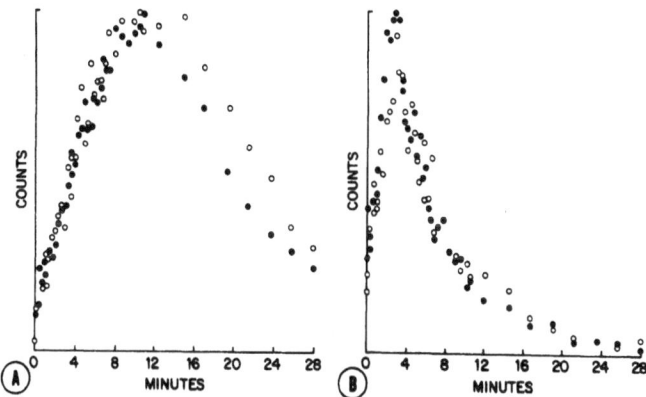

Fig. 2. *A.* Hippuran renogram performed prior to supplementing formula with NaCl. The curve is symmetrically abnormal. The mean transit time is delayed to ten minutes; the normal mean transit time is four to six minutes. The descending portion of the curve is delayed. The 25- to 30-minute image showed excessive intraparenchymal retention. *B.* Hippuran renogram performed after supplementing formula with NaCl. The curve is now normal. Open dots are left kidney and closed dots, right kidney.

A hippuran renogram showed bilateral equal uptake with moderate intra parenchymal retention and delayed excretion when the child was alkalotic while ingesting the NeoMullsoy formula prior to the addition of supplemental salt. In contrast, repeat hippuran renograms obtained after sodium chloride supplementation were normal. Upon withdrawal of the additional dietary salt, the hippuran curves reverted to a pattern identical to that observed when the child was alkalotic.

We measured the electrolyte content of NeoMullsoy and found it to contain 8 mEq/l of sodium, 28 mEq/l of potassium and 2 mEq/l of chloride. The potassium citrate content of NeoMullsoy according to the product label was 240 mg/dl of formula.

The patient was discharged from the hospital weighing 9 kilograms. Follow-up two weeks later while on NeoMullsoy plus supplemental sodium chloride revealed normal serum pH and serum electrolyte values. His urine chloride was measured to be 178 mEq/l. At this time NeoMullsoy was withdrawn from the market. We then fed the child Prosobee, a formula which according to its product label had a potassium citrate content of 140 mg/dl of formula. After one week on Prosobee plus supplemental sodium chloride, the child continued to grow, was nonalkalotic, and was excreting 186 mEq/l of chloride in his urine. At this time we discontinued the supplemental salt. The child's venous pH and electrolytes remained normal, but his urine chloride concentration decreased to 3 mEq/l. In the absence of alkalosis we wondered if the low urine chloride might indicate that Prosobee also had insufficient dietary chloride, but lack the necessary load of base needed to generate an alkalosis. However, the chloride content of Prosobee was measured and found to be 13 mEq/l. At this time the child was home perspiring slightly in the hot Kansas weather. We, therefore, wondered if the chloride content of the Prosobee might be sufficient but simply lack the necessary citrate to generate the alkalosis despite some subcutaneous salt loss through sweating. With this in mind we performed the following experiment: Since the product label indicated the potassium citrate content of NeoMulsoy to be greater than that of Prosobee by 100 mg/dl of formula, we added to the child's diet 100 mg of potassium citrate per 100 ml of Prosobee ingested. This would provide approximately 1.5 mEq/kg of a potential bicarbonate load for the volume of formula ingested by this infant. Within four days the infant became irritable, began to resist feeding, and his venous pH rose to 7.44. The child became normal after stopping the supplemental citrate.

Follow-up some fifteen months after initial evaluation shows the child to be normotensive and to have normal growth and development with no evidence of alkalosis or renal dysfunction.

Under normal circumstances the addition of 1.5-2 mEq/kilo of sodium bicarbonate to a normally hydrated patient would result in volume expansion and urinary excretion of the additional bicarbonate.[3] However, in a state of volume depletion, addition of bicarbonate will generate an alkalotic state. Since our patient demonstrated avid urinary chloride retention, mild hyperuricemia, and abnormal renal hippuran renogram, it would have appeared that this child was clearly chloride depleted and volume contracted despite the lack of clinical evidence of dehydration. Thus, it would not be difficult to explain the mechanism for the maintenance of the child's alkalosis since volume depletion is known to impair excretion of bicarbonate.[4]

The generation of the alkalosis, however, is another matter. It would not appear that the degree of volume contraction observed in this infant is sufficient to explain the severe alkalosis observed since he was only moderately ill. Loss of acid was unlikely since mouth pH measurements by litmus paper were consistently 6.0 or higher and urine pH was not acid. Although the slight decrease in potassium observed on admission might contribute to the loss of bicarbonate, this finding probably is of little importance in the generation of the alkalosis since the child remained virtually normokalemic during the time of his study. Nonreabsorbed anion in the formula, perhaps sulfates or nitrates, might have led to increased urinary loss of acid, but we have not measured the formula content of these anions. On the other hand, it would appear that there was sufficient citrate provided in the NeoMullsoy formula capable of generating alkalosis either through its metabolism or through its nonreabsorbed anion effect. In this regard it is of interest that the alkalosis only developed when the NeoMulsoy intake was increased. This maneuver probably increased the citrate load sufficiently to generate the alkalosis.

We believe that NeoMullsoy formula generated a metabolic alkalosis because it had a citrate content too high for its chloride load, and when given in sufficient volumes without additional food or supplemental sodium chloride, resulted in the syndrome of metabolic alkalosis.

Illustrations are reproduced with permission of the Journal of Pediatrics, 96:4, pp. 635-640, 1980. Prosobee (Mead Johnson)

The authors express their appreciation for secretarial assistance provided by Shirley Habberfield.

REFERENCES

1. Linshaw MA, Harrison HL, Gruskin AB, et.al.: Hypochloremic Alkalosis in Infants Associated with Soy Protein Formula. J. of Pediatrics, 96:4, pp. 635-640, April, 1980.
2. Davis JO, Freeman RH: Mechanism regulating renin release Physio Rev., 56:1, 1976.
3. Sanderson PH: Renal Response to Massive Alkali Loading in the Human Subject. In Ciba Foundation Symposium on the Kidney. Little, Brown, and Company, Boston, p. 165, 1954.
4. Seldin DW: Metabolic Alkalosis. In Brenner BM, Rector FC (ed). The Kidney, Vol. I, Chapter 17, pp. 661-702, 1976. WB Saunders Company.

METABOLIC ALKALOSIS FROM A CHLORIDE DEFICIENT FORMULA: RENAL HISTOLOGY

Shane Roy, III

1. INTRODUCTION

Renal histopathologic changes have previously been described in chloride deficient syndromes such as pyloric stenosis, serruptitious vomiting, congenital chloride losing diarrhea (CCD), laxative abuse and Bartter's syndrome. The similarity of the renal histologic changes in these varied clinical conditions suggests that the changes may represent a renal response to biochemical and physiological changes that the disorders have in common. Renal histologic changes in these clinical disorders, in experimentally chloride deprived animals and in 2 of our patients who received chloride-deficient Neo-Mull-Soy[R] (NMS[R]) will be discussed.

2. HUMAN STUDIES

Six unrelated infants were evaluated at the University of Tennessee Center for the Health Sciences during the same month of 1979 because of failure to thrive (1). Each infant had hypochloremic, hypokalemic, metabolic alkalosis, hyperaldosteronism, elevated plasma renin activity, normal blood pressure and hematuria in 4 of 6 patients. Anorexia for solid foods, delayed motor development, muscular weakness, severe constipation, polyuria and polydipsia were also observed. NMS[R] had been the primary source of nutrition for each infant for 2 to 5 months prior to their evaluation. Mean Na^+ intake for the infants was 2.1 mEq/kg/day, mean K^+ intake 3.2 mEq/kg/day and mean chloride intake was <0.3 mEq/kg/day. Twenty-four hour urinary chloride excretion was <1.0 mEq/kg in 1 infant and <0.1 mEq/kg in 5 infants.

Since chloride loss could not be documented in vomitus, urine, stool or sweat, an analysis of their NMS[R] formula revealed that, contrary to product information, the chloride concentration was less than 2 mEq/L. The volume of formula intake provided each infant less than 0.3 mEq/kg/day of chloride as opposed to the recommended 3 to 5 mEq/kg/day. The sodium and potassium contents of the formula were 17 and 25 mEq/L respectively. NMS[R] also contains 240 mg/dl of citrate and provided an equivalent bicarbonate load of approximately 2 mEq/kg/day to these infants.

Plasma electrolytes, blood urea nitrogen and weight gain were measured during 4 periods of observation for 2 affected infant girls at age 6 and 5.5 months. Hypochloremia, hyponatremia, hypokalemia, elevated plasma bicarbonate and elevated blood urea nitrogen were present in both infants when they were receiving NMS[R] alone. During the second period of observation, when KCl (3 to 4 mEq/kg/day) was added to NMS[R], plasma electrolytes returned to normal. Hypochloremic, hypokalemic metabolic alkalosis recurred promptly when KCl was discontinued and NMS[R] was fed. The electrolyte abnormalities were again corrected when Nutramigen[R] (Cl^- = 23 mEq/L) and Similac[R] (Cl^- = 18 mEq/L) were substituted for the chloride-deficient NMS[R].

Similar electrolyte abnormalities in 4 other infants who were receiving NMS[R] were also corrected by feeding a different formula with a chloride concentration of at least 13 mEq/L. Elevated plasma renin activity (PRA) of 30 to 81 ng/ml/hour was observed in the 4 infants tested. PRA decreased to 16, 13.6 and 38.6 ng/ml/hour in 3 patients one week after feeding a chloride-sufficient formula and to 0.5 and 3.3 ng/ml/hour 6 months later in 2 patients. Initial plasma aldosterone (PA) values in 4 patients of 12, 35, 41 and 119 ng/dl decreased one week after feeding chloride-sufficient formula to 28, 34, and 34 ng/dl in the latter 3 patients. During 12 months of follow-up, hematuria has disappeared and plasma electrolytes have remained normal.

Because of unexplained metabolic alkalosis in association with hematuria, proteinuria and elevation of plasma creatinine, renal biopsies were performed in the first 2 index patients at a time when hypochloremic, hypokalemic metabolic alkalosis was present and before the formula deficiency was proven. No histologic changes and no juxtaglomerular hyperplasia were observed in 65 glomeruli from one patient. Slight interstitial fibrosis without tubular atrophy or tubular vacuolization were noted. Immunofluorescence (IF) microscopy was negative. Focal foot process effacement of epithelial cells was observed on electronmicroscopy (EM). Interstitial collagen was increased and a few fibroblasts, plasma cells and lymphocytes were identified in the interstitium. The tubules were unremarkable. In the second patient's biopsy 66 glomeruli were unremarkable. No juxtaglomerular hyperplasia was observed and IF was negative. Focal foot process effacement of epithelial cells was noted on EM. Tubules were also unremarkable. Areas of increased interstitial collagen and a focal area of interstitial calcification were observed.

When our findings in the first 3 infants (2) were made known to the formula manufacturer, local public health authority, Center for Diasese Control and the Food and Drug Administration, 28 additional cases of unexplained metabolic alkalosis were rapidly identified by the CDC in a telephone survey of selected pediatric nephrology training programs (3). Twenty-seven of these 28 infants were receiving NMS[R] when their metabolic alkalosis was diagnosed. Both NMS[R] and CHO-Free[R] were subsequently recalled from the market on August 2, 1979. The CDC has subsequently identified at least 150 infants who developed metabolic alkalosis while receiving the 2 formulas between late 1978 and August 1979 (4).

Longitudinal growth data in our 6 infants revealed a significant decrease in weight during NMS[R] feeding and a significant increase in weight and head circumference when NMS[R] was discontinued and chloride adequate formula was fed. Delayed onset of expressive language has been noted in 6 of 31 infants who received NMS[R] and have been followed for a mean of 7 months. Receptive language skills were normal but expressive language skills were 6 to 18 months behind their chronological age (5).

Learning disabilities, mental retardation, and developmental delays have been described in children with metabolic alkalosis and hypochloremia secondary to pyloric stenosis (6), Bartter's syndrome (7) and familial chloride-losing diarrhea (8). It seems appropriate, therefore, to advise that infants, who received the chloride-deficient NMS[R], be evaluated prospectively with special attention to language skills and the possible appearance of perceptual problems by school age.

3. RENAL STRUCTURAL ABNORMALITIES

Much has been written describing renal structural changes associated with potassium deficiency in animals and humans. Conversely, very few studies describing renal structural changes secondary to hypochloremia are available.

Holliday et al (9) first described extensive changes in the cortex of rats acutely depleted of chloride and later (10) showed that extensive cell damage and hyperplasia was confined to the mid-portion of the proximal convoluted tubule. Furthermore, the severity of histologic changes was increased by concomitant potassium deficiency. In another group of rats, depleted of chloride and given phosphate, calcification and hyperplasia of the terminal half of the proximal convoluted tubule were observed similar to that which follows massive phosphate ingestion.

Sequential light microscopic and ultrastructural renal changes in chloride depleted rats have been described (11). Small masses of calcification in proximal tubules were evident by the third day of chloride deprivation. The deposits rapidly increased in amount with time, so that, by the sixth day grossly visible calcified streaks were evident involving the entire lower cortex. Satellite deposits coalesced forming large, lobulated liths with laminations, which first disrupted and then destroyed the brush border, finally eroding into the cytoplasm of epithelial cells. Lysosome-like bodies and mitochondria contained electron dense deposits consistent with calcification. Basement membranes and the interstitium were not involved.

Striking nephrocalcinosis was reported in rats fed a chloride deficient diet containing 8.2% sulfate when they drank a neutral phosphate solution (12). Nephrocalcinosis could be prevented by adding chloride initially to the drinking solution, accentuated by furosemide-induced chloriuresis and partially reversed if chloride was subsequently ingested. Nephrocalcinosis has also been described in fatal cases of pyloric stenosis (13), in congenital chloride diarrhea (14) and in Bartter's syndrome (15).

Severe glomerular and interstitial nephritis with mild juxtaglomerular (JG) hyperplasia and progressive renal failure have also been reported in Bartter's syndrome. Other features of glomerulonephritis such as enlarged hypercellular glomeruli, membranous thickening of glomerular capillar walls, mesangial hypercellularity, crescent formation, concentric periglomerular fibrosis, glomerulosclerosis and thickening and sclerosis of arteries and arterioles have also been associated with JG hyperplasia in Bartter's syndrome. The presence of some of these renal histopathologic features in extrarenal disorders which have clinical findings similar to Bartter's syndrome suggest that these changes may not be unique to Bartter's syndrome but may represent a renal response to biochemical and physiologic changes which the disorders have in common (16). The specificity of any of these histologic changes in Bartter's syndrome will await further clarification of the nature of the abnormality in tubular chloride transport. The description of a sibship with clinical and biochemical features of Bartter's syndrome in association with thickening of the proximal tubular basement membrane and no JG hyperplasia (17) adds further confusion to our knowledge of renal changes in metabolic alkalosis.

4. DATA FROM PILOT ANIMAL STUDY

Several studies have examined the effects of dietary chloride depletion in various animal species. Rats, which were chloride deprived, developed a depressed appetite, retarded growth, increased water consumption, increased heat production, decreased energy stores and a smaller proportion of weight gain as fat and water (18).

Two month old Holstein calves fed a chloride-deficient diet (0.038% Cl^-) for 7 weeks showed a decrease in plasma chloride concentration from 104.7 to 92 mEq/L after 2 weeks (19). Chloride was barely detectable in the urine by the 3rd week of chloride deprivation. Blood pH, pCO_2 and bicarbonate concentrations increased significantly but severe alkalosis did not develop. Plasma potassium decreased to 80% of control values by the 7th week of the study. Decrease in extracellular fluid volume was evidenced by increase in total plasma solids and hematocrit. Symptoms of polydipsia and polyuria became progressively more pronounced with time.

We have fed the chloride-deficient NMS[R] (<2 mEq/L) to 3 mongrel canine puppies 2 to 3 months of age for 11 weeks in an attempt to examine the pathophysiology and pathology resulting from the chloride-deficient formula. Control and weekly blood samples for electrolytes, pH, pCO_2, hematocrit, PRA, PA, creatinine and ECFV were obtained. Formula intake, urinary output, urinary electrolyte excretion and weight were measured daily. PGE_2 was measured in selected urine samples. After 11 weeks of chloride-deficient (CD) formula, dog A continued to receive CD formula, dog B received chloride adequate (CA) NMS[R] (Cl^- = 14.4 mEq/L) and dog C received CA Isomil[R] (Cl^- = 11 mEq/L) for 3 additional weeks.

Dog A's average weight gain was 36.8 gm/day. During CD feeding dog B lost an average of 3.31 gm/day and dog C, after losing 580 gm during the first 10 days, gained at a rate of 3.8 gm/day. When CA formula was fed, dog B gained 10 gm/day, and dog C gained 39 gm/day, a 13 and 10 fold increase in rate of weight gain.

Sodium and potassium intakes were similar between dog A and dogs B and C during CD feeding. Dogs B and C however, ingested slightly more chloride 0.295±0.004 mEq/kg/day than dog A 0.26±0.004 mEq/kg/day (P<0.05) during CD feeding. Chloride intake for dogs B and C was significantly greater during CA than CD feeding (1.77±0.14 vs 0.295±0.004 mEq/kg/day; P<0.005).

Twenty-four hour urinary chloride excretion was similar in the 3 dogs during CD feeding (0.13±0.08 mEq/kg/day), however, dog A excreted significantly more sodium (2.06±0.14 vs 1.615±0.004 mEq/kg/day; P<0.005) and more potassium (2.28±0.17 vs 1.625±0.025 mEq/kg/day; P<0.025) than dogs B and C. Urine chloride excretion increased from 0.135±0.11 to 0.605±0.08 mEq/kg/day (P<0.025) in dogs B and C during CA feeding. There was no difference in sodium and potassium excretion between the dogs.

During 11 weeks of CD formula, mean plasma potassium and chloride decreased significantly while plasma bicarbonate and pH increased significantly. Plasma potassium, chloride, bicarbonate and pH returned to control levels during 3 weeks of CA formula in dogs B, and C.

Plasma creatinine was increased significantly above control values at 4 weeks, was below control values at 5 weeks and similar to control values each week thereafter.

Mean PRA increased significantly from 1.0±0.51 ng/ml/hour to 7.93±2.9 ng/ml/hour after 11 weeks of CD feeding. PRA in dogs B and C after 3 weeks of CA feeding (0.4±0.14 ng/dl) was significantly lower (P<0.01) than PRA in dog A (8.1 ng/dl) fed CD formula.

Initial PA concentrations were not obtained. Mean PA after 2 weeks of CD feeding was 36.4±9.12 ng/dl and increased to 44.9±8.06 after 11 weeks. Mean PA in dogs B and C during CA feeding decreased to 23 ng/dl but this difference was not statistically significant.

Control mean ECFV decreased from 341.8±51.7 to 284.8±34.7 ml/kg after 11 weeks of CD feeding. ECFV decreased further in dog A to 180.3 ml/kg at 14 weeks but increased in dogs B and C, fed CA formula, to 321 ml/kg. These differences were not statistically different. Urinary PGE_2 during CD formula progressively decreased in dog A, decreased and then increased in dog B, and increased in dog C. As plasma chloride and potassium increased during CA formula in dogs B and C, urinary PGE_2 increased strikingly during the 14th week. Plasma PGE_2 concentrations at the end of the study were higher in the recovered dogs B and C than in dog A.

Samples of liver, heart, skeletal muscle and cartilage as well as whole kidney and brain were weighed immediately and then oven dried to a stable weight. Values for each tissue were compared as follows: wet weight-dry weight ÷ dry weight x 100. There were no differences in percent water content of heart muscle, brain and cartilage between dog A and dogs B and C.

The liver of dog A contained more water than the liver of dogs B and C
(298.9% vs 239.6±3.4%; P<0.025). Both skeletal muscle (374.2±0.14% vs
83.4%; P<0.005) and kidney (386±0.67% vs 333.7%; P<0.005) from dogs B and C
contained a higher percent water per gram of dry tissue than dog A.

Sodium, potassium and chloride concentrations of liver, skeletal muscle,
heart muscle, kidney and brain were measured and expressed as milliequivalents
per gram of dry tissue weight. Sodium concentration of liver was significantly
higher in dog A than in dogs B and C (0.265 vs 184.5±0.001 mEq/gDW; P<0.005).
Sodium content in skeletal muscle and kidney of dogs B and C was significantly
higher than dog A (SM - 0.273±0.02 vs 0.122 mEq/gDW; P<0.05; K - 0.428±0.01
vs 0.363 mEq/gDW; P<0.025). There was no difference in sodium content of
heart muscle or brain between dog A and dogs B and C.

Skeletal muscle potassium of dogs B and C was significantly greater than
dog A (0.435±0.011 vs 0.169 mEq/gDW) but there were no differences in
potassium content of liver, heart muscle, kidney or brain.

Chloride content of skeletal muscle (0.14±0.004 vs 0.07 mEq/gDW; P<0.025)
and kidney (0.35±0.004 vs 0.25 mEq/gDW; P<0.01) were significantly greater
in dogs B and C fed CA formula. There were no differences in chloride content
of liver, heart muscle or brain between dog A and dogs B and C.

Samples of kidney obtained from cortex, cortico-medullary junction and
medulla from each animal were studied histologically and showed no changes
by light microscopy.

This preliminary study did not reveal a mechanism to explain the hematuria
observed in the chloride deprived infants. It is possible, however, that
the canine kidney is as resistant to the changes resulting from chloride
deprivation as it is to the changes observed with potassium deficiency.
Future studies in younger puppies or in a different animal species may
reveal a mechanism for the hematuria. It has been suggested that the citrate
content of NMS[R] (240 mg/dl) played a significant role in producing metabolic
alkalosis in the chloride deprived infants. Correction of the biochemical
abnormalities in dog B fed CA NMS[R] was as prompt as in dog C fed CA Isomil[R]
suggesting that chloride deficiency was the sole mechanism causing the
metabolic alkalosis in the animals. Biochemical correction in the infants,
obtained by adding chloride to their deficient formula, appears to justify
a similar conclusion.

Our knowledge of the effects of chloride deficiency upon renal structure
and function and upon somatic and brain growth and function in the maturing

infant is far from complete. Follow-up studies of the infants involved in this deficient syndrome as well as studies of chloride deficiency produced in various animal species hopefully will provide answers to some of these questions.

REFERENCES

1. Roy S III, Arant BS Jr. 1980, in press. Hypokalemic metabolic alkalosis in normotensive infants with elevated plasma renin activity and hyperaldosteronism: the role of dietary chloride deficiency. Pediatrics.
2. Roy S III, Arant BS Jr. 1979. Alkalosis from chloride deficient Neo-Mull-Soy^R. N Engl J Med 301:615.
3. Center for Disease Control. 1979. Infant metabolic alkalosis and soy-based formula-United States. Morbidity and Mortality Weekly Report 28:358.
4. Center for Disease Control. 1980. Follow-up on formula-associated illness in children. Morbidity and Mortality Weekly Report 29:124.
5. Roy S III, Stapleton FB, Arant BS Jr. 1980. Hypochloremic metabolic alkalosis in infants fed a chloride-deficient formula. Pediatr Res 14:509.
6. Klein PS, Forbes GB, Hader PR. 1975. Effects of starvation in infancy (pyloric stenosis) on subsequent learning abilities. J Pediatr 87:8.
7. Simopoulos AP. 1979. Growth characteristics in patients with Bartter's syndrome. Nephron 23:130.
8. Holmberg C, Perheentupa J, Laumiala K, Hallman N. 1977. Congenital chloride diarrhea: Clinical analysis of 21 Finnish patients. Arch Dis Child 52:255.
9. Holliday MA, Schulz D. 1954. The renal lesion in acute metabolic alkalosis. AJDC 88:629.
10. Holliday MA, Bright NH, Schulz D, Oliver J. 1961. The renal lesions of electrolyte imbalance. J Expl Med 113:971.
11. Sarkar K, Tolnai G, Levine DZ. 1973. Nephrocalcinosis in chloride depleted rats: an ultrastructural study. Calc Tiss Res 12:1.
12. Levine DZ, Roy D, Tolnai G, Nash L, Shah BG. 1974. Chloride depletion and nephrocalcinosis. Am J Physiol 227:878.
13. Cooke AM. 1933. Calcification of the kidneys in pyloric stenosis. Quart J Med 2:539.
14. Holmberg C, Perheentupa J, Pasternack A. 1977. The renal lesion in congenital chloride diarrhea. J Pediatr 91:738.
15. Arant BS Jr, Brackett NC, Young RB, Still WJS. 1970. Case studies of siblings with juxtaglomerular hyperplasia and secondary aldosteronism associated with severe azotemia and renal rickets-Bartter's syndrome or disease? Pediatrics 46:344.
16. Gill JR. 1980. Bartter's syndrome. Ann Rev Med 31:405.
17. Gullner HG, Gill JR, Bartter FC, Chan JCM, Dickman PS. 1979. A familial disorder with hypokalemic alkalosis, hyperreninemia, aldosteronism, high urinary prostaglandins and normal blood pressure that is not "Bartter's syndrome," Trans Assoc Am Phys 92:175.
18. Voris L, Thacker EJ. 1941. The effects of the substitution of bicarbonate for chloride in the diets of rats on growth, energy and protein metabolism. J Nutr 23:365.
19. Burkhalter DL, Neathery MW, Miller WJ, Whitlock RH, Allen JC, Gentry RP. 1980. Influence of a low chloride practical diet on acid-base balance and other factors of blood in young dairy calves. J Dairy Sci 63:269.

METABOLIC ALKALOSIS, PROSTAGLANDINS, LOW CHLORIDE, OR SOMETHING ELSE?

JOSE R. SALCEDO, M.D.

The recent epidemic of metabolic alkalosis in a large number of infants fed soy protein isolate [1-3] which was deficient in chloride has prompted a renewed interest in this pathophysiological state. These infants were characterized by having an elevated blood pH, increased serum bicarbonate concentration, and a slight compensatory increase in pCO_2. Under experimental [4, 5] and clinical conditions, metabolic alkalosis can result from either the gain of base or the loss of acid from extracellular fluid associated with chloride and potassium deficits. Thus, two phases of this disorder can be considered: 1) the mechanisms which produce the metabolic alkalosis, i.e. increased alkali intake, or acid loss through vomiting, and 2) the processes responsible for subsequent maintenance of the alkalosis, i.e. hypochloremia, sodium avid state, etc. The clinical and laboratory evaluation of the infants fed soy formula failed to show the first phase in the development of metabolic alkalosis. Therefore, the composition of the formula itself was considered, namely, the low chloride, high citrate, phytate phosphorus, soy bean protein as well as the hypothetical consideration of prostaglandin precursors or enhancers. Chloride, in current views of acid base physiology, is considered a very weak base due to its low affinity to combine with hydrogen ions and the fact that it does not donate hydrogen ions to body fluids. However, it seems that chloride depletion is the most critical factor in clinically occurring metabolic alkalosis. This is substantiated by experimental data where metabolic alkalosis is produced by loss of gastric acid or by treatment with commonly used diuretics. But its major role seems to be in the second phase.

The citrate content was found to be 240 mg/100 grams of formula (each 324.4 mg of citrate is equal to 1 mEq) so that a liter of formula would provide 7.5 mEq of citrate. The metabolic oxidation of 1 mkg of citrate would produce an equivalent of 3 moles of bicarbonate. This amount of base could be excreted readily under normal circumstances. However, since 70% of the phosphorus in soy isolates is present as phytate phosphorus [6] one can speculate that these can act as a non-reabsorbable anion. Furthermore, previous investigators have found soy isolates to be deficient in several nutrients. Fung in the Singapore Medical Journal [7] evaluated the effect of soya bean milk as an antacid in a lactose intolerant population and concluded that significant gastric acid neutralization occurs with its use. Later, the same author [8] reported that soya bean milk was equally as efficacious as aluminum hydroxide in promoting the healing of gastric ulcers. In the meantime, Gardiner, et al, [9] reported in British Poultry Science the interesting observation that broiler chicks fed wheat soya bean diet had a high chloride requirement. This finding prompted us to speculate as to whether soy isolate formula contained a natriuretic factor that would act concomitantly with the baseload creating a sodium avid state. Because of the clinical and laboratory resemblance to Bartter's syndrome, prostaglandin-like substances or precursors were considered.

It is known that biologically active prostaglandins (PG) are synthesized from essential fatty acids. [10-12] Prostaglandin E_1 and F_1 groups are synthesized from DI-Homo linolenic acid, and PGE_2 and F_2 from arachidonic acid. Both DI-Homo linolenic and arachidonic acid are derived from linoleic acid. The precursors of prostaglandins are the free, unesterified fatty acids and their availability as precursors are one of the important controlling factors of PG biosynthesis in essential fatty acid deficient rats.

The precursors of essential fatty acids (EFA) are stored as a moiety of the phospholipids in the cell membrane. Since the most abundant EFA in the body is arachidonic acid the majority of tissue contains mostly PGE_2 and PGF_2. Unlike biogenic amines PG's are not stored in the body but rather are formed immediately prior to release. A variety

480

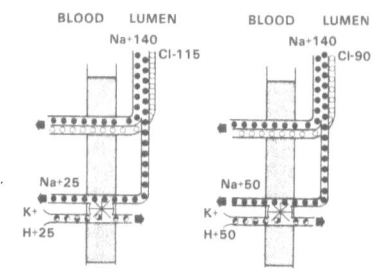

From KASSIRER and SCHWARTZ

of physiological, pharmacological and pathological stimuli
trigger the activation of phospholipase "A" which splits the
precursors of EFA's from the phospholipids in the cell
membrane with resultant cleavage of arachidonic acid and
rapid synthesis of PGE. Once synthesized, PGE exercises its
pharmacological actions which include increased blood flow,
induction of natriuresis, kaliuresis, and water diuresis and
its potent renin releasing properties. [13] This action can
indirectly be assessed by the significantly high levels of
renin found in these infants - levels which are not accounted
for by the infant's body fluid depletion. Furthermore, the
persistent natriuresis, normal blood pressure, and high
renin and aldosterone levels mimic those seen with the use
of loop diuretics and/or prostaglandin infusions.

As mentioned above, chloride depletion is the most
critical factor in clinically occurring metabolic alkalosis.
However, its major role seems to be in the second phase or
as one of the processes responsible for the subsequent
maintenance of the alkalosis. The significance of chloride
depletion can best be considered in view of the theory
proposed by Kassirer and Schwartz in the mid sixties. These
authors proposed that in the normal state [4] (Figure 1)
sodium enters the glomerular filtrate at a concentration of
140 mEq/L and chloride at a concentration of 115 mEq/L. As
sodium is removed from the filtrate electroneutrality is
maintained by the parallel reabsorption of anion, in this
case chloride. Hence, 115 mEq/L of sodium is reabsorbed
with chloride while 25 mEq/L is reclaimed by exchange for

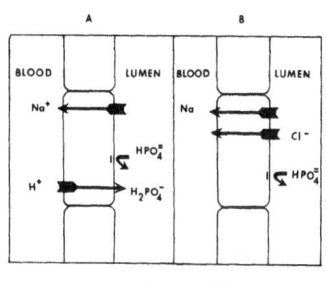

potassium or hydrogen. [4]

When hypochloremia is present the concentration of chloride in the filtrate sets a new limit on the quantity of sodium which can be reabsorbed paired with an anion. As shown, if the chloride concentration is 90 mEq/L, only 90 mEq/L of sodium can be reabsorbed. In the circumstance of a sodium avid state, the kidney opts for reabsorbing the sodium deprived of chloride by accelerating sodium-potassium and/or sodium-hydrogen exchange. This alteration accounts for the rise in bicarbonate threshhold and for the negative potassium balance.

Furthermore, to emphasize the role of anion reabsorbability in acceleration of sodium-hydrogen exchange, in a sodium avid state, the schematic representation [5] in Figure 2, was presented wherein the sodium salt of a non-reabsorbable anion is administered to subjects ingesting a low sodium diet. Under these circumstances sodium reabsorption is accelerated at a time when poorly reabsorbable anions, i.e. sulfate, phosphate are available. The requirement for electroneutrality is met by acceleration of hydrogen ion secretion. By contrast, when there is a readily reabsorbable anion there is a prompt decrease in the rate of hydrogen ion secretion. These observations were made during a short steady state and no significant changes in pH were observed unless significant volume depletion was accomplished either by the use of diuretics or by constant hydrochloric acid drainage.

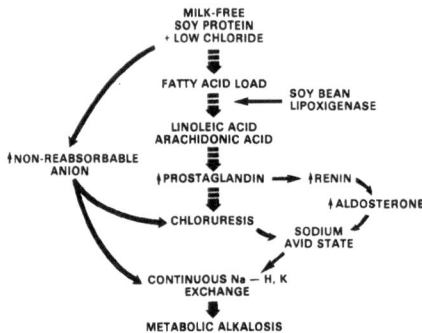

Finally, Figure 3 depicts the proposed hypothetical mechanisms by which patients could develop metabolic alkalosis. All of them remain to be demonstrated by prospective studies. As mentioned initially, an increased fatty acid load could increase the precursors of prostaglandins which in turn could cause chloruresis (either renal or intestinal) creating a sodium avid state. A sodium avid state in the presence of a low chloride could then promote continuous exchange of sodium for hydrogen/potassium with continuous metabolic alkalosis. Furthermore, the addition of a non-reabsorbable anion could then worsen the suppression of the low chloride in the formula.

In summary, the following speculations can be made:

1) Metabolic alkalosis cannot be explained by a low chloride diet alone.

2) Low chloride can perpetuate metabolic alkalosis.

3) Soy bean isolates may contain large amounts of non-reabsorbable anions, polyunsaturated fatty acids and/or prostaglandin precursors.

4) The low chloride, relative high citrate, and soy bean alkalinization properties may constitute a large baseload.

REFERENCES
1. Roy S, III, Arant BS Jr: Alkalosis from chloride-deficient Neo-mullsoy, Letter to the Editor. N. Eng. J. Med. 301:615, 1979.
2. Infant Metabolic alkalosis and soy based formula - United States. Morbidity and Mortality Weekly Rep. 28:358, 1979.

3. Grossman H, Dugan E, McCamman, et al: The dietary chloride deficiency syndrome. Pediatr. 66:366, 1980.
4. Kassirer JP and Schwartz WB. The response of normal man to selective depletion of hydrochloric acid. Amer. J. of Med. 40:10, 1966.
5. Schwartz WB, Ypersele deStrihou CV, Kassirer JP: Role of anions in metabolic alkalosis. N. Eng. J. Med. 279:630, 1968.
6. O'Dell BL, Savage JE: Effect of phytic acid on zinc availability. Proc. Soc. Exp. Biol. Med. 103:304, 1960.
7. Fung WP: Effect of soyabean milk on the healing of gastric ulcers, a controlled endoscopic study. Med. J. of Aust. 1:717, 1975.
8. Fung WP, Tye CY: Evaluation of soya bean milk as an antacid. Sing. Med. J. 14:515, 1973.
9. Gardiner EE, Dewar WA: Dietary chloride requirement of broiler chicks fed on a wheat-soyabean diet. Br. Poult. Sci. 17:337, 1976.
10. Weber PC: Renal prostaglandins in the control of renin. Contr. Nephrol. Vol. 12, p 92, Karher Basel, 1978.
11. McGiff JC, Crowshaw K, Itskowitz HA: Prostaglandins and renal function. Fed. Proc. Fed. Am. Soc. Exp. Biol. 33:39, 1974.
12. Horton R, Zipser R: Prostaglandins: Renin release and renal function. Contr. Nephrol. Vol. 14, p 87, Karher Basel, 1978.
13. Weming C, Vetter W, Weidmann P, et al: Effect of prostaglandin E_1 on renin in the dog. Am. J. Physiol. 220:852, 1971.

Figures 1 & 2 reproduced by permission of the publishers.

UREMIC POISONING

R.A. CAMPBELL, F. BARTOS, D. BARTOS

Present knowledge of intracellular polyamines (PAs) suggest
they play a critical role in cell cycle processes at the
molecular level (1,2,3,4,5). Key enzymes and organelles
involved in transcription, translation and numerous post-
translational events would appear to result from alterations
of form and function of highly susceptible molecules by
regulative manipulation of PA profiles and concentrations
(6,7,8,9,10, 11,12,13,14). Rather stereotypic PA pathway
activation responses have been identified with a great variety
of hormones directed at particular target cell types (15). The
vital requirements of PAs for accomplishing such basic biological phenomena as embryogenesis, differentiation, hypertrophy,
hyperplasia and wound-healing are now well documented (16,17).

A pharmacological toxicology for these aliphatic polycations
has been established and it is now clear that with manipulation
of PAs in in vitro and in vivo test systems a wide variety of
deleterious effects on cell metabolism and physiological
function result (18,19,20,21). It is reasonable to suggest the
experimental findings share some degree of equivalence with
extracellular space (ECS) changes found in hyperpolyaminemic
states in man. The hyperpolyaminemic states of various etiologies and clinical expressions, i.e., cancer, pregnancy, Reye's
syndrome, systemic lupus erythematosus, transplant rejection
and various forms of cell trauma, all have distinctive features
in common with uremia (18,22,23,24,25,26,27,28,29). Even when
compared alone, the congruence of experimental PA research
findings and the characteristics of the uremic syndrome are
truly remarkable (see Table).

Table. Uremic Poisoning and Polyamines.

OBSERVATION	UREMIA (Refs.)	PAs (Refs.)
Vomiting	28,30,31	32
Peripheral neuropathy, paralysis	33,34,35	36,18,37
Convulsions	38,35	37,39
Coma and death	38,35	37,39
Depressed O_2 consumption	40,35	41,42
Hypothermia	38,43	44,36
CHO and fat transpt. and metab.	45,46,47,48	49,50
Electrolyte and organic ion transpt.	51,52,53	54,55
Diuretic action	52,53,56	57
Cell proliferation; immunity	58,59,60,61,62	63,64,65,66

In terms of mathematical probabilities, it is remote that this scientific verisimilitude could be casual. Pernicious vomiting is a cardinal feature of the hyperpolyaminemic conditions of terminal uremia, Reye's syndrome and early pregnancy (hyperemesis gravidarum). We and others have induced paralysis in animals with PAs. Depressed O_2 consumption occurs in uremic tissues such as brain and liver. PAs also depress tissue O_2 consumption, i.e., the brain.

Coma and death are features common to both PA toxicity and uremia. Uremic patients may have dialysis-correctable hypothermia. Either uremic serum fractions or PAs administered to experimental animals induce hypothermia.

Pseudodiabetes mellitus occurs in such hyperpolyaminemic states as uremia, cancer and pregnancy (67,68,69,70). PAs block transcellular glucose transport. Spermidine (SPD) peptide binds insulin and decreases lipoprotein lipase activity of adipocytes in vitro (71).

Na^+, K^+-ATPase activity is seriously deranged in uremic tissues. PAs inhibit ATPase activity. Abnormal electrolyte and organic ion transport are features common to uremia and experimental PA toxicity. Uremic serum (naturetic factor) and PAs administered to rats are both diuretic.

Uremic serum (fractions) inhibits lymphocytes and erythroblastic cell systems. PAs have been demonstrated to do the same (64). It has now been demonstrated that specific anti-PA antibodies (ABs) prevent inhibition of erythroblastic cell proliferation by uremic serum, its fractions, or PAs. Where studied, hyperpolyaminemic states identified to date have depressed cellular immunity. Uremic peptidic fractions inhibit lymphocyte blast transformation and formation of rosettes. Most all of these fractions partially characterized to date have been reported to be basic (cationic) or contain excess non-amino acid nitrogen (72). PAs inhibit lymphocyte blast transformation in tissue culture. Uremic dialytic therapy comparing hemo- and peritoneal dialysis reveals the latter to be much more efficacious in restoring cellular immunity. The peritoneal membrane, more permeable than cuprophane, we suggest, facilitates PA peptide egress.

PA dysmetabolism in uremia was first identified by us (18). Conventional hemodialysis reduced radioimmunoassay (RIA) values in 16 patients only 32% and none fell to the upper limits of normal. Our bench studies demonstrated free PAs readily passed across cuprophane membranes; this was paradoxical. We then proceeded to study undialyzed uremic sera with highly specific SPD AB RIA before (native) and after silica gel column (SGC) treatment. Free SPD levels, 6 times normal before, dropped into the normal range indicating the bulk of the SPD immunoreactive substances were bound and not adsorbed on SGC (73). The poor diffusibility of the substance(s) and binding of SPD or spermine (SPM) in an exteriorized immunoreactive site suggested we might be dealing with one or several of the biologically active basic uremic peptides described over the years (72). At this time, a basic PA containing peptide was identified in plasma, and shortly thereafter several others were identified in amniotic fluid (74,75). We then discovered an overlooked paper in the Polish literature describing a SPD-containing peptide (1400 dalton) in peritoneal dialysis fluid which bound insulin and inhibited lipoprotein lipase activity (76). It is of no small moment that this PA-peptide also contains arginine and lysine. Such composition would suggest the capacity for strong non-specific binding to anionic structural components such as glycoproteins and phospholipids. This peptide has since been identified in uremic serum (50).

In the interim we were studying the effects of PAs on proximal tubule morphology (naturetic factor?), the action of PAs on in vitro arterial smooth muscle cells (ASMC) (77,78), which we suspected might be altered in their proliferation propensity in the presence of PAs. In view of our hemodialysis PA findings and the reports of increased cardiovascular disease in dialysis patients, this seemed potentially productive. Finally, the effect of PAs on in vitro erythroblastic activity was undertaken as a joint effort (79,80). Not only did PAs induce distinct morphological changes in the proximal tubule but the animals developed hind-leg paralysis (78). The arterial cells proliferated in the presence of PAs and the erythroblastic clot cells were inhibited. Silica gel treatment of uremic serum reduced the ASMC activity. The addition of anti-PA AB to erythroblastic clot cultures restored cell production after inhibition by any one of several treatments, i.e., crude uremic serum, fractions thereof, or free SPM or SPD.

These preliminary findings are consistent with widely held theoretical constructs on the pathogenesis of atherosclerosis and the anemia of uremia (81,82,83,84,85,59). It should be pointed out that the differences in various in vitro cell line responses to feeding, i.e., fibroblasts and ASMCs versus lymphocytes, are well known. The inhibitory effects of uremic cationic peptides on a number in vitro cell lines, however, have been considered disruptive and anti-anabolic (72).

That PA metabolism is disturbed in dialysis patients has been confirmed and extended using other methods (86). Hemodialysis failed to significantly reduce red blood cell PA concentration. In uremic animals, PAs accumulate in tissues (87). Dialyzing liver homogenates failed to restore activity (88). It is evident that both efficiency of anabolism and absence of messenger misreading are subject to intracellular space (ICS) PA concentrations (89). SPD appears to be critical and the optimal range is narrow (90). Tissue wasting in uremia

488

may be further explained by the recent observations that polyribosome formation is reduced in uremic muscle obtained from rats (91). Reduced synthetic activity was attributed to anabolic inefficiency secondary to ribosomal disaggregation. The role of ICS PAs in connection with $[mg++]$ in polyribosome formation is also well known (13).

Why the alterations in ECS and ICS? The kidney is a major organ for metabolizing and excreting PAs (18). The host must employ new PA strategies in renal failure. As one of the 13 failsafes we have, PA receptors on cell membranes may be of particular importance in shutting down the PA pathway (92). Under appropriate circumstances PAs are actively transported into the cells (93). The observation of reduced PA excretion in steady state urine is consistent with uremic hypometabolism (86).

There are many gaps in our knowledge. Much is known about peptide hormone levels in uremia. The same cannot be said for PA peptides. We need to identify the spectrum of PA peptides in blood and urine, their physicochemical and biological properties. Nothing is known about SPM and putrescine (PTC) peptides in end-stage renal disease. Nothing has been done to clarify ECS PA values, free and bound, in the interdialysis period. Finally, the isolation, identification and quantification of PA peptides in hemo- and peritoneal dialysis fluids will help close some of the gaps in the PA-uremia story with respect to effectiveness of therapy.

Creatinine, urea and uric acid poorly correlate with uremic toxicity. Other small putative toxins have, in their overall impact, failed to stand up to scrutiny (94). In contrast to PAs, none of these compounds play central roles in cell anabolism and growth (95). In addition, they lack potent cationic characteristics of the PAs and PA congeners which can confer profound influence on biological structures and properties. Despite changes in certain serum peptides with infection, malnutrition, neuropathy, pericarditis and fluid retention, reduction in middle molecules (MM) with

conventional hemodialysis and reported improvements in neuropathy, carbohydrate intolerance and anemia with aggressive
dialysis, identification of specific family of poisons has
not been achieved (19,96,97,98,99). MMs not only possess some
intrinsic toxicity but also must be considered as substances
serving as markers for higher M.W. poisons exerting their
adverse effects (100). This view is supported by the evidence
that an 18,000 dalton fraction of uremic serum inhibits
macrophage function (101,102). Since the PA peptides reported
to date include several fractions of far greater weight than
the MMs, i.e., 30,000 daltons, evaluation of biological
activity of higher M.W. PA containing substances is important
to close gaps in our knowledge (103).

AB development and RIA of suspect peptidic substances will
ultimately accelerate uremia/dialysis research, allow specific
detection in the picomole range on 20-40 ul patient samples
in batch quantities. Should our views concerning PAs and
uremia prevail, the availability of cost-effective RIA peptide
monitoring at the bedside will be a consequent spin-off of
this research effort.

ACKNOWLEDGMENT

We wish to express our appreciation to Mary Pitkin, Norma Fritz
and Faith Cory for expert assistance with this manuscript. We
acknowledge the generous support of the M. J. Murdock Charitable
Trust and an NIC Research Grant Award #CA16328.

REFERENCES

1. Cohen SS. 1971. Introduction to the Polyamine. New Jersey,
   Prentice-Hall.
2. Bachrach U. 1973. Function of Naturally Occurring Polyamines. New York, Academic Press.
3. Campbell RA, Bartos D, Morris DR, Bartos F, Daves GD, Jr.
   1978. Advances in Polyamine Research, Vol. 2. New York,
   Raven Press.
4. Campbell RA, Bartos D, Morris DR, Bartos F, Daves GD, Jr.
   1978. Advances in Polyamine Research, Vol. 2. New York,
   Raven Press.
5. Gaugas JM. 1980. Polyamines in Biomedical Research. New
   York, J. Wiley & Sons.

6. Das R, Kanunga MS. 1979. Biochem Biophys Res Commun 90(3):708-14.
7. Lipetz PD, Boyle SM, Mhaskar D, Lowney DS, Modak SD, Stevens R, Hart R. Submitted for publication in Nucleic Acid Res.
8. Lipetz PD, Lowney DS, Mhaskar D. 1981, to be published. Gene Structure and Expression, Ed., D.H. Dean et al.
9. Loftfield RB, Pastuszyn A, Eigner EA. 1981, in press. In: Perspectives in Polyamine Research, Eds., D. Morris, L. Marton. New York, Marcel Deckker.
10. Cohen SS, Lichtenstein J. 1960. J Biol Chem 235:2112-16.
11. Garcia-Patrone M, Algranati D. 1976. FEBS lett 66(1):39-43.
12. Ikemura T. 1969. Biochim Biophys Acta 195:389-95.
13. Raina A, Janne J. 1975. Med Biol 53:121-47.
14. Atkins J, Lewis J, Anderson C, Gesteland R. 1975. J Biological Chem 250(14):5688-95.
15. Bachrach U. 1980. In: Polyamines in Biomedical Research, Ed., J.M. Gaugas. New York, John Wiley & Sons, pp. 81-107.
16. Luk GD, Marton LJ, Baylin SB. 1980. Science 210:195.
17. Raina A, Eloranta T, Pajula RL, Mantyjarvi R, Tuomi K. 1980. In: Polyamines in Biomedical Research, Ed., J.M. Gaugas. New York, John Wiley & Sons, pp. 35-49.
18. Campbell R, Talwalkar Y, Bartos D, Bartos F, Musgrave J, Harner M, Puri H, Grettie D, Dolney AM, Loggan B. 1978. In: Advances in Polyamine Research, Vol. 2, Eds., R.A. Campbell et al. New York, Raven Press, pp. 319-43.
19. Campbell RA, Bartos F, Bartos D, Grettie DP. 1979. In: Controversies in Nephrology, Vol. 1, Eds., G.E. Schreiner et al, Georgetown University Press, pp. 435-47.
20. Shaw GG. 1979. Biochem Pharmacol 28:1-6.
21. Campbell RA, Grettie DP, Bartos D, Bartos F. 1981, in press. In: Polyamines in Normal and Malignant Cells, Ed., V. Zappia et al. New York, Raven Press.
22. Russell DH, Durie BGM. 1978. Polyamines as Biochemical Markers of Normal and Malignant Growth. New York, Raven Press, pp. 162-64.
23. Russell DH. 1971. Nature 233:144-45.
24. Puri H, Campbell RA, Puri V, Harner MH, Talwalkar YB, Musgrave JE, Bartos F, Bartos D, Loggan B. 1978. In: Advances in Polyamine Research, Vol. 2, Eds., R.A. Campbell et al. New York, Raven Press, pp. 359-67.
25. Musgrave JE, Campbell RA, Bartos D, Bartos F, Harner MH, Talwalkar YB, Puri H, Grettie DP, Loggan B. 1978. In: Advances in Polyamine Research, Vol. 2, Eds., R.A. Campbell et al. New York, Raven Press, pp. 351-58.
26. Desser H. 1980. In: Polyamines in Biomedical Research, Ed. J.M. Gaugas. New York, Wiley & Sons, pp. 415-33.
27. Nishioka K, Romsdahl MM, McMurtrey MJ. 1977. J Surg Oncol 9:555-62.
28. Campbell RA, Isom JB, Bartos D, Bartos F. 1978, abstract. Ped Res 12(4):550.
29. Schreiner GE, Maher JF. 1961. Uremia: Biochemistry, Pathogenesis and Treatment. Springfield, Ill., Charles C. Thomas, pp. 331-47.
30. Reye RDK, Morgan G, Boral J. 1963. Lancet ii:749.

31. (As many pregnant women know.)
32. Risetti U, Mancini G. 1954. Acta Neurol (Napoli) 8:911-15.
33. Ibrahim MM, Crosland JM, Honigsberger L, Barnes AD,
     Dawson-Edwards P, Newman CE, Robison BHB. 1974. Lancet
     ii:739-42.
34. Asbury AR, Victor M, Adams R. 1963. Arch Neurol 8:413-28.
35. Fishman RA, Raskin NH. 1967. Arch Neurol 17:10-12.
36. Friedman AH, Rodichok LD. 1970. Fed Proc 29:617.
37. Shaw GG. 1979. Biochem Pharmacol 28:1-6.
38. Schreiner GE, Maher JF. 1961. Uremia: Biochemistry,
     Pathogenesis and Treatment, Springfield, Ill., Charles C.
     Thomas.
39. Anderson DJ, Crosland J, Shaw GG. 1975. Neuropharmacology
     14:571-77.
40. Rinando JB, Gallice P, Crevat A, Saingra S, Murisasco A.
     1979. Biomedicine 30:215-18.
41. Evans EA, Vennesland B, Schneider JJ. 1939. Proc Soc Ex
     Biol Med 41:467-70.
42. Chaffee RRJ, Arine RM, Rochelle RH, Walkar CD. 1978. In:
     Advances in Polyamine Research, Vol. 2, Eds. R.A. Campbell
     et al. New York, Raven Press, pp. 123-28.
43. Feher I, Desi I, Szold E. 1958. Experientia 141:292.
44. Anderson DJ, Crosland J, Shaw GG. 1975. Neuropharmacology
     14:571.
45. Myers VC, Bailey CV. 1916. J Biol Chem 24:147.
46. Bagdade JD, Porte D, Jr., Bierman LL. 1968. NEJM 269:181.
47. Dzurik R, Hupkova V, Holman J, Valvovicova E. 1971. Int
     Urol Nephrol 3(4):409-13.
48. Dzurik R, Spustova V, Cernacek P. Presented 5th Symposium
     on "Metabolic Aspects of Kidney Function," Oxford, England.
     To be published in Internat J Biochem.
49. Arvanitakis S, Mangos J, McSherry NR, Rennert O. 1976. Tex
     Rep Biol Med 34:175-86.
50. Lutz W. 1980, in press, Physiol Chem Phys.
51. White AG, Nachev P. 1975. Am J Physiol 228:436-40.
52. Bricker NS, Bourgoignie JJ, Klohr S. 1970. Arch Intern Med
     126:860-64.
53. Weber H, Bourgoignie JJ, Bricker NS. 1974. Am J Physiol
     226:419-25.
54. Quarfoth G, Ahmed K. 1977. Fed Proc 36(3):360.
55. Tashima Y, Hasegawa M. 1975. Biochem Biophys Res Commun
     66(4):1344-48.
56. Henderson LW, Nolph KD, Puselett JB, Goldberg M. 1968.
     NEJM 278(9):467-73.
57. Tabor CW, Rosenthal SM. 1956. J Pharmacol Exp Ther 116:139-55.
58. Schreiner GE, Maher JF. 1961. Uremia: Biochemistry,
     Pathogenesis and Treatment. Springfield, Ill., Charles C.
     Thomas, pp. 375-79.
59. Rege AB, Ohno Y, Barona J, Fisher JW. 1978, abstract. 8th
     Ann Clin Dial Transpl Forum, pp. 34.
60. Elves MW, Israels MCG, Collinge M. 1966. Lancet i:682-85.
61. Harris R. 1972. J Urol 108:312-13.
62. Selroos D, Pasternack A, Virolainen M. 1973. Clin Exp
     Immunol 14:365-70.

63. Gaugas JM. 1980. In: Polyamines in Biomedical Research, Eds. J.M. Gaugas. New York, John Wiley & Sons, pp. 343-62.
64. Byrd WJ, Jacobs D, Amoss MS. 1978. In: Advances in Polyamine Research, Vol. 2, Eds., R.A. Campbell et al. New York, Raven Press, pp. 71-83.
65. Allen JC, Smith CJ, Curry MC, Gaugas JM. 1977. Nature 267(5612):623-25.
66. Gahl WA, Changus JE, Pitot HC. 1976. Ped Res 10:531-35.
67. Muck BR, Trotnow S, Hommel G. 1975. Arch Gynaekol 220(1): 73-81.
68. Holroyde CP, Gabuzda TG, Putnam RC, Paul P, Reichhard GA. 1975. Cancer Res 35:3710-14.
69. Campbell N, Pyke DA, Taylor KW. 1971. J Ob Gyn Brit Commonwealth 78:498-504.
70. Carrington ER, McWilliams NB. 1966. Am J Ob Gyn 96:922-27.
71. Lutz W. 1981, in press. Physiol Chem Physics.
72. Bergstrom J, Furst P, Zimmerman L. 1979. Clin. Nephrol. 11(5):229-38.
73. Campbell RA, Grettie DP, Bartos F, Bartos D, Marton LJ. 1979. Proc 8th Ann Clin Dial Transpl Forum, pp. 194-98.
74. Lutz W. 1976. Acta Med Pol 17:2.
75. Seale TW, Chan WY, Shukla JB, Rennert O. 1979. Clin Chim Acta 95:461-72.
76. Lutz W. 1976. Acta Med Pol 1:1.
77. Bagdade JD, Campbell RA, Grettie DP, Bartos D, Bartos F. 1978. In: Advances in Polyamine Research, Vol. 2, Eds., R.A. Campbell et al. New York, Raven Press, pp. 345-59.
78. Campbell RA, LaBerge T, Brooks RE, Campbell-Boswell MC, Talwalkar YB. 1976. Clin Res 24(2):199A.
79. Radtke HW, Rege AB, LaMarche MB, Bartos D, Bartos F, Campbell RA, Fisher JW. 1980, abstract. 18th Congress ISH and 16th Congress ISBT, Montreal, Canada.
80. Radtke HW, Rege AB, LaMarche MB, Bartos D, Bartos F, Campbell RA, Fisher JW. 1980, submitted for publication. J Clin Invest.
81. Ross R, Glomset JA. 1976. Eng J Med 295:369-77.
82. Ross R, Glomset JA. 1976. Eng J Med 295:420-32.
83. Eschbach TW, Jr., Funk D, Adamson J, Kulm I, Schribner BH, Finch CA. 1967. N Eng J Med 276(12):653-58.
84. Wallner SF, Ward HP, Vantim R, Alfrey AC, Mishall J. 1975. Proc Soc Exp Biol Med 149:939-44.
85. Gral T, Schroth P, Maxwell MH. 1972. Trans Am Soc Artif Intern Organs 18:291-94.
86. Swendseid ME, Panaqua M, Kopple JD. 1980. Life Sci 26(7):533-3
87. Wang M, Kopple JD, Swendseid ME. 1980. Metabolism 29(8):733.
88. Shibata S, Auvenshine P. Kopple JD, Swendseid ME. 1980, abstract. Fed Proc, Vol. 39, pp. 728.
89. Atkins JF, Lewis JB, Anderson CW, Gesteland RF. 1975. J Biol Chem 250(4):5688-95.
90. Jelenc P. 1979, personal communication. University of Uppsala.
91. Wassner SJ, Li JB, Schlitzer J. 1980. Ped Res 14(8):1004, and personal communication.

92. Canellakis ES, Heller JS, Kyriakidis D, Chen KY. In:
     Advances in Polyamine Research, Vol. 1, Eds. R.A. Campbell
     et al. New York, Raven Press, pp. 17-30.
93. Kano K, Oka T. 1976. J Biol Chem 251(9):2795-2800.
94. Bergstrom J. 1978. In: Replacement of Renal Function by
     Dialysis, Eds. Drukker et al, Martinus Nijhoff.
95. Janne J. 1978. Biochim et Biophys Acta 473:241-93.
96. Funck-Brentano JL, Cueille GF, Nam NK. 1978. Kid Int, Vol.
     13 (S8) 531.
97. Babb AL, Popovich RP, Christopher TG, Scribner BH. 1971.
     Trans Am Soc Artif Int Organs 17:81-89.
98. Dzurik R, Bozek P, Reznicek J, Obornikova A. 1973. Proc
     Eur Dial Transpl Assoc 10:263-70.
99. Bozek P, Erben J, Zahradnik J, Dzurik R. 1979. Int Urol
     Nephrol 11(3):223-28.
100. Ravid M, Lang R, Robson M. 1980. Dial Transpl 9(8):763-65.
101. Jorstad S, Smeby LC, Wideroe TE, Berg KJ. 1980. Clin
     Nephrol 13(2):85-92.
102. Jorstad S, Smeby LC, Wideroe TE, Berg KJ. 1979. Clin
     Nephrol 12(4):168-73.
103. Rennert OM, Chan WY, Griesmann G. 1981, in press. Physiol
     Chem Physics.

ON GOING PROTOCOLS IN END STAGE RENAL DISEASE - 1. HEIGHT GROWTH
FOLLOWING RENAL TRANSPLANTATION. 2. ZINC SUPPLEMENTATION IN PREDIALYSIS
PATIENTS. 3. RENAL TRANSPLANTS IN CHILDREN <6 YEARS OF AGE.

G.S. ARBUS, E. WOLFFE, V. WILLIAMS, C.C. McCUAIG, T. KRAMREITHER,
S. SOLDIN, H. HUROWITZ, F.J. HOLLAND, I.C. RADDE, D. HILL, B.E. HARDY,
J.W. BALFE, B.M. CHURCHILL, B.T. STEELE, C.P. RANCE. HOSPITAL FOR SICK
CHILDREN, TORONTO, ONTARIO, CANADA.

1. HEIGHT GROWTH FOLLOWING RENAL TRANSPLANTATION

Over 70% of growing children in our program were at or below the third
percentile for height at the time of renal transplantation. More than 8
years ago we initiated a program of low-dose alternate-day prednisone
therapy (Table 1), in part, to maximize growth.

Table 1. Standard Post-Transplant Therapy

Prednisone -	Week 1:	3 mg/kg body weight (b.wt.) (maximum 120 mg)
	Week 4:	40-60 mg q̄2 days
	6 months:	5-20 mg q̄2 days

Thus by 6 months post-transplant, most of our patients were on an
alternate day prednisone dosage approximately equal in number of mg to
the patient's age in years.

We studied the 51 children in our program who had long term transplants over the past 8 years and were capable of height growth from the
time of transplant. The majority (Table 2) were able to manifest some
"catch-up" growth or sustain normal growth (i.e., growth parallel to the
growth curve). Poor growth was usually seen when the patient's serum
creatinine was >2 mg/dl or when the patient was over 11 years old at the
time of transplant.

Table 2. Height Growth Post-Transplantation in Children

	No	%
Catch-up growth	27	53
Parallel to growth curve	7	14
Poor growth: serum creatinine >2 mg/dl	5	10
: >11 years old	8	15
: unexplained	4	8
	51	100

Despite these apparently encouraging results, 60% of our patients were still below the third percentile for height at the time of study. Thus it appears that the best means of preventing growth retardation in end stage renal disease is to maintain a normal growth pattern in the predialysis and dialysis periods.

2. ZINC SUPPLEMENTATION IN PREDIALYSIS CHILDREN

Zinc deficiencies are known to cause anorexia secondary to hypogeusia and hyposmia. Consequently, we gave zinc supplements to determine whether they would increase appetite, thereby raising caloric intake and promoting growth.

Ten children with renal disease who were less than the 10th percentile for height and were not growing were given daily supplements of 1-4 mg Zn^{++}/kg body weight. Five received supplements for 12 months and 5 for 6 months. Patients were assessed before beginning zinc, 6 months after starting zinc and again at the end of one year.

Patients on zinc tended to have increased plasma and red cell zinc but no consistent change was noted in hair zinc (Table 3). Red cell zinc levels returned to normal when the zinc supplement was discontinued after 6 months.

Table 3. Zinc Status (Mean Values)

Time of starting Zn/ time on Zn	Plasma Zn mg/dl		RBC Zn µg/dl		Hair Zn ppm	
	12 mos	6 mos	12 mos	6 mos	12 mos	6 mos
Control	113	99	891	1043	144	171
6 months	140	96	1646	1700	107	152
12 months	180	144	1663	1217	155	172

Alkaline phosphatase levels increased in both groups over the 12 month period, apparently in response to ongoing deterioration of renal function (Table 4). Radiographs showed similar or increased renal osteodystrophy in all 10 patients one year after they started receiving zinc supplements.

Table 4. Renal Function and Hemoglobin Levels (Mean Values)

Time of starting Zn/ time on Zn	BUN mg/dl		Creat. mg/dl		Hb gm/100 ml	
	12 mos	6 mos	12 mos	6 mos	12 mos	6 mos
Control	36	26	1.6	1.5	12.1	13.4
6 months	40	25	1.5	1.6	12.5	12.4
12 months	41	32	1.8	1.7	12.1	-

Mean caloric intake (based on intake for three days) did not show appreciable changes with zinc supplementation (Table 5).

Table 5. Mean Caloric Intake

Time of starting Zn/ time on Zn	Kcal		Kcal/kg b.wt.		Kcal/M^2	
	12 mos	6 mos	12 mos	6 mos	12 mos	6 mos
Control	1180	1348	97	84	2091	1898
6 months	1170	1411	88	99	1881	2253
12 months	1215	-	87	-	1880	-

The 3 patients in whom taste acuity could be determined showed no change with zinc supplementation.

There were no appreciable changes in height and weight growth velocities (Tables 6 & 7) during zinc supplementation.

Table 6. Height Growth Velocities (Percentiles) One Year Before and One Year After Starting Zinc Supplementation

Patient with 12 mos supplementation		Patient with 6 mos supplementation	
Prior to Zn	During Zn	Prior to Zn	During Zn
<3	50	50	50-75
50	10-25	50	50
97	3	10-25	3-10
25-50	90-97	50	25-50
97	90	50-75	90-97

Table 7. Weight Velocities (Percentiles) One Year Before and One Year After Starting Zinc Supplementation

Patient with 12 mos supplementation		Patient with 6 mos supplementation	
Prior to Zn	During Zn	Prior to Zn	During Zn
25-50	70	50-75	50-75
25	25-50	50	10
25	>97	25	3
25-50	75-90	3	50
50	50	50	50

There were no changes in somadomedins, growth hormone or insulin levels with zinc supplementation.

It is concluded that zinc supplementation does not appreciably improve growth in predialysis children who have growth retardation secondary to renal failure.

3. RENAL TRANSPLANTS IN SMALL CHILDREN

We have done 33 cadaveric renal transplants in 23 recipients <6 years of age. At present, 17 transplants are still functioning up to 6 years (mean 2.5 $\pm$ 1.97 yrs) after transplantation.

Of the 33 transplants, 16 failed for various reasons (Table 8). Of the 5 storage failures (i.e., transplanted kidneys that never functioned in cases where rejection and vascular thrombosis were eliminated as causes of the failure), 4 occurred in donor kidneys <6 months of age (8 days, 8 days, 2.5 mos, 6 mos).

Table 8. Cause of Graft Failure

No of failures	
5	Storage failure (primary nonfunction)
4	Renal artery and/or vein thrombosis
4	Recurrence of hemolytic-uremic syndrome (1 pt)
2	Recurrence of Wilm's tumor
1	Rejection
16	

Of 8 kidneys from donors over 10 years old transplanted into children <6 yrs old, 3 renal artery and/or vein thromboses occurred. The fourth episode of thrombosis in a small child occurred when a donor kidney from a 1-year-old was placed on the common iliac artery of a 2-year-old; the artery went into spasm and subsequently thrombosed. In the past 3 years, no other patient in our program has experienced a renal artery/vein thrombosis.

In the past year, 7 transplants were done in children <10 kg (all over 1 year of age) and 4 are functioning; there were 3 graft failures, 2 from vessel thrombosis and 1 from primary nonfunction.

Thus, it appears that renal transplants can be performed successfully in young children, including those <10 kg. However, donor kidneys ≤ 6 months old have a poor chance of functioning and there is a high risk of renal artery and/or vein thrombosis when a large kidney is placed in a small child, possibly as a result of poor blood perfusion.

CLINICAL DISORDERS OF CALCIUM METABOLISM IN CHRONIC RENAL FAILURE IN CHILDREN

JAMES C. M. CHAN, M.D., C.M., F.A.A.P.
Professor of Pediatrics and Director of Nephrology, Medical College of Virginia, Health Sciences Division of Virginia Commonwealth University, Richmond, Virginia, U.S.A.

1. INTRODUCTION

In 1883, Lucas (1) noted the coincidence of late-onset rickets and albuminuria, but it was Fletcher (2) who first recognized the association between chronic renal failure and the development of metabolic bone disease. In 1937, Albright (3) as well as others (4) demonstrated a connection between hyperplasia of the parathyroid gland and the development of renal rickets. Finally, in 1943, Liu and Chu (5) characterized the malabsorption of calcium and "resistance" to vitamin-D therapy in chronic renal failure and proposed the term "renal osteodystrophy" for this constellation of metabolic and clinical disorders involving the bone.

2. GROWTH FAILURE IN CHRONIC RENAL DISEASE

The etiology of growth failure in chronic renal disease involves a combination of the following factors: (1) metabolic acidosis; (2) a deficiency in calorie-protein; (3) deficient production of the renal hormone 1,25-dihydroxyvitamin-D_3 and perhaps other such metabolites; (4) azotemia; (5) hyposthenuria; (6) hormonal disorders, such as insulin and glucose malfunctions; and (7) defective metabolism of trace minerals.

McSherry et al (6), among others (7, 8), demonstrated the growth failure associated with persistent metabolic acidosis in children with renal tubular acidosis, and the reversal of growth failure when their metabolic acidosis was adequately counteracted by bicarbonate therapy. During the 1970's, Holliday and his associates (9) underscored the role of calorie-protein malnourishment in causing growth failure in chronic renal diseases. In the late 1970's, Chan et al (10) and Chesney et al (11) demonstrated that growth failure in chronic renal disease was reversed by treatment with vitamin-D metabolites.

From the Nephrology Section, Department of Pediatrics, Medical College of Virginia, Richmond, Virginia, U.S.A.

Key Words: 1,25-dihydroxyvitamin-D_3, renal function, accelerated growth, chronic renal failure.

Reprints: James C. M. Chan, M.D., MCV Station Box 498, Richmond, Virginia 23298, U.S.A.

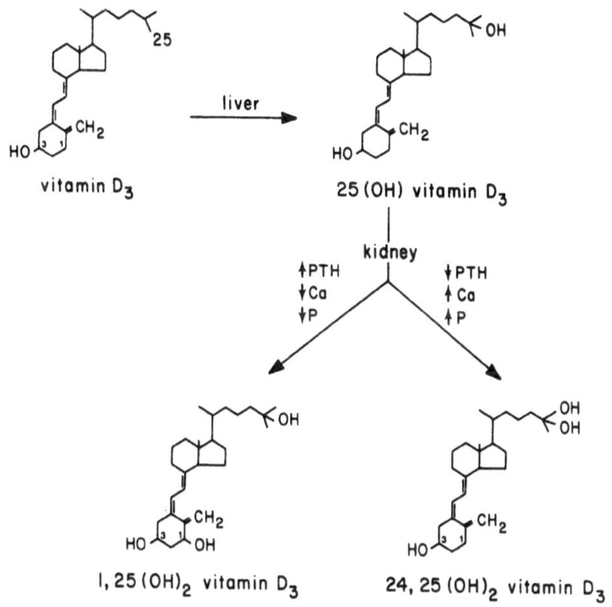

Figure 1: Metabolic Pathway of Vitamin D. Approximately 3 to 6 hours after it is ingested, vitamin-D is metabolized in the liver with the addition of a hydroxyl molecule at the carbon 25 position to form 25-hydroxyvitamin-D. In 4 to 6 more hours, the kidney activates 25-hydroxyvitamin-D to 1,25-dihydroxyvitamin-D (1,25-(OH)$_2$-D$_3$) or to 24,25-dihydroxyvitamin-D$_3$ (24,25-(OH$_2$-D$_3$), the path depending on the serum concentrations of parathyroid hormone (PTH), calcium (Ca), and phosphorus (P). From Chan, JCM and Hsu AC: Vitamin-D and Renal Diseases. Adv Pediatr 27:117, 1980. Reproduced by permission.

3. VITAMIN-D METABOLISM

To be metabolically active, vitamin-D from diet or sunlight must undergo hydroxylation first in the liver to form 25-hydroxy-vitamin-D$_3$ and then in the kidney to form either 1,25-dihydroxy-vitamin-D$_3$ or 24,25-dihydroxyvitamin-D$_3$ (Figure 1). Usually, normal serum calcium concentrations or hypercalcemia promote the formation of 24,25-dihydroxyvitamin-D$_3$, which has an additional function of inhibiting parathyroid hormone secretion (12), whereas hypocalcemia stimulates production of 1,25-dihydroxyvitamin-D$_3$ in increasing concentrations to restore normal serum calcium concentrations.

The intensity of the research leading to the discovery of 1,25-dihydroxyvitamin-D$_3$ is exemplified by the simultaneous publications in 1970 by Fraser and Kodicek (13) of Cambridge, England; DeLuca and associates (14) in Madison, Wisconsin; and Norman and associates (15) in Riverside, California. By 1972 Brickman and his co-workers (16) had developed an intravenous 1,25-dihydroxyvitamin-D$_3$ therapy for hypocalcemia in the hemodialysis patients, and two years later the first short-term report (17) of oral administration of 1,25-di-hydroxyvitamin-D$_3$ appeared. A preliminary description of the reversal of calcium malabsorption in the intestinal tract in children treated with 1-alpha-hydroxyvitamin-D was published in 1975 (18),

500

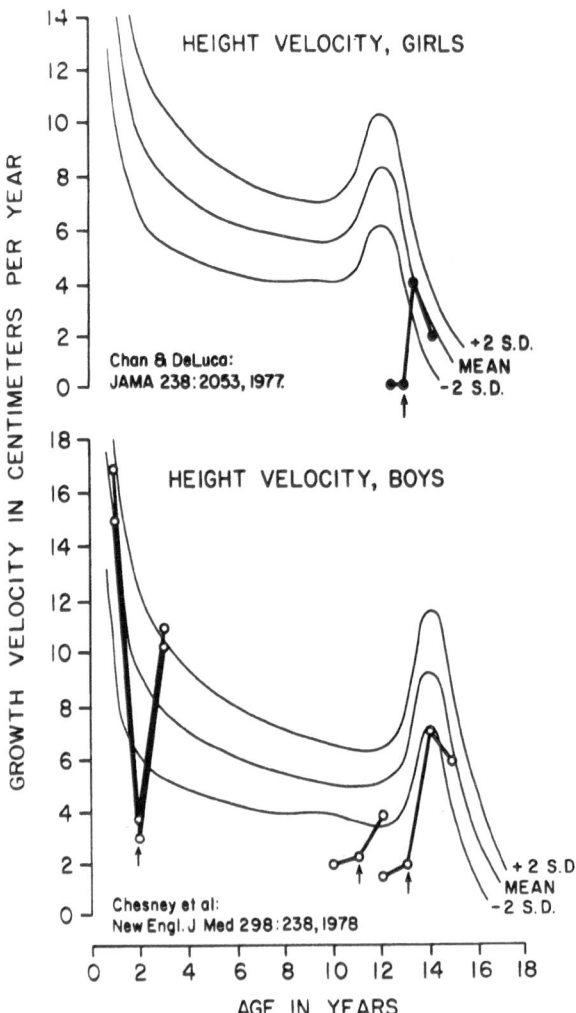

Figure 2: The reversal of growth failure in a 12-year-old girl
(upper panel) on hemodialysis for one year, whose complete growth
arrest yielded to essentially a mean height velocity after one year
of 1-alpha-hydroxyvitamin-D$_3$ therapy. Similar findings are shown
for 4 children with chronic renal insufficiency not yet requiring
hemodialysis (lower panel). Re-drawn from data of Chan and DeLuca
(10) and Chesney et al (11). Normal growth velocity curves for age
and sex are re-drawn from data of J. M. Tanner and R. H. Whitehouse
(Archive Dis Child 51:170, 1976)

succeeded by a long-term follow-up study in 1977 documenting sustained reversal of renal osteodystrophy (19). To date, 57 patients with chronic renal failure and 208 patients (20) including 28 children have been treated with 1,25-dihydroxyvitamin-D_3.

4. GROWTH FAILURE: REVERSAL WITH 1,25-DIHYDROXYVITAMIN-D_3

The first documentation that growth failure can be reversed by vitamin-D metabolite therapy for chronic renal disease was the accelerated growth after a year of complete arrest, displayed by one 12-year-old girl on hemodialysis (10) after a 12-month course of l-alpha-hydroxyvitamin-D_3 at 2 mcg/day (Figure 2, upper panel). Later, four children with chronic renal disease (11) manifested similar accelerated growth velocities after treatment with 14 ng/kg/day of 1,25-dihydroxyvitamin-D_3 (Figure 2, lower panel).

By 1980, eleven children at the Medical College of Virginia, (mean age 8 $\pm$ 5 years at first treatment with chronic renal insufficiency) with glomerular filtration rate 18% $\pm$ 13% of normal, had been treated for up to three years with 1,25-dihydroxyvitamin-D_3. (21) The height velocity of six of the eight children (75%) under 12 years of age, markedly surpassed that expected for chronologic and bone ages after one year of treatment with orally-administered 1,25-dihydroxyvitamin-D_3 at 15-35 ng/kg/day. Growth velocity was unimproved in two of the three children over 12 years of age at initiation of 1,25-dihydroxyvitamin-D_3.

The serum creatinine concentrations in four of the patients, available for retrospective and prospective analyses to 32 months of 1,25-dihydroxyvitamin-D_3 treatment, revealed that renal failure progressed at rates linearly identical to those before treatment (21), a fact indicating that the treatment did not accelerate the rate of deterioration (Figure 3). Indeed, one patient manifested a slight improvement in renal function (p<0.05).

Mineral balance data on these treated patients (21) showed significant mean retention of calcium, phosphorus, magnesium and zinc (357, 250 and 23 mg/m^2/day and 1157 mcg/m^2/day, respectively) after treatment with 1,25-dihydroxyvitamin-D_3 at 15-35 ng/kg/day. In addition, serum calcium, alkaline phosphatase and parathyroid hormone concentrations returned to normal. Healing of renal osteodystrophy (21) was radiologically evident after therapy (Figure 4).

5. RENAL FUNCTION STUDIES

In 1976, Tougaard et al (22) and later Christiansen et al (23) disclosed a possible deterioration of renal function with 1,25-dihydroxyvitamin-D_3 therapy. However, their conclusions were challenged because the reliability of single determinations of creatinine clearances performed only before and after initiation of 1,25-dihydroxyvitamin-D_3 therapy was questioned (24). Moreover, Massry et al (24) in an editorial commentary observed that deterioration of renal function had actually been observed only when the patients had been allowed to become hypercalcemic. In 1976, Mitch et al (25) and later Rutherford et al (26) demonstrated that a mathematical and linear correlation of the reciprocals of serial serum creatinine concentrations across time permits estimation of the progression of renal failure as the slope of the plot of these two variables. Thus, when reciprocal serum creatinine concentrations (dl/mg) before initiation of 1,25-dihydroxyvitamin-D_3 (vide supra)

502

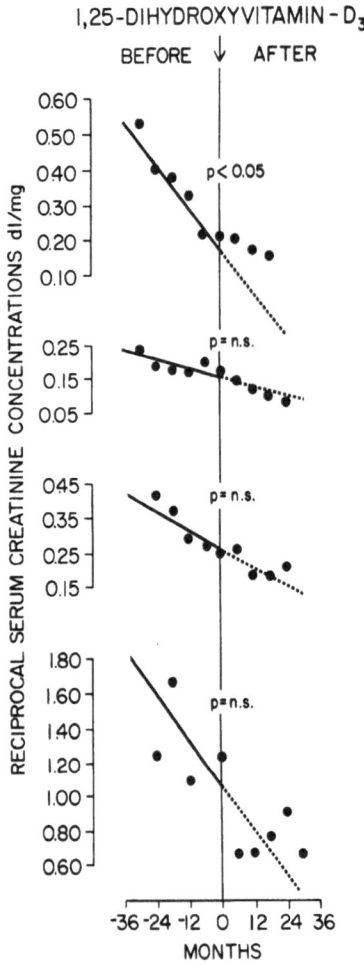

Figure 3: The progression of renal failure in 4 children, represented for each by a plot of reciprocal serum-creatinine concentrations (in dl/mg) versus months of observation before and after initiation of 1,25-dihydroxyvitamin-D$_3$ (arrow). Renal functions were declining at constant rates before therapy (solid linear regression line). When those rates were extrapolated to the post-treatment plot (interrupted linear regression line) it became evident that in those patients 1,25-dihydroxyvitamin-D$_3$ effected no change in the rate of renal failure progression whereas in one patient the rate of deterioration was actually reversed (p<0.05).

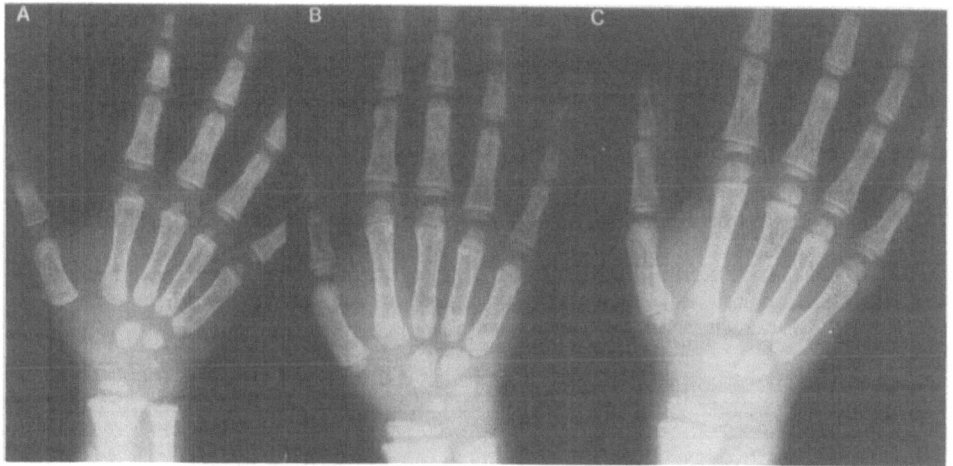

Figure 4: A, radiographic examination of the hand in a patient
with chronic renal insufficiency (creatinine clearance 50 ± 14 ml/min
per 1.73m²)at 3 years of age demonstrated very minimal irregularity
of the provisory zone of calcification of the distal ulna and slight
coarsening of the trabecular pattern. These findings represented
very early changes of rickets and hyperparathyroidism, respectively.

B, at age 5 years and 5 months there was marked subperiosteal bone
resorption particularly along the proximal and middle phalanges
and a very coarse trabecular pattern typical for hyperparathyroidism. In addition, there had been progression of the rickets involving both the distal radius and distal ulna. Shortly after this
radiograph was taken, therapy with 1,25-dihydroxyvitamin-D$_3$ was initiated.

C, at 8 years of age, there had been healing of rickets and reversal
of hyperparathyroidism.

It is important to note that the bone age progressed only a year
and a half between the examinations in A and B which span a three-
year interval, whereas the bone age increased three and one-half
years between the radiographs in B and C, a period which spans
two years.

therapy are plotted over time, the progression of the patient's renal failure can be established (Figure 3). A similar plot after initiation of 1,25-dihydroxyvitamin-D_3 therapy, compared to the extrapolation of the pre-therapy data will determine whether the rate of deterioration has changed and, if so, in which direction. These data indicate that no compromise of renal function (21) is occasioned by the vitamin-D therapy.

6. SUMMARY

Growth potentials of children with chronic renal failure appear to be significantly enhanced by 1,25-dihydroxyvitamin-D_3 therapy, especially when it is initiated early. Accelerated deterioration of renal function, once proposed as a hazard, is not a risk, as long as hypercalcemia is avoided.

Compared with the meager partial reversal of renal osteodystrophy by conventional treatment with vitamin-D_2, phosphate-binders and calcium supplementation, the often dramatic and sustained response to 1,25-dihydroxyvitamin-D_3 therapy, as documented by mineral balances and radiography, implies that true control and possibly even prevention of the dystrophic process may now be at hand.

REFERENCES

1. Lucas RC. 1883. Form of late rickets associated with albuminuria, rickets of adolescents. Lancet 1:993.
2. Fletcher HM. 1911. Case of infantilism with polyuria and chronic renal disease. Proc Royal Soc Med 4:95.
3. Albright F, Drake TG, Sulkowitch HW. 1937. Renal osteitis fibrosa cystica: Report of a case with discussion of metabolic aspects. Bull. Johns Hopkins Hosp 60:377.
4. Barber H. 1920-21. Renal dwarfism. Quart J Med 14:205.
5. Liu SH, Chu HI. 1943. Studies of calcium and phosphorus metabolism with special reference to pathogenesis and effects of dihydrotachysterol (A.T. 10) and iron. Medicine 22:103.
6. McSherry E, Morris RC, Jr. 1978. Attainment and maintenance of normal stature with alkali therapy in infants and children with classic renal tubular acidosis. J Clin Invest 61:509.
7. Chan JCM. 1979. Acid-base, calcium, potassium and aldosterone metabolism in renal tubular acidosis. Nephron 23:153-159.
8. Chan JCM. 1980. Renal acidosis. Chapter 12 in Laboratory Diagnostic Procedures for Renal Function. Edited by C. G. Duarte, Little Brown and Co. Publ. Boston. p. 239-268
9. Simmons JM, Wilson CJ, Potter DE et al: 1971. Relation of calorie deficiency to growth failure in children on hemodialysis and the growth response to calorie supplementation. N Eng J Med 285:653.
10. Chan JCM, DeLuca HF. 1977. Growth velocity in a child on prolonged hemodialysis: Beneficial effect of 1-α-hydroxyvitamin-D_3. J Am Med Assoc 238:2053.
11. Chesney RW, Moorthy AV, Eisman JA, et al. 1978. Increased growth after long-term oral 1-α-25-vitamin-D in childhood renal osteodystrophy. N Eng J Med 298, 238.

12. Canterbury JM, Lerman S, Claflin AJ, et al. 1978. Inhibition of parathyroid hormone secretion by 25-hydroxycholecalciferol and 24,25-dihydroxycholecalciferol in the dog. J Clin Invest 61:1375.

13. Fraser DR, Kodicek E. 1970. Unique biosynthesis by kidney of a biologically active vitamin-D metabolite. Nature (Lond)288:764.

14. DeLuca HF. 1979. Vitamin D: metabolism and function. Monographs on endocrinology, vol 13. Edited by F. Gross, et al. Springer-Verlag, NY.

15. Coburn JW, Brickman AS, Sherrard DJ, et al. 1977. Clinical efficiency of 1,25-dihydroxyvitamin-D3 in renal osteodystrophy; in Norman, Schaefer, Coburn, Grigoleit and V. Herrath, vitamin-D, biochemical, chemical and clinical aspects related to calcium metabolism, p. 657-666 (DeGruyter, Berlin).

16. Brickman AS, Coburn JW, Norman AW. 1972. Action of 1,25-dihydroxycholecalciferol, a potent, kidney-produced metabolite of vitamin-D, in uremic man. N Eng J Med 287:891.

17. Brickman AS, Coburn JW, Massry SG. 1974. 1,25-dihydroxyvitamin-D_3 in normal man and patients with renal failure. Ann Intern Med 80:161.

18. Chan JCM, Oldham SB, Holick MF, et al. 1975. 1-α-hydroxyvitamin-D3 in chronic renal failure. A potent analog of the kidney hormone, 1,25-dihydroxycholecalciferol. JAMA 234:47.

19. Chan JCM, Oldham SB, DeLuca, HF. 1977. Effectiveness of 1-α-hydroxyvitamin-D_3 in children with renal osteodystrophy associated with hemodialysis. J Pediatr 90:820.

20. Massry SG, Goldstein DA, Malluche HH. 1980. Current status of the use of 1,25-dihydroxyvitamin-D_3 in the management of renal osteodystrophy. Kidney Int 18:409.

21. Chan JCM, Kodroff MB and Landwehr DM. 1980. Effect of 1,25-dihydroxyvitamin-D_3 on renal function, mineral nutrition and growth in children with severe chronic renal failure. Proceedings Am Soc Neph 13:15A.

22. Tougaard LE, Sorensen E, Brochner-Mortensen J, et al. 1976. Controlled trial of 1-α-hydroxycholecalciferol in chronic renal failure. Lancet 1:1044.

23. Christiansen C, Rodbro P, Christensen MS, et al. 1978. Deterioration of renal function during treatment of chronic renal failure with 1,25-dihydroxycholecalciferol. Lancet 2:700.

24. Massry SG, Goldstein DA. 1979. Is calcitriol (1,25-dihydroxyvitamin-D_3) harmful to renal function? JAMA 242:1875.

25. Mitch WE, Walser M, Buffington GA, et al. 1976. A simple method of estimating progression of chronic renal failure. Lancet 2:1326.

26. Rutherford WE, Blondin J, Miller JP, et al. 1977. Chronic progressive renal disease: Rate of change of serum creatinine concentration. Kidney Int 11:62.

ACKNOWLEDGEMENTS. The author would like to thank Mrs. Martha Wellons and Mrs. Marilyn Reilly for their expert research and secretarial assistance.

THE NEONATAL STRESSED KIDNEY

J.-P. Guignard

Department of Pediatrics
Centre Hospitalier Universitaire Vaudois
Lausanne, Switzerland

A. PHYSIOLOGY OF THE DEVELOPING KIDNEY

1. Fetal maturation

The human kidney develops through three sequential embryo-logic stages: the pronephros, the mesonephros and the meta-nephros. The latter appears at the fifth week of gestation and forms the definitive kidney. Nephrogenesis proceeds in a centri-fugal pattern, achieving the full complement of 1.2 million nephrons per kidney by the 35th week of gestation. During the last 20 weeks of gestation, there is a linear increase in renal mass, kidney weight bearing a linear relationship to gestational age, body weight and the body surface area (1). The fetal kidney does not carry any homeostatic responsibility, and fetal growth consequently does not relate to functional requirements. Urine formation already starts around the 9-12th week of gestation. By the 32nd week, fetal urine production rate approaches 12 ml/h. It reaches 28 ml/h shortly before birth (2).

Maturation of glomerular filtration rate (GFR) and effective renal plasma flow (ERPF) have been assessed in premature and term neonates during the last 12 weeks of gestation. GFR in-creases rapidly from the 28th to the 35th week of gestation (Fig. 1). This probably reflects functional changes in existing nephrons as well as the appearance of new nephrons. From the 35th week of gestation, the increase in GFR reaches a plateau up to the time of birth, reflecting a parallel increase in kidney size and renal function (3). The development of renal blood flow appears to follow the same pattern (4).

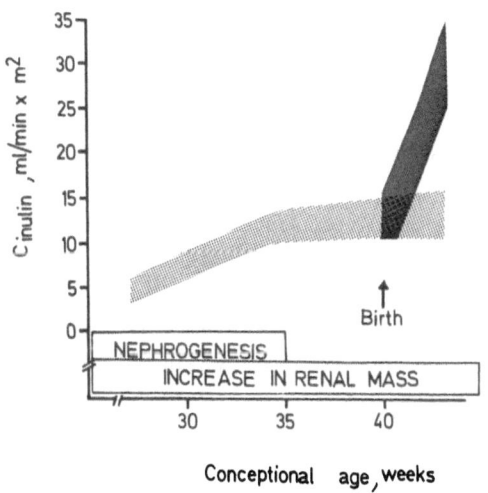

FIGURE 1. Maturation of GFR in relation to conceptional age.

The progressive increase in systemic blood pressure observed in the last 3 months of gestation (3), as well as the striking decrease in renal vascular resistance occurring during this period, are probably responsible for the development of renal blood flow and glomerular filtration.

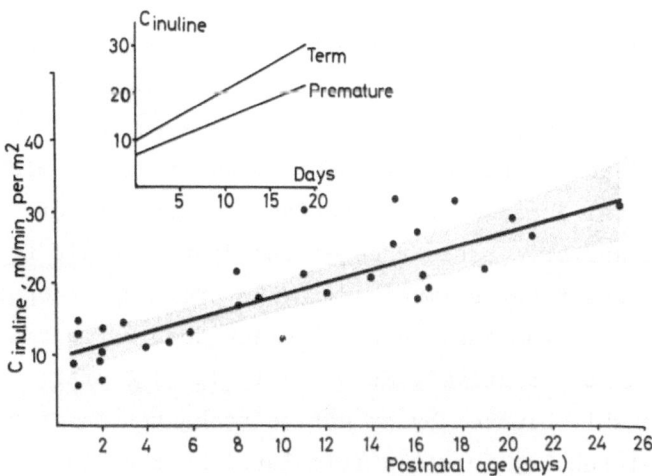

FIGURE 2. Postnatal maturation of GFR in term and preterm neonates.

2. Postnatal maturation

During gestation the placenta acts as hemodialyser perfectly adapted to the fetal needs. At birth removal of the placenta is the signal for a striking increase in renal function (Fig. 2). From a low value of 10 ml/min per m^2 at term, GFR increases to 20 ml/min per m^2 during the second week of life (4). The postnatal increase in GFR is similar in both preterm and term neonates, the former starting at lower values. Development of renal blood flow follows the same pattern, its values doubling during the first two weeks of life. The striking postnatal increase in GFR and renal blood flow has been explained by an increase in effective filtration pressure (5), an increase in the glomerular filtering area, an increase in basement membrane permeability and a decrease in intrarenal vascular resistance (6).

Tubular functions are either fully effective at birth or rapidly mature after birth. The neonatal kidney is able to dilute the urine maximally, reaching urinary osmolalities as low as 50 mosm/kg H_2O, and to regulate the acid-base balance (7). Concentrating ability is slightly impaired, the defect being explained a) by the lack of availability of osmotically active solutes, mainly urea, to deposit in the renal medulla (8), b) by the immaturity of the ADH-adenylate cyclase-cyclic AMP system. The regulation of Na balance is also somewhat vulnerable in newborn infants. Because of a functional immaturity of the proximal tubule and/or a resistance of the distal tubule to aldosterone, Na retention is impaired in the premature neonate (9). On the other hand the term newborn infant does not eliminate a sodium load as effectively as an adult (10). Overall natriuresis is probably blunted by an active reabsorption of sodium in the distal tubule, possibly stimulated by the high serum aldosterone levels present at this age.

The neonatal kidney is well adapted to the current needs of a normal infant. It has however a limited capacity to maintain homeostasis under pathological conditions, and is more vulnerable to abnormal stresses. Some of these stresses are endogenous, others are iatrogenic.

B. THE STRESSED KIDNEY

1. Perinatal asphyxia and hypoxemia

Perinatal anoxia, or post-natal hypoxemia, as seen during severe respiratory distress syndrome, profoundly affects renal function (11, 12). These two conditions are often associated with hypotension, hypovolemia, metabolic and respiratory acidosis. Hypoxemic neonates present with decreased water excretion, and a correlation has been observed between decreased urine output, expressed in percent of fluid intake and the lowest plasma oxygen tension recorded during the urine collection period. Urine dilution is impaired as is urine acidification (Figs 3, 4, 5). Glomerular filtration rate and effective renal plasma flow are

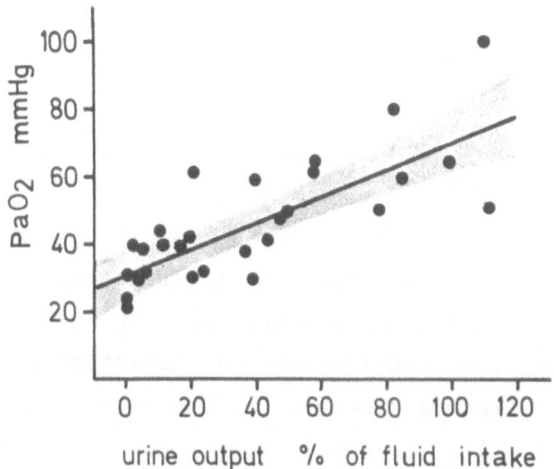

FIGURE 3. Urine output in relation to the plasma oxygen tension.

510

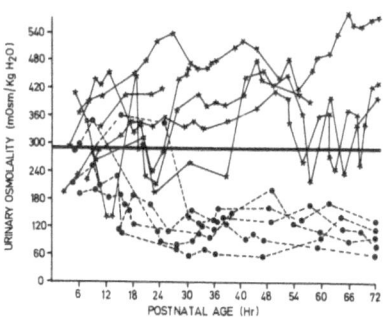

FIGURE 4. Urine osmolality during the first 72 hours of life in control (•) and hypoxemic (⁕) newborn infants presenting with respiratory distress syndrome.

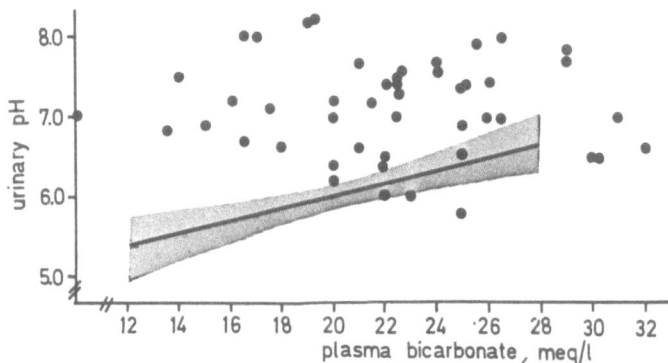

FIGURE 5. Urine pH in relation to plasma bicarbonate during the first 72 hours of life of control (regression line) and hypoxemic (•) newborn infants presenting with respiratory distress syndrome.

significantly depressed (11). The low glomerular filtration rate in severely hypoxemic neonates probably explains the impairment in free-water excretion. Intravenous administration of hypertonic mannitol can improve diuresis, and raise GFR and ERPF toward normal levels (11). The renal defects are reversible upon restoring normoxemia, extracellular fluid volume and cardiac output.

Pathogenesis:

The pathogenesis of the hypoxemia/asphyxia-induced renal failure
is not yet clear. Prerenal factors are probably involved (11);
a stimulation of the renin-angiotensin system has been demonstrated in human neonates with respiratory distress syndrome (13).
The role of the renin-angiotensin system has been studied in an
experimental model. Acute experiments in the anesthetized rabbit show that moderate hypoxemia (PaO_2 = 45 mmHg) induces a
state of renal hypoperfusion secondary to increased renal
vascular resistance, with consequent oliguria, decreased GFR and
decreased solute excretion.

Table 1. Renal changes during acute hypoxemia.

	CONTROL	30'	60'
BP, mmHg	94,3 ± 4,2	88,0 ± 5,0	83,4 ± 3,7
PO2, mmHg	70,5 ± 2,0	43,9 ± 1,6	42,0 ± 1,7
V̇, ml/kg·min	0,91 ± 0,11	0,33 ± 0,03	0,37 ± 0,04
GFR, ml/kg·min	3,90 ± 0,46	1,66 ± 0,23	1,74 ± 0,20
ERPF, ml/kg·min	23,2 ± 2,7	9,3 ± 1,2	10,7 ± 1,4
Resistance	4,8 ± 0,5	11,8 ± 1,8	12,0 ± 2,2

Intrarenal distribution of blood flow is not affected (14) and
the hemodynamic disturbances are rapidly reversible upon restoring normoxemia (14). The hypoxemia-induced increase in renal
vascular resistance is associated with an elevated plasma renin
activity (Fig. 6) (15).

Administration of saralazin, a competitive inhibitor of
angiotensin II, prior to inducing hypoxemia, prevents the renal
effects of moderate hypoxemia. In this condition no changes in

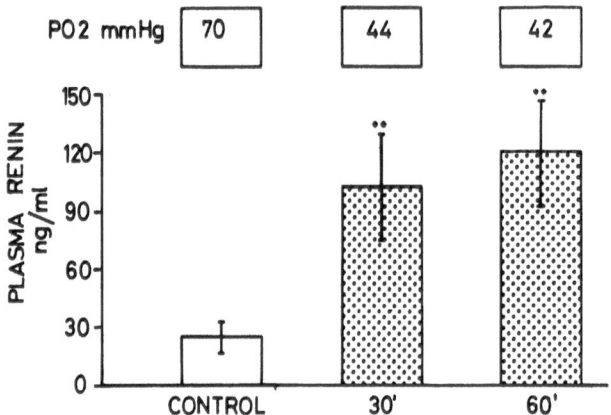

FIGURE 6. Changes in plasma renin activity induced by acute hypoxemia.

urine flow, solute excretion, GFR and ERPF occur in response to
hypoxemia (16).

The role of the renin-angiotensin in mediating the renal
effects of hypoxemia in the anesthetized rabbit is further demonstrated by the use of verapamil (17), a potent antagonist of
transcellular calcium ion transport. Calcium ion appears to be
an important modulator for the expression of angiotensin II on
the renal cortical microcirculation. Pretreatment of rats with
verapamil indeed prevented the vasoconstrictor effect of angiotensin II on the glomerular circulation (17). Verapamil was thus
administered to anesthetized rabbits before and during hypoxemia.

Administration of verapamil (1.0 µg/kg x min) to control
animals slightly increased sodium excretion without changes in
systemic blood pressure, GFR and ERPF. Decreasing PaO₂ in vera-
pamil-infused rabbits did not produce any of the renal defects
normally associated with hypoxemia. Renal vascular resistance
remained unchanged. So did urine output, electrolyte secretion,
GFR and ERPF. This is best explained by an inhibition by verapamil of the effect of angiotensin II on the mesangial glomerular
smooth muscle (17).

2. Iatrogenic stresses

The function of the neonatal kidney can be affected by iatrogenic manipulations, in addition to the endogenous stress:

a) Artificial ventilation: In infant primates, intermittent positive pressure ventilation decreases cardiac output and renal blood flow, and increases renal vascular resistance (18). It also induces a redistribution of intrarenal blood flow. Whether this effect applies to the human newborn is unknown.

b) Diazepam: Intravenous diazepam, frequently used to control out of phase respiration by the infant on the ventilator, can depress both glomerular filtration and effective renal plasma flow (19).

c) Indomethacin: This inhibitor of prostaglandin synthesis is sometimes used to achieve pharmacological closure of the patent ductus arteriosus in premature infants. It can induce a transient, but significant decrease in glomerular filtration rate and free-water excretion. Its long-term effects are not known (20).

d) Tolazoline: Persistent pulmonary hypertension of the newborn causes right-to-left blood shunting through the foramen ovale and ductus arteriosus. This leads to severe hypoxemia. Tolazoline, an α-adrenergic blocking agent has been used as a pulmonary vasodilator. Side effects such as oliguria and transient renal failure have been described in infants receiving this drug (21). Experiments in the pentobarbitone-anesthetized rabbit demonstrate that tolazoline, 1.0 mg/kg followed by 1.0 mg/kg per hour, increased systemic blood pressure, and decreased urine flow, sodium excretion, GFR and ERPF (Fig. 7). The depression of ERPF was accompanied by a redistribution of blood flow to the inner cortex (22). The increase in renal vascular resistance induced by tolazoline seems to represent a partial α-agonist action of tolazoline. Whether tolazoline

514

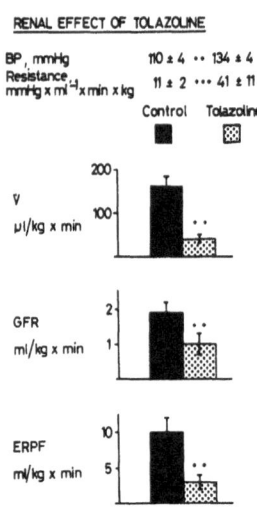

RENAL EFFECT OF TOLAZOLINE

BP, mmHg   110 ± 4 ** 134 ± 4
Resistance mmHg x ml⁻¹ x min x kg   11 ± 2 *** 41 ± 11

FIGURE 7. Changes in renal function following tolazoline administration, 1.0 mg/kg and per kg x h, to the anesthetized rabbit.

retains such an action in the hypoxemic neonate remains to be determined.

CONCLUSIONS

Because it operates close to its maximal capacity, the new-born kidney is very vulnerable to endogenous and pharmacological stresses. Hypoxemia and asphyxia represent a frequent and danger-ous stress for the neonatal kidney. Great care should conse-quently be taken to prevent and treat these conditions. And, when doing so, the physician should make sure that the drugs or the methods he is using do not add another stress to the neonatal kidney.

Acknowledgements: The author is grateful to Mrs B. Bailly and Miss C. Walliman for valuable technical assistance. This work was supported by the Swiss National Science Foundation (Grant Nos 3.361.74 and 3.917.78).

REFERENCES

1. Schulz D M, Giordano D A, Schulz D H. 1962. Weights of organs of fetuses and infants. Arch. Pathol. 74: 244-250.
2. Campbell S, Wladimiroff J W, Dewhurst C J. 1973. The antenatal measurement of fetal urine production. J. Obstet. Gynaec. Brit. Cwlth. 80: 680-686.
3. Fawer C L, Torrado A, Guignard J-P. 1979. Maturation of renal function in full-term and premature neonates. Helv. Paediat. Acta 34: 11-21.
4. Guignard J-P, Torrado A, Da Cunha O, Gautier E. 1975. Glomerular filtration rate in the first three weeks of life. J. Pediat. 87: 268-272.
5. Spitzer A, Edelmann C M. 1975. Maturational changes in pressure gradients for glomerular filtration. Amer. J. Physiol. 221: 1431-1435.
6. Gruskin A B, Edelmann C M, Tuan S. 1970. Maturational changes in renal blood flow in piglets. Pediat. Res. 4: 7-13.
7. Torrado A, Guignard J-P, Prod'hom L S, Gautier E. 1974. Hypoxemia and renal function in newborns with respiratory distress syndrome (RDS). Helv. Paediat. Acta 29: 399-405.
8. Edelmann C M, Barnett H L. 1960. Role of the kidney in water metabolism in young infants: physiologic and clinical considerations. J. Pediat. 56: 154-179.
9. Sulyok E, Varga F, Györy E, Jobst K, Csaba I F. 1979. Postnatal development of renal sodium handling in premature infants. J. Pediat. 95: 787-792.
10. Aperia A, Broberger O, Thodenius K, Zetterström R. 1972. Renal response to an oral sodium load in newborn full term infants. Acta Paediat. Scand. 61: 670-676.
11. Guignard J-P, Torrado A, Mazouni M, Gautier E. 1976. Renal function in respiratory distress syndrome. J. Pediat. 88: 845-850.
12. Dauber I M, Krauss A N, Symchych P S, Auld P A M. 1976. Renal failure following perinatal anoxia. J. Pediat. 88: 851-855.
13. Broughton-Pipkin F, Smales O R C. 1977. A study of factors affecting blood pressure and angiotensin II in newborn infants. J. Pediat. 91: 113-119.
14. Guignard J-P, Filloux B. 1979. Pathophysiologic renal changes during hypoxemia in the rabbit. Kidney Int. 15: 585.
15. Guignard J-P, Wallimann C, Gautier E. 1981. Prevention by verapamil of the hypoxemia-induced renal vasoconstriction. Kidney Int., in press.
16. Guignard J-P, Filloux B. 1978. Renal effect of hypoxemia during angiotensin II inhibition. Kidney Int. 13: 537-538.
17. Ischikawa I, Miele J F, Brenner B M. 1979. Reversal of renal cortical actions of angiotensin II by verapamil and manganese. Kidney Int. 16: 137-147.
18. Moore E S, Galvez M B, Paton J B, Fisher D E, Behrmann R E. 1974. Effect of positive pressure ventilation on intrarenal blood flow in infant primates. Pediat. Res. 8: 792-796.

19. Guignard J-P, Filloux B, Lavoie J, Pelet J, Torrado A. 1975. Effect of intravenous diazepam on renal function. Clin. Pharmacol. Ther. 18: 401-404.
20. Catterton Z, Sellers B, Gray B. 1980. Inulin clearance in the premature infant receiving indomethacin. J. Pediat. 96: 737-739.
21. Goetzman B W, Sunshine P, Johnson J D, Wennberg R P, Hackel A, Merten D F, Bartoletti A L, Silvermann N H. 1976. Neonatal hypoxia and pulmonary vasospasm: response to tolazoline. J. Pediat. 89: 617-621.
22. Naujoks S, Guignard J-P. 1979. Renal effects of tolazoline in rabbits. Lancet ii: 1075-1076.

RESTING SUPINE AND SEATED BLOOD PRESSURE INTERRELATIONS IN ADOLESCENCE*

S.H. KATZ, B. ZEMEL, M.L. HEDIGER, J.I. SCHALL, J.R. COLEMAN JR., E.J. BOWERS, L. VALLEROY, W.F. BARKER, P.B. EVELETH, A.B. GRUSKIN, J. PREBIS, J.S. PARKS. KROGMAN GROWTH CENTER UNIVERSITY OF PENNSYLVANIA AND CHILDREN'S HOSPITAL OF PHILADELPHIA, PHILADELPHIA, PA. 19104

Over the last decade there has been increasing interest in the measurement of blood pressure during childhood and adolescence. Generally, a number of investigators have hypothesized that elevated blood pressure during childhood and adolescence may be predictive of elevated blood pressure and/or hypertension in adulthood. This hypothesis is supported by the evidence that elevated blood pressure in early adulthood tends to track or positively correlate over time with elevated and hypertensive blood pressures in older adults.(10)

Although there are virtually no longitudinal data linking childhood blood pressures with those of adults, it is likely that some significant relationship exists. Therefore there has been considerable interest in establishing norms for childhood and adolescence so that effective preventive and interoceptive techniques can be instituted before any significant end organ damage can occur as a result of significantly elevated blood pressure. However, before such standards can be effectively used to assess risk for the later development of hypertension, a number of questions need resolution. Among the most important of these problems is the postural position to be used in establishing blood pressure norms. A variety of reports on postural hypotension and hypertension indicate that significant changes in blood pressure occur from the supine to the upright postural positions.(5,6,9,13) Currently, the standards developed by the Task Force on Blood Pressure Control in Children are for the casual seated postural position (2). Also recent reports by our group (8) and Voors et al (15) indicate that resting seated blood pressures are less variable and more reproducible over short periods of time than supine pressures.

However the differences in an individual's supine and seated blood

*Supported by NIH HLBI Grant no. 19869.

pressure measures may provide important insights into their cardiovascular status. This is because, like standing blood pressures and/or upright passive tilting, the gravitational effects of upright sitting produce a significant pooling of blood below the level of the heart and therefore produce an orthostatic stress which should be measureable. Moreover the differences between supine and seated blood pressure may vary according to the ability of the cardiovascular system to respond normally to this change. Thus assessing blood pressure in the two most common postural positions for its measurement may yield important information on the regulation and control of resting blood pressure that neither measure if taken alone might provide.

In order to investigate the significance of these differences in standard postural position, we measured resting seated and supine blood pressures as a part of the Philadelphia Blood Pressure Project (PBPP). Specifically, this paper presents our first report of results on blood pressure responses to postural change using the data from a three—year mixed longitudinal study of blood presure variation in over 600 black adolescents aged 12-17 who are members of the Philadelphia population of the National Collaborative Perinatal Project (NCPP).

METHODS

The population of adolescents assessed for this study consisted of a representative sample from the population of children originally enrolled in the Philadelphia branch of the NCPP. The NCPP was a comprehensive, longitudinal study of pregnancy and neurological disorders of childhood, which was begun in 1959 by the National Institute of Neurological and Communicative Disorders and Stroke. The Philadelphia CPP, between 1959 and the end of 1965, registered nearly 10,000 women into the study. The courses of the women's pregnancies were followed carefully, and medical, neurological, and psychological data were collected on their children through age seven. Overall, the Philadelphia CPP population was 87% black, 10% white, and 3% Puerto Rican. The Philadelphia CPP families were of relatively low socioeconomic status. Although, in general, the blacks were slightly above and the whites were slightly below their respective national averages. Additional information on the Philadelphia CPP and NCPP populations can be found in Niswander and Gordon (11).

The PBPP was initiated in 1976 and was designed initially to be a three year follow-up study of the Philadelphia CPP population as they reached adolescence. The primary sample reported in this paper was a representative sample of over 600 black adolescents, stratified by age and sex. Age cohorts were selected to represent +/-0.5 years from the nearest whole year of age, that is, for example, chronological age 12 represents the age interval 11.5 to 12.4 years. Over 100 adolescents were enrolled from each of the five Philadelphia cohorts born and registered between 1961 and 1965, so that in the first year of this study the adolescent were 11 to 15 years of age and by its conclusion they were 13 to 17 years of age.

Blood pressure and pulse rates (30 second radial arterial pulses) were assessed after at least 10 minutes of rest in the supine postion and then again in the seated position after at least 5 minutes of rest. In order to determine the reliability of these blood pressure measurements, we conducted a number of studies of intra and inter observer error using a mercury gravity sphygmomanometer and a series of cuffs calibrated for variation in adolescent arm circumference. Correlation coefficients for the serial intra-observer readings were over 0.90 for systolic blood predsure and over 0.80 for diastolic phase IV (DBP4) and phase V (DBP5) blood pressures indicating a high degree of reliability for these readings among observers (8,10).

Also in order to determine if the duration of resting time in either the supine or the seated position affected the blood pressure levels, one way analyses of variance were computed by age and sex for blood pressure levels versus duration of time at rest in each position. Resting time ranged from 10 to 25 minutes in the supine position and from 5 to 20 minutes in the seated position. Overall, there were no consistant statistically significant trends in the data due to the duration of resting in either the supine or seated position. Thus the data reported in this paper reflect baseline resting blood pressures and/or pulse rates in each postural position.

We have defined the response to postural change as, simply, the difference in blood pressure or pulse rate (calculated as rate/minute) that results from the change from resting supine to resting seated position. This is calculated as: seated blood pressure (or pulse) minus supine blood pressure (or pulse).

RESULTS

The pooled blood pressure means for all adolescents are presented on Table 1. These results are combined across all five age groups for both males and females. We and others have demonstrated, particularly among males, that systolic blood pressure does increase during this period. However the results for diastolic blood pressure do not show any age trends over this age range, and therefore we have pooled the data across ages for this publication. A more complete manuscript presenting all of the data by each individual age is in preparation.

Overall, for both males and females, there are small mean decreases in systolic blood pressure (SBP). In the case of diastolic pressures there were more substantial rises in mean DBP4, and even larger mean rises in DBP5 upon change from resting supine to seated posture. There is also a mean difference in the minute pulse rates taken in the supine and seated postural positions. For males in the supine position the mean and standard deviation pulse rate/minute was 68.6 +/-9.12 (n=794) and for females, 72.8+/-9.66 (n=755); and for the seated position the pulse rates/minute were 72.5+/-9.82 (n=708) and 77.1+/-9.96 (n=659) for males and females, respectively. Although there are statistically significant age trends in the data for males (16), these data were pooled here merely to show the range and variation of the data for pulse.

In order to determine the relationship of initial supine blood pressure to the subsequent change in blood pressure in the resting seated position, the individual's supine data were divided into three categories based upon percentiles calculated at each age and sex for each supine blood pressure. These percentiles groupings were selected to examine the effects of "low", "normal", and "high" supine blood pressure upon the degree of change in the seated position. The three groups represent the percentiles from 0-15% (low), 15-85% (normal), and 85-100% (high). The degree of change from supine to seated (seated minus supine) was analysed among these three groups using one-way analyses of variance (ANOVAS), and the results are presented on Table 2. Data on pulse change from supine to seated were calculated in the same manner and are presented on Table 2.

TABLE 1: BLOOD PRESSURE MEANS REPRESENTATIVE BLACK ADOLESCENTS AGES 12-17

		MALES				
		SUPINE			SEATED	
	N	MEAN	S.D.	N	MEAN	S.D.
SYSTOLIC (SBP)	798	114.2*	10.2	709	112.6*	10.0
DIASTOLIC IV (DBP4)	793	70.4	10.2	708	74.7	8.1
DIASTOLIC V (DBP5)	776	58.4	12.5	708	68.6	10.0
		FEMALES				
SYSTOLIC	750	112.0	8.7	658	109.8	8.4
DIASTOLIC IV	744	71.0	9.1	658	75.4	8.4
DIASTOLIC V	740	60.7	11.1	656	70.2	9.2

*Significant age trends were found only for SBP among males, both supine and seated. For supine SBP, there was a mean rise from 110.3+/-10.2 mmHg at age 12 to 119.3+/-10.5 at age 17. Likewise, for seated blood pressure, mean SBP levels rose from 107.7+/-9.4 at age 12 to 118.9+/-9.9 at age 17. These trends were highly significant ($p < .001$) by one way analyses of variance.

TABLE 2: BLOOD PRESSURE AND PULSE RESPONSES TO POSTURAL CHANGE FROM RESTING SUPINE TO SEATED POSTURAL POSITIONS IN BLACK ADOLESCENTS*

MALES	Low Supine: 0-15%			Normal Supine:>15-85%			High Supine:>85-100%		
	MEAN BP	MEAN BP CHANGE	N	MEAN BP	MEAN BP CHANGE	N	MEAN BP	MEAN BP CHANGE	N
SBP	100.3	+2.8	92	114.0	-1.9	428	131.4	-6.2	99
DBP4	53.4	+15.1	111	70.8	+4.1	481	85.4	-2.3	93
DBP5	38.5	+21.9	100	58.4	+10.6	497	77.2	-0.2	102
FEMALES									
SBP	88.7	+2.0	99	111.7	-2.3	494	125.7	-5.9	95
DBP4	56.4	+12.9	100	71.3	+4.2	450	84.5	-0.2	56
DBP5	43.1	+19.8	101	61.5	+9.3	457	76.6	+2.2	87

60 SEC	MEAN P (PULSE)	MEAN P CHANGE	N	MEAN P (PULSE)	MEAN P CHANGE	N	MEAN P (PULSE)	MEAN P CHANGE	N
MALE	55.0	+7.0	97	68.2	+5.4	477	84.2	+0.8	95
FEMALE	58.2	+9.2	100	72.6	+5.2	426	88.4	+0.6	85

* All blood pressure and pulse changes were analysed by one way analyses of variance. The significance of the differences in responses to change from the resting supine to the seated postural position was at $p < 0.0001$ for all blood pressure changes in all cases. Moreover, the pulse changes from supine to seated also varied significantly at $p < 0.005$ for both males and females when grouped according to initial pulse levels in the supine position.

In contrast to the overall data presented on Table 1, these data on Table 2 indicate highly significant differences ($p < 0.0001$) in response pattern from the resting supine to seated postural position. In both males and females those groups whose supine blood pressures were in the low category responded with the greatest positive response with over a 2mm Hg change in systolic blood pressure, over a 12-15mm Hg change in DBP4 in females and males, and over 19-22mm Hg change in DBP5 for females and males. This result was in sharp contrast to the high group which demonstrated a mean decrease in bood pressure for SBP, DBP4, and DBP5 in the males and similarly in the females with only the small exception of a rise of 2mm HHg for DBP5. The middle group varied consistantly between the two extremes for all measures. Likewise, the pattern of change in the 30 second pulse percentile groups followed the same pattern as for blood pressure with the low group evidencing the greatest change from the resting supine to seated position.

Further preliminary analyses were conducted by two-way ANOVA to determine if the relation between blood pressure change in SBP and DBP4 percentile groups was significantly associated with the pulse changes upon assumption of the upright seated position. In this case the data were divided by sex and by age grouped to the nearest year. These analyses indicated that there were no significant associations between the variation in pulse responses to the postural change and the three percentile groupings of supine SBP and DBP4 or degrees of change in these pressures. Thus the data indicate that while there is a significant change in pulse with seated posture, the degree of change at these ages is not associated with the variation in blood pressure. Finally, preliminary studies of change in blood pressure responsiveness over age indicates that in both males and females there are significant declines in responsiveness to the change in postural position over ages 12-17 (this data will be published in greater detail elsewhere).

DISCUSSION

The results indicate that, as expected, in normal individuals shifting from the supine position to an upright postural position produces a series of cardiovascular adjustments that incompletely restore blood pressure to previous levels. With the assumption of upright posture, there is a pooling of blood in the lower extremities below the level of the heart and into the splanchnic vascular bed. This results in a fall in central venous pressure, a decrease in right and left ventricular filling pressures and a decrease in stroke volume. This, in turn, stimulates the aortic and carotid baroreceptors resulting in reflex vasoconstriction, an increased heart rate, and increases in norepinephrine and renin levels (7). Our overall blood pressure results seen on Table 1 reflect these changes for both males and females at these ages (12-17), and the responses were in the same direction as reported for standing in adults (6,12,14).

However the results of categorizing the supine blood pressures into low, normal and high groups (see Table 2) yielded a completely different pattern. The normal group, as might have been expected, tended to follow the overall pattern established above. In the case of the low blood pressure group, however, the response to upright seated posture was quite exaggerated with some individuals increasing up to 30mm Hg in DBP5 going from the supine to the seated postion. Preliminary analyses of this highly significant response indicate that it tends to decrease with age for the low group as well as for the normal groups. This may mean that the cardiovascular regulatory system undergoes a decrease in responsivity to orthostatic stress through adolescence. Since this phenomenon to our knowledge is previously unreported, further analyses will have to be conducted in order to interpret this aging trend. Nevertheless, the fact that this exaggerated response occurs raises, among others, questions about the tracking of this response. It has been reported that labile and sustained hypertensives tend also to have upon assumption of upright posture an exaggerated increase in blood pressure (5). Hence it is possible that, although this population as a whole is within the normal range for baseline blood pressures, there may be some significant fraction of these adolescents whose over-responsiveness will continue to track upward into labile and sustained hypertension of adulthood. The same suggestion may be the case for the other patterns of response to change in postural position and therefore become useful predictors in the tracking of blood pressure from adolescence to adulthood.

The results for the high blood pressure group are also very striking, since the expected blood pressure responses to change in postural position did not occur. Furthermore, the results are not merely diminished, they are opposite from those that are expected from the reports in the literature on orthostatic testing (12,13,14). Specifically, the fact that mean DBP4 and DBP5 actually slightly decrease in the seated position of the high group suggests a decreased responsiveness to the postural stimulation. While it is not known what would cause this decreased compensatory response in all three blood pressure measures, it is likely that it either involves some expansion and/or decreased responsiveness of the venoconstrictor tone or some generalized decrease in the sympathetic responsiveness to the expected response to postural stimulation (4,12). In other studies of borderline hypertension there have been reports of marked increases of systolic blood pressure upon assumption of upright posture (5). Since marked increases in the mean systolic blood pressure in the seated position did not occur in the case of the high groups, it is possible that further analyses of the individual responses in these groups will yield both postural hypotensives and hypertensives.

Although the blood pressure among the high group of males declines, the decrease in pressure is probably not sufficient to be termed postural hypotension (9). However, a sufficient number of postural hypotensives in this group could have brought the overall averages into the lowered levels particularly for the diastolic pressures. Several sources for postural hypotension have been suggested in the literature and one or more may be reponsible in part or in some combination for the observed response pattern. These posssible sources include: decreased baroreceptor activity, increased venous pooling in the splanchnic vascular bed and lower extremities, and inadequate increases in antidiuretic hormone, plasma renin and/or catecholamine levels (1,7). While it is not possible in this case to rule out any one of these possible causes, it is worth noting that there were no significant associations between pulse rate changes and the blood pressure changes. This suggests that the parasympathetic mechanisms controlling heart rate and possibly renin secretion (3,12) may not be linked to these results. Also the degree to which volume expansion secondary to elevated sodium intake combined with the potential of excessive venoconstriction in the supine position as a result of over stimulation of the sympathetic nervous system response mechanisms also requires careful investigation as a possible source of the response (1,4,14).

Furthermore, since the correlates of elevated supine blood pressure in these adolescence are becoming increasingly well documented (10), it is reasonable to suggest that such factors as obesity, increased muscle mass, and early maturation be investigated further for their possible associations with these responses to postural stimulation. Finally, the degree to which the blood pressure response to postural change tracks or is predictive of blood pressure variation in either postural position from one year to the next remains to be determined.

In summary, there are striking and highly significant differences between supine and seated blood pressure in normal individuals throughout adolescence. Furthermore, analyses of these differences strongly suggests that the degree of change in blood pressure from the resting supine to the resting seated position is closely associated with the level of blood pressure in the supine position. Since the ease and reliability of assessing blood pressure in the two most common postural positions reported in the clinical literature yields highly signicant differences in response patterns in normal adolescents, the analyses of both blood pressures under conditions similar to those described in this paper may provide a valuable diagnostic tool in the prediction of the risk of various types of hypertension.

REFERENCES

1. Abelmann, W.H. and Fareeduddin, K.: Increased Tolerance of Orthostatic Stress in Patients with Heart Disease. Am. J. of Cardiology 23:354-363, 1969.

2. Blumenthal, S. et al: Report of the Task Force on Blood Pressure Control in Children. Pediatrics 59(5 Supplement): 797-820.

3. Dampney, R.A.L., Stella, A., Golin, R., and A. Zanchetti: Vagal and Sinoaortic Reflexes in Postural Control of Circulation and Renin Release. Am. J. Physiol. 237(2): H146-H152, 1979.

4. Ellis, C.N., and Julius, S.: Role of Central Blood Volume in Hyperkinetic Borderline Hypertension. Brit. Hrt. J. 35: 450-455, 1973.

5. Franco-Morselli, R., Baudouin-Legros, M., and P. Meyer: Plasma Adrenaline and Noradrenaline in Essential Hypertension and After Long Term Treatment with Beta-androrecptor-blocking Agents. Clinical Sci. and Molec. Med. 55:97s-100s,1978.

6. Frohlich, E.D., Kozul, V.J., Tarazi, R.C., and H. Dustan: Physiological Comparison of Labile and Essential Hypertension. Circulation Research 26&27(Supplement 1):I-55-I-69, 1970.

7. Guyton, A.C.: Textbook of Medical Physiology. 5th edition, Philadelphia, Saunders, 1976.

8. Hediger, M.L., Schall, J.I., Barker, W.F., Bowers, E.J., Gruskin, A.B., and S.H. Katz: Variability and Reliability of Diastolic Blood Pressure during Adolescence: The Philadelphia Blood Pressure Project. Prev. Med. 10: (in press, 1981)

9. Hilsted, J.: Decreased Sympathetic Vasomotor Tone in Diabetic Orthostatic Hypertension. Diabetes 28:970-973, 1979.

10. Katz, S.H., Hediger, M.L., Schall, J.I., Bowers, E.J., Barker, W.F., Aurand, S., Eveleth P.B., Gruskin, A.B., and J.S. Parks: Blood Pressure, Growth and Maturation from Childhood Through Adolescence. Hypertension 2(4 Supplement 1):I-56-I-69, 1980.

11. Niswander, K.R., and R. Gordon: Women and Their Pregnancies. Philadelphia, Saunders, 1972.

12. Messerli, F.H., DeCarvalho, J.G.R., Christie, B., and E.D. Frohlich: Systemic and Regional Hemodynamics in Low, Normal and High Cardiac Output Borderline Hypertension. Circulation 58:441-448, 1978.

13. Sannerstedt, R., Julius, S., and J. Conway: Hemodynamic Responses to Tilt and Beta-andronergic Blockade in Young Patients with Borderline Hypertension. Circulation 42:1057-1064, 1970.

14. Ulrych,M., Frolich,E.D., Tarazi,R.B., Dustan,H.P., and I.H. Page: Cardiac Output and Distribution of Blood Volume in Central and Peripheral Circulation in Hypertensive and Normotensive Man. Brit. Heart J. 31:570-574, 1969.

15. Voors, A.W., Webber, L.S., and G.S. Berenson: A Choice of Diastolic Korotkoff Phases in Mercury Sphygmomanometry of Children. Prev. Med. 8:492-499, 1979.

16. Schall, J.I., Hediger, M.L., Bowers, E.J., Eveleth, P.B. and S.H. Katz: Pulse Rate and Blood Pressure During Adolescence. Ped. Res.14:1011(209), 1980.

LIST OF ADDRESSES OF FIRST-NAMED AUTHORS

Aperia, A.
Karolinska Institute
Pediatriska Kliniken
St. Gorans Barnkliniker
Box 12500
112 81 Stockholm

Arbus, G.S.
Hospital for Sick Children
Toronto, Ontario
Canada

Arant, B.S.,Jr.
Department of Pediatrics
University of Texas Health
Science Center at Dallas
5323 Harry Hines Boulevard
Dallas, Texas 75235

Arneil, G.C.
University of Glasgow
University Department
 of Child Health
Royal Hospital for Sick Children
Yorkhill, Glasgow G3 8SJ

Baluarte, H.J.
Section of Nephrology
St.Christopher's Hospital
 for Children
5th and Lehigh Avenue
Philadelphia, PA 19133

Barnett H.L.
International Study of
 Kidney Disease in Children
Albert Einstein College
 of Medicine
1410 Pelham Parkway North
Bronx, NY 10461

Barratt, T.M.
Department of Nephrology
Institute of Child Health
30 Guilford St.
London W.C. 1, U.K.

Bergstein, J.M.
James Whitcomb Riley
Hospital for Children
1100 West Michigan Street
Indianapolis, IN 46223

Bernstein, J.
William Beaumont Hospital
3601 West 13 Mild Road
Royal Oak, Michigan 48072

Brodehl, J.
Department of Pediatric Nephrology
 and Metabolic Disorders
Kinderklinik
Medizinische Hochschule
9 Karl Wicchort Allee
D-3000 Hannover-61, F.R.G.

Broyer, M.
Hopital des Enfants Malades
149 Rue de Sevres
75730 Paris Cedex 15, France

Calcagno, P.L.
Department of Pediatrics
Georgetown University Medical Center
3800 Reservoir Road, N.W.
Washington, DC 20007

Cameron, J.S.
Renal Unit
Department of Medicine
Guy's Hospital
London SE1 9RT, U.K.

Campbell, R.A.
Department of Pediatrics
University of Oregon
Health Sciences Center
Portland, Oregon 97201

Chan, J.C.
Section of Nephrology
Department of Pediatrics
Medical College of Virginia
MCV Station
Richmond, Virginia 23298

Chesney, W.R.
Department of Pediatrics
University of Wisconsin Medical School
Madison, WI 53711

Chantler, C.
Evelina Department of Pediatrics
Guy's Hospital
London SE1 9RT, U.K.

Couser, W.G.
Evans Memorial
Department of Clinical Research
Department of Medicine
University Hospital
Boston University Medical Center
Boston, MA 02118

DeSanto, N.G.
University degli studi di Napoli
1st Facolta de Medicine
Cattedra di Nefrologia Medica
Naples, Italy

Dillon, M.J.
The Hospital for Sick Children
Great Ormond Street
London WC1N 3JH

Drukker, A.
Division of Pediatric Nephrology
Shaare Zedek Medical Center
Jerusalem, Israel

Duckett, J.W.
Children's Hospital of Philadelphia
34th and Civic Center Boulevard
Philadelphia, PA 19104

Edelmann, C.M., Jr.
Department of Pediatrics
Albert Einstein College of Medicine
Bronx Municipal Hospital
Pelham Parkway South and
Eastchester Road
Bronx, NY 10461

Elfenbein, I.B.
Temple University School of Medicine
Department of Pathology
Philadelphia, PA 19140

Elzouki, A.Y.
Department of Pediatrics
Faculty of Medicine
University of Garyounis
Benghazi, Libya

Foreman, J.W.
Children's Hospital of Philadelphia
34th and Civic Center Boulevard
Philadelphia, PA 19104

Giordano, C.
University degli studi di Napoli
1st Facolta de Medicine
Cattedra de Nefrologia Medica
Naples, Italy

Guignard, J.-P.
Department of Pediatrics
Centre Hospitalier
Universitaire Vaudois
11011 Lausanne, Switzerland

Harcke, H.T.
Department of Radiology
St.Christopher's Hospital for Children
5th and Lehigh Avenue
Philadelphia, PA 19133

Harrison, H.L.
Department of Pediatrics
University of Louisville
School of Medicine
Louisville, KY 40202

Holliday, M.A.
Children's Renal Center
Department of Pediatrics
University of California at
San Francisco
San Francisco, CA 94143

Houston, I.B.
Royal Manchester Children's Hospital
Department of Child Health
Pendlebury, Manchester M27 1HA, U.K.

Inglefinger, J.R.
Children's Hospital Medical Center
Division of Nephrology
300 Longwood Avenue
Boston, MA 02115

Jose, P.A.
Department of Pediatrics
Georgetown University Hospital
3800 Reservoir Road N.W.
Washington, DC 20007

Katz, S.
School of Dental Medicine
University of Pennsylvania
Philadelphia, PA 19104

Koskimies, O.
Department of Pediatrics
Children's Hospital
University of Helsinki
Stenbackinkatu 11
SF-00290 Helsinki 29
Finland

Krohn, H.P.
Medizinische Hochschule Hannover
Kinderklinik
Karl-Weichert Allee 9
3000 Hannover, Germany

Leumann, E.P.
Universitats-Kinderklinik
University Zurich
Steinwiesstr 75
CH-8032 Zurich
Switzerland

Lewis, E.J.
Section of Nephrology
Rush-Presbyterian
St. Luke's Hospital
1753 West Congress Parkway
Chicago, Ill. 60612

Lewy, J.E.
Department of Pediatrics
Tulane University Medical School
1430 Tulane Avenue
Room 4536
New Orleans, LA 70112

Lewy, P.R.
Children's Memorial Hospital
Chicago, Ill. 60614

Linshaw, M.A.
Department of Pediatrics
University of Kansas Med.Center
39th at Rainbow Boulevard
Kansas City, KS 66103

McAdams, A.J.
Children's Hospital Research Foundation
Elland and Bethesda Avenue
Cincinnati, Ohio 45229

McSherry, E.
University of California, San
Francisco, 1203 M
San Francisco, CA 94143

Mehls, O.
Universitatis-Kinderklinik
Im Neuenheimer Feld 150
69 Heidelberg, F.R.G.

Meinert, C.
Johns Hopkins University
615 North Wolf Street
Baltimore, MD 21205

Mendoza, S.A.
Department of Pediatrics
University of California School of Med.
La Jolla, CA 92093

Mongeau, J.G.
Department of Pediatrics
University of Montreal
St. Justine Hospital
3175 St. Catherine Road
Montreal H3T1C5
Canada

Moore, E.S.
Department of Pediatrics
Michael Reese Medical Center
2901 South Ellis Avenue
Chicago, Ill. 60616

Murray, T.G.
Department of Medicine
University of Pennsylvania
School of Medicine
Hospital of the University of Penna.
Philadelphia, PA 19104

Norman, M.E.
Section of Nephrology
Children's Hospital of Philadelphia
34th and Civic Center Boulevard
Philadelphia, PA 19104

Oetliker, O.
Division of Pediatric Nephrology
University Children's Hospital
Berne, Switzerland

Olbing, H.
Universitatskinderklinik
Hufelandstr. 55
D-4300, Essen 1
F.R.G.

Ooi, B.S.
Department of Medicine
University of Cincinnati
Medical Center
231 Bethesda Road
Cincinnati, OH 45267

Prebis, J.W.
Department of Pediatrics
Section of Nephrology
St. Christopher's Hospital
 for Children
5th and Lehigh Avenue
Philadelphia, PA 19133

Proesmans, W.
A.Z. Gasthuisberg
3000 Leuven, Belgium

Roy, S., III
Le Bonheur Children's Med.Center
848 Adams Avenue
Memphis, TN 38103

Salcedo, J.R.
Children's Hospital
National Medical Center
Department of Nephrology
111 Michigan Avenue N.W.
Washington, DC 20010

Segal, S.
Children's Hospital of Philadelphia
34th and Civic Center Boulevard
Philadelphia, PA 19104

Smeilie, J.M.
Department of Pediatrics
University College Hospital
Huntley Street
London WC1E 6A, U.K.

Soriano-Rodriguez, J.
Department of Pediatrics
Hospital Infantil de la Seguridad
 social and University School of Medicine
Bilbao, Spain

Spitzer, A.
Division of Pediatric Nephrology
Albert Einstein College of Medicine
Rose F. Kennedy Center
Bronx, NY 10461

Strauss, J.
Department of Pediatrics
Jackson Memorial Hospital
University of Miami School of Medicine
P.O.Box 01690
Miami, FL 33101

Turner, D.R.
Department of Pathology
Guy's Hospital Medical School
London Bridge, SE1 9RT, U.K.

West, C.D.
Children's Hospital Medical Center
The Children's Hospital Research Foundation
Elland and Bethesda Avenue
Cincinnati, OH 45229

White, R.H.R.
The Children's Hospital of Birmingham
Ladywood Middleway
Birmingham B16 SET, U.K.

Yamashita, F.
Department of Pediatrics and Child Health
Kurume University Medical Center
67 Asahi-machi
Kurume City, Japan 830